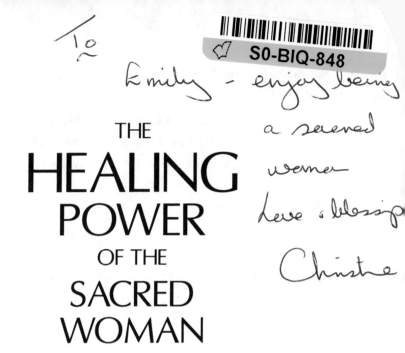

To
Emily — enjoy being
a sacred
woman
Love & blessings
Christine

THE
HEALING
POWER
OF THE
SACRED
WOMAN

"A brilliant contribution to health and consciousness literature . . . every reader will benefit enormously from Dr. Christine Page's knowledge and wisdom."

CAROLINE MYSS, AUTHOR OF THE NEW YORK TIMES
BESTSELLING *ANATOMY OF THE SPIRIT*

"Showing that a woman's purpose is to give birth not only to new life but also to new levels of consciousness, *The Healing Power of the Sacred Woman* is a wake-up call for both humanity and every woman on the planet. I love this book."

DONNA EDEN, COAUTHOR OF *ENERGY MEDICINE:*
BALANCING YOUR BODY'S ENERGIES FOR OPTIMAL HEALTH,
JOY, AND VITALITY AND *ENERGY MEDICINE FOR WOMEN*

"After 4,000 years the true role of women, as the essential foundation for human life itself and for the sacred rituals of life, is reintroduced to our society. Dr. Page has given us a tremendous gift through the embodiment of the Sacred Woman. Essential reading for all conscious individuals!"

C. NORMAN SHEALY, M.D., PH.D., PRESIDENT
OF HOLOS INSTITUTES OF HEALTH AND AUTHOR OF
ENERGY MEDICINE: PRACTICAL APPLICATIONS AND SCIENTIFIC PROOF

"In her book *The Healing Power of the Sacred Woman,* Christine R. Page, M.D., asks a question of timeless importance: 'How do we really connect with the feminine essence?' It's clear she has also lived the question, in both ordinary and extraordinary ways, making this more than an ordinary book, but a pure expression of the search for the most authentic answer. You'll discover insights and ancient wisdom on every page, because it is all within you, waiting for your inevitable embrace."

ANAIYA SOPHIA, AUTHOR *SACRED SEXUAL UNION* AND
COAUTHOR OF *WOMB WISDOM*

"*The Healing Power of the Sacred Woman* is filled with ancient wisdom that activates conscious awareness while simultaneously nourishing and renewing our souls."

LINDA STAR WOLF, FOUNDER OF VENUS RISING
ASSOCIATION FOR TRANSFORMATION AND AUTHOR OF
SHAMANIC BREATHWORK

THE
HEALING
POWER
OF THE
SACRED
WOMAN

HEALTH, CREATIVITY, AND FERTILITY FOR THE SOUL

CHRISTINE R. PAGE, M.D.

Bear & Company
Rochester, Vermont • Toronto, Canada

Bear & Company
One Park Street
Rochester, Vermont 05767
www.BearandCompanyBooks.com

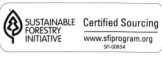

Text stock is SFI certified

Bear & Company is a division of Inner Traditions International

Library of Congress Cataloging-in-Publication Data
Page, Christine R.
  The healing power of the sacred woman : health, creativity, and fertility for the soul / Christine R. Page.
        p. cm.
  Includes bibliographical references and index.
  Summary: "How to enhance well-being by reconnecting to sacred womanhood"— Provided by publisher.
  ISBN 978-1-59143-144-2 (pbk.) — ISBN 978-1-59143-802-1 (e-book)
  1. Feminist therapy. 2. Feminist spirituality. 3. Women—Identity. 4. Indian philosophy—North America. I. Title.
  RC489.F45P34 2012
  613.04244—dc23

                                                                              2012010888

Printed and bound in the United States by Lake Book Manufacturing, Inc.
The text stock is SFI certified. The Sustainable Forestry Initiative® program promotes sustainable forest management.

10   9   8   7   6   5   4   3   2   1

Text design by Priscilla Baker and layout by Brian Boynton
This book was typeset in Garamond Premier Pro with Legacy Sans, Gill Sans, Myriad Pro, and Omni as display typefaces.

To send correspondence to the author of this book, mail a first-class letter to the author c/o Inner Traditions • Bear & Company, One Park Street, Rochester, VT 05767, and we will forward the communication, or contact the author directly at **www.christinepage.com**.

*This book is dedicated to all women presently in the world,
from babies to crones;*

*To all women who have walked this way before
and those still to come;*

To my beloved mother, sister, aunts, and grandmothers;

*To all the soul sisters I have met along the path, who have showered
me with love, hugs, laughter, and wisdom;*

*To the Great Mother in all her forms, especially Mother Earth
and the silvery Moon;*

*To all men who love the women in their lives,
supporting them on their journey of living from their sacred
and essential identity, now;*

*And especially to my darling Leland:
I offer love, gratitude, and celebration.*

CONTENTS

Part Four
The Queen Bee

PREFACE

Life has an amazing way of attracting our attention when important issues are at stake. During the writing of this book, I came face to face with some of the wounds that had been subconsciously driving many of my decisions and ways of thinking. Behind a kind and compliant facade, I unearthed layers of resentment and frustration that had built up from years of denying my true feelings. It soon became clear how much these hidden emotions had influenced the quality of my relationships. However, I was scared to allow the angry woman, my inner "bitch," out of the cellar for fear of the turmoil she would cause in my life. And yet, she had just as much right to be seen and acknowledged as the compassionate and considerate part of me.

Fortunately, my soul took the lead, manifesting these suppressed feelings in the form of abnormal and unruly cellular changes in my breast: I developed breast cancer. The diagnosis propelled me into the chaos I most feared, but instead of devastating me, the turmoil released untapped sources of assertiveness and inner strength, leaving me stronger and more self-assured than ever before. My husband is delighted, for as he has always said, there is nothing more beautiful in the universe than a woman in her power.

Deep healing begins when we agree to be true to our heart and recognize that we have the power and choice to change our circumstances, even if it starts in very small ways. Emotions such as irritation, frustration, disappointment, hurt, and sadness are warning signs that things are not okay and, as I have learned, should not be denied, dishonored, or drugged. Indeed, the first step in healing oneself is recognizing that there is a problem. For most of us, the number-one concern is whether we are loved just for being ourselves; as Mother Teresa commented, "There is more hunger for love and appreciation in this world than for bread."

For more than twenty years, the focus of my teaching has been to show that illness is not merely a physical problem but represents a message sent from the soul. Disease offers us the opportunity to step back, review life, and make the appropriate adjustments that will bring us closer to our heart's desire. This understanding is based on the spiritual teachings I have received since I was a child as well as my own personal experiences and professional insights from both allopathic and complementary medicine, where I witnessed many people undergoing positive transformation in the presence of illness.

Like other major events in our lives, such as divorce or losing our job, illness opens a door to reveal the potential for change, directing us toward greater joy and contentment. Whether we hear the message and step through the doorway is up to us; we have free will to choose our path. If we choose not to heed the message, the illness may well disappear, we may remarry, and we will probably find another job, but the door to this particular opportunity for growth will close. By grasping these golden opportunities to release old, unsatisfactory patterns of behavior and ways of thinking, our consciousness can expand, moving us toward the love, health, and fulfillment we all basically seek.

Equipped with this kind of knowledge, when I was diagnosed with cancer I couldn't go along with the popular belief that I was being attacked by an outside invader. I refused to go to battle against my own body or soul. Instead, I remembered that nothing had ever happened in my life, however painful, that hadn't changed me for the better. I have never doubted that my soul loves me and created the cancer for my own good. All I needed to do was to hear its message and make the most of the possibilities it was affording me. For instance, as news of my illness spread, I was overwhelmed by the depth of love shown to me by my family and friends; this is something I may never have known without the cancer.

I did receive a few comments expressing surprise that I, with all my medical and spiritual knowledge, should become sick. This reminded me of the stigmatization of illness, which is sometimes erroneously believed to happen only to the unfortunate or to those who fail to take care of themselves. I thought of remarks I had heard, like, "She didn't deserve to get ill," which has always made me want to ask, "Who do you think *does* deserve illness?" This blame-and-shame game is especially well developed in those who are always well and who can't wait to give you their personal health tips.

It also became clear that my approach to disease is very different from that of many of my colleagues, whose focus is on offering a variety of ways to rid the client or patient of the "intruder" and thus return them "back to normal," to life before cancer. Among such professionals, there seems to be little appreciation of the opportunity being presented by an illness; there is simply a desire to fix the problem as quickly as possible. If illness carries a message from the soul, why would we want to shoot the messenger? Having worked and taught in both complementary and allopathic medical fields, it saddens me to see how little space is given for the needs of the soul, with nearly all of the attention firmly focused on physical wellness and not spiritual growth.

I was also surprised to see that it was often people who claim to practice holistic medicine who couldn't wait to launch into trying to heal me, without ever asking for my permission or considering that I may have developed the illness for a purpose. It made me think of the old adage *Don't give advice unless you're asked* and reminded me that integrative practitioners can be just as reductionist as some of those who work within the mainstream medical profession.

I was often given assurances that other people had gone through the same cancer treatment and were now well, several years later. While I was happy for their good health, I wanted to ask, "How did they change because of the cancer? What gifts did they take away from the experience?"

For a time, I felt isolated except for close family members and friends. Cancer is among a small group of illnesses that both are life threatening and appear out of the blue, their origins unclear, even to the medical profession. Because of this, such diseases evoke deep emotions, especially fear and helplessness around death, deformity, and incapacity. It is therefore easy to be persuaded to grasp onto anything that will improve your chances of survival and your prognosis, a situation I have seen all too often during my career, especially in cases of multiple sclerosis, motor neuron disease, and cancer. I consider myself fairly tuned in to the needs of my body, but even I found myself questioning whether I should change my diet, go on a fast, or exercise more, based often on the unsolicited advice of do-gooders.

Even more insidious were those who dabbled in religious superstition, imploring me to have more faith, pray more fervently, or call on my "guidance," which presumably had forsaken me. It was that final comment that shook me awake from my downward-spiraling confusion and made me actually laugh out loud, for in that moment I saw my soul family in the spirit world, celebrating my development of cancer with great enthusiasm, for they knew that nothing else would have stopped me in my tracks so effectively.

Moments like these, which cause us to question our beliefs and our intuitive insights, also make us stronger. The diagnosis gave me the opportunity to test my ideals in the fire of truth, and they returned to me intact. I know deep down inside that I am not deluding myself and am prepared to take full responsibility for my healing choices, listening to my heart's inner guidance. The only thing that matters is knowing that everything I do, I do because I love and care for myself. With this in mind, and with the best experts within the field of cancer care looking after me, I am listening to the call of my soul, whose words are expressed through the message of my dis-ease.

Illness does not arise merely from a poor diet or lack of exercise; it is highly influenced by the perceptions and beliefs we hold about ourselves and those around us, usually passed down through the generations. If we receive distorted ancestral beliefs about ourselves as women, then this will definitely influence the potential for disease, not because it is in our genes but because of the messages in our heads. During my childhood in the 1950s, my family held the belief, common in that era, that girls were less important than boys and therefore should be prepared for marriage, motherhood, and a possible occupation (as long as the husband's career took precedence). This balance of power has obviously changed over the decades, although ancestral concepts die hard, as experienced by the many women today who attempt to pass through the glass ceiling or who try to juggle too many roles just to stay ahead.

As a girl I was taught to be kind, selfless, and grateful for any advice and attention I received, even if it went against my intuition. My mother often reproached me for forming too quick an opinion about someone, always telling me to give them a second chance. So I did. In many of my relationships, both male and female, I disregarded my intuitive urges and gave the person a third, fourth, and fifth chance, while my self-esteem and self-respect fell through the floor.

I prided myself on being seen as adaptable and easygoing until the wake-up call of breast cancer. Within weeks of the diagnosis, I realized that in my desire to fit in and be accepted, I had become disconnected from my own true feelings and had fallen out of love with myself. It became clear that many of my decisions were based on the desires of others, while my own needs often seemed irrelevant, even to me. Because of my poor sense of self for most of my life, I had listened to other people tell me how to dress, what to eat, and how to act, especially if I wanted to be their friend. I remembered being five years old when two girls told me they would only play with me if I spent my precious bus money to buy them sweets. Fortunately, I only complied with this demand once, because I wasn't that desperate for friendship and it was a long walk home!

However, I have to admit that over the years the concept of self-love and self-nurturing has all too often been an enigma to me. I do partake in pleasurable massages, enjoy luxurious baths, and spend fun time with loved ones—but when the sense of self or "I" has been hiding in a cave for so long, it's often hard to know what part of me is actually receiving the loving or nurturing. During the early weeks after the diagnosis, as I swam in the depths of discovery, I realized that although Christine, the wise, caring, and charismatic teacher, was alive and well, my more personal self was often missing in relationship. I came to see that from childhood I had honed my intuitive gifts to read the needs of others so as not to hurt their feelings or attract their displeasure. I had become a pleaser. The diagnosis of cancer has given me the courage—for the first time in my life—to be self-centered and even what I used to think of as selfish.

Strengthened at the core of my being, my deep healing has begun. When faced with choice, instead of deferring to my perception of the emotional needs of others, I now allow my own feelings, coming from my heart and my body, to provide the answer, bringing a much-welcomed honesty to all my relationships. I am much more content with being who I am, nurturing my unique qualities and needs. Surrounded by loving friends, it is clear that I no longer have to take care of people or put up with emotional blackmail to know that I belong or that I am accepted. I now follow my initial instincts and can say no without justifying my response or needing to add sweetly "but maybe some other time." As I let go of the burden of always thinking of others' feelings before I think of my own, my mind has become quieter and I'm much more present to the beauty of the world all around me. I also know that my story, my journey, is not so very different from that of many women around the world.

ACKNOWLEDGMENTS

As an author who trusts implicitly in my inner guidance when it comes to writing a new book, I am deeply indebted to the many people who have supported my vision and who have helped in the birthing of this work. This includes:

Jon Graham of Inner Traditions • Bear & Company whose own dedication to the empowerment of men and women enabled him to recognize the vision of my book proposal, filling my heart with joy.

Eran Cantrell, for her beautiful and creative illustrations.

Jamaica Burns and Margaret Jones, whose skillful, knowledgeable, and sensitive editing brought emphasis and clarity to my words and thoughts.

And especially Leland Landry, my husband, who has loved, nurtured, and supported me during the writing of this book. He was my constant companion during every moment of my journey with cancer, holding my hand, listening to my fears, attending hospital appointments, cooking my meals, and never questioning any of my decisions. Thank you for being by my side and for your beautiful photography, represented by the many pictures you took that are used throughout this book.

PART ONE

Reconnecting with the Great Mother

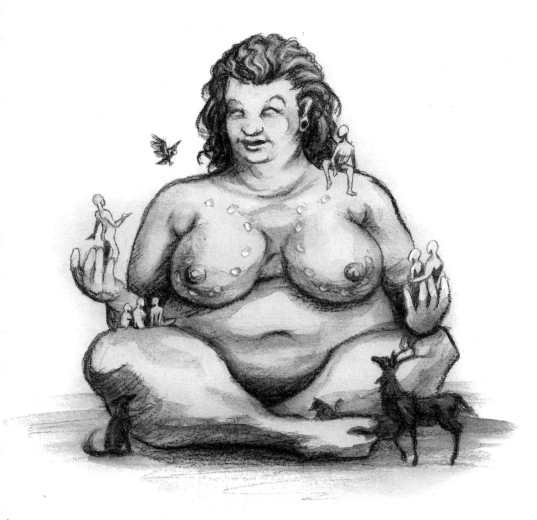

1
WOMAN, KNOW THYSELF

Once again, I find myself sitting in a large auditorium during a conference, where most of the people in the audience are women listening to a panel of experts—mainly men—telling us how to connect with the feminine side of our nature. In solemn tones they instruct us in the intricate rituals that must be performed before we will be allowed to connect with the essence of Mother Earth, our archetype. As I listen to their seductive words and watch their reverent posturing, my mind conjures up images of past boyfriends who, with comparable charm along with tempting chocolates, hoped to gain access to the succulent soil of my own feminine abode. I find myself chuckling out loud at the similarities between the two scenarios—resulting in quizzical looks from my fellow participants.

Then, as humor gives way to mild indignation, I realize that men telling women how to live their lives is not a new phenomenon; it has been the pattern for thousands of years, with women often only too happy to go along with their game. Indeed, we have only to look at the Catholic Church, where male priests are required to be unmarried and women are still not allowed to perform Mass, to know that any recommendations about womanhood that arise from this lopsided source must be taken with a grain of salt.

As I continue to listen to the words of veneration for the Great Mother from the male speakers on the panel, I hear echoes of the same words spoken by male priests of the ancient past who performed elaborate ceremonies to gain access to her ocean of creative and inspirational abundance. Indeed, these priests were even known to drink menstrual blood, believing it to have mystical qualities that would heighten their state of consciousness and allow them to sit in the very lap of the Divine Mother. From that exalted position, their duty was to share the wisdom and insights they received with the general populace so that all the people could thrive. Unfortunately, over time, the temptation by a few to possess such power over the many became overwhelming; the journey to the Mother's source of inspiration and wealth became a way of serving the ambitions of the priests and leaders, while the common people were misled by this powerful elite group into believing that they needed an intermediary to receive such a blessing.

As I reflect on the scenario in the auditorium where I now sit, I experience an epiphany that may sound strange coming from a medical doctor with more than thirty years of experience: men and women are not the same! Yes, it is true that within every man is an anima, or female counterpart, and within every woman an animus, or masculine aspect. But the sacred vessel—the physical body—through which the soul expresses itself is quite different in each gender, causing me to know on a deeply intuitive level that men and women have diverse and specific functions here on earth.

With respect to my male colleagues, such differences mean that as a woman it would be impertinent and impractical for me to believe that I could instruct men in *their* purpose and process, as I have no concept of what it feels like to have male levels of testosterone pulsing through my bloodstream twenty-four hours a day. Yet for the past three millennia, during which the patriarchy has dominated and polarized the world, men have believed it is their right to tell women how to look, act, speak, and behave, and women, for the most part, have simply gone along with the deception.

Unlike men, women do not need to kneel down at the feet of the Great Mother. Instead, we should stand tall and honor her as living examples of this feminine archetype. Why is this so? Because women physically embody this powerful divine presence, our bodies conform to her expression through their qualities of juiciness, softness, curvaceousness, and voluptuousness, to name just a few. Like Mother Earth, we experience cycles and seasons, not just within a year or a lifetime but every twenty-eight days. During the time it takes for the moon to orbit around the Earth, we give birth to life, cultivate the egg until it is ripe, nurture its fertility, and then allow it to die. However, for centuries women have been enmeshed in an archaic and no doubt patriarchal belief that the only purpose of these monthly cycles is for a woman to become pregnant and thus ensure the continuation of the species. Yet if we look at the figures, it is clear that this is grossly inaccurate. On average, a woman has 420 cycles during her reproductive years. Today, the global mean number of children born to a woman has been calculated to be only 1.2. If the menstrual cycle is thus solely an aspect of procreation, it is a remarkable waste of potential in a natural world that abhors excess.

Children are indeed our future, but what seeds of belief and awareness are we planting in their minds? What if the purpose of a woman's monthly cycle is to nurture not only physical life but also the seeds of inspiration that encourage the consciousness of her family to thrive? What if, in a perfect world, once a woman has completed her approximately 420 cycles, she no longer requires the physical changes to give birth to wisdom and inspiration, becoming the wise crone at menopause? Such a hypothesis would change the way a woman views not only her menstrual cycle but in particular her periods or menses. Though it is often known as the "curse" of womanhood, menstruation is in fact the time during which she is at her most powerful and creative.

This sacred and unique role of women has always been known by indigenous peoples around the world. During the menses, or moon time, a woman enters into the symbolic valley of death and, in service to humanity, sheds her blood, which carries with it not only the unfertilized egg but also unfertilized dreams, painful emotions, and the remnants of grief. She performs this cleansing for herself and for her family or tribe. This is the reason why women brought up in traditional ways refrain from cooking and taking care of their families during this period of purification, reluctant to contaminate the food with energies that are toxic or dead. At the same time, because of their body's ability to undergo such processes of transformation, women are recognized as extremely powerful during their moon time and therefore isolate themselves from others, where possible, in a desire to do no harm.

Toward the end of her menses, with the cleansing complete, a woman's intuitive awareness is heightened. She can then access the Great Mother's realm of creative ideas, delivering back to her family and tribe fresh dreams that collectively can be manifested. When a woman really understands that this unique and intimate knowledge of death and rebirth that occurs on a monthly basis is preparing her to have no fear of either, she becomes a truly formidable figure. I wonder if this was one of the reasons why the patriarchy decided to suppress the feminine energies, for when there is no fear of death, people cannot be easily manipulated or controlled.

But then when I read advertisements offering pills, injections, and patches so that women don't have to be bothered with their "inconvenient" feminine cycles, I realize that the disconnect from a woman's true source of power and purpose has reached a critical level. By denying our monthly moon cycles, women negate the very essence of our sacred feminine identity. The conversion of women into mini-men is almost complete. Yet there is no future for humanity if we're all expressing the same masculine qualities such as competitiveness, independence, logical reasoning, and ambition. Without the powerful transformative feminine qualities of sensitivity, creativity, nurturing, and purification, along with a deep desire to connect, our bodies, minds, and environment will become unproductive and barren, leading to the extinction of our species.

Historically, this disconnect can be traced back almost 4,000 years, to ancient societies that had, in earlier times, been egalitarian and polytheistic. Here women were considered sacred for their inherent link to the divine, Mother Earth was honored for her abundant fertility, and cyclical episodes, such as seasons, were respected as essential for life to evolve. Such cultures existed between 7000 and 1700 BCE in what archaeologist Marija Gimbutas termed Old Europe or Neolithic Europe, with people of both genders and all ages being treated with equal respect.[1] From 4500 to 2500 BCE there were increasing waves of infiltration of people from the Russian steppe who brought with them attitudes that were warlike and patriarchal—the prototype of the ensuing Indo-European culture. Such a culture believed not in equality but rather in stratification and hierarchy dominated by male divinities, the majority of which lived high in the sky, away from the common man or woman. Over time increasing power and authority were given to priesthoods who were seen as intermediaries between the deities and the people, enacting laws that were deemed to represent the word and the will of the gods.

From around 2000 BCE onward there was increasing vilification of anything feminine, whether this was goddess worship, respect for the female body, or honoring of Mother Earth. It is often said that this suppression was in response to the power previously bestowed on the matriarchy in earlier societies. However, as mentioned above, most cultures of Old Europe were egalitarian. So why did the patriarchy feel the need to subdue the feminine? It is my hypothesis that they knew that women possessed powers far more potent than physical strength, financial wealth, and man-made laws. These forces include fearlessness in the face of death, the ability to purify and transform, the power to create life, the gift of inspiration, and, most importantly, the power of love.

In essence, these qualities mirrored those of the Great Mother, who had been worshipped for tens of thousands of years before the appearance of the patriarchy. Her message has always been clear. When we fully believe in her love for us, celebrate all the gifts she offers, and completely accept the necessity of the cycles of life, which include death and birth, then we will know ourselves as eternal beings. Such concepts did not completely disappear with the appearance of the patriarchy but were repackaged and delivered by teachers, such as Jesus Christ, who also spoke about love and resurrection into an eternal life. However, by the early part of the first millennium CE, religious dogma had created so many hoops a person had to jump through before reaching such an enlightened state that the sense of a loving deity who truly offered unconditional love had become a far distant memory.

Despite courageous attempts by women to hold on to their historical and intuitive connection to the power and compassion of the Great Mother, by 500 CE women in cultures all over the world had succumbed to patriarchal dogma. As human minds were reprogrammed over the span of generations and the new way of thinking became absorbed into the deep unconsciousness, women collectively developed amnesia as to what it was to be a sacred woman. Over time, women were programmed and patterned to perpetually strive to satisfy the needs of men while denying their own inner urges and inner feminine guidance.

This brainwashing continues to the present day, with the media bursting with images of the ideal female figure: thinness achieved through constant dieting, exercise, slimming tablets, injections, and the occasional nip and tuck. Let's get real; I will never be six feet tall or a size 0! It is time for each woman to worship the body she has, and for all women to take charge of their own images of womanhood, remembering that the natural contours of Mother Earth take many shapes and sizes. Only then will we see a reduction in the number of women with body-image issues, who are often desperately trying to be something they are not, seeking the approval of others whose opinions they think matter more than whether they love themselves. Since we are all created in the image of the Great Mother, like every flower in the garden, all are perfect and beautiful just as they are.

LET ME INTRODUCE MYSELF

As my indigenous friends always say, when you know someone's background and ancestry, you know the source of the wisdom they have to share. My insights do not come simply from books or from the Western educational system; they arise from my personal experience. I am a great believer in walking my talk, and that only happens when you're willing to do your own inner work.

I was raised in a village just east of London, England, with the benefit of both the countryside and the city at my doorstep. Three of my four grandparents had died before I was born, and yet I was surrounded by wonderful aunts, uncles, and family friends who kept the ancestral energy alive. I was a bright child with a natural curiosity, which probably infuriated my teachers, as I never took anything at face value and was always asking questions. My mind could quickly grasp the bigger picture, plus I was gifted with a photographic memory and a natural ease at mental arithmetic. This made learning enjoyable for me as a child, although one of my most valuable life lessons has been to develop tolerance for those who are slower at such things.

While that logical, rational side of my life came relatively easy, I struggled with my equally strong intuitive gifts, which were both a curse and a blessing. From a very early age I was in constant communication with spiritual beings whose wisdom and universal knowledge I have learned to trust over the years. It felt completely natural to me to travel between the dimensions to meet those I consider my soul family. These spirit beings have always offered me love, encouragement, and wisdom, so that I have rarely ever had to ask for advice outside this inner counsel. And as various members of my family and close friends have died, my "team" has grown in size, meaning there is never a lack of spiritual guidance.

On the downside, my lack of boundaries between the different dimensions of awareness caused me, as a child, to be extremely sensitive to the energy of other people. I could easily sense the energies in another's auric field, but I wasn't able to protect myself from any pain and suffering they held within their emotional body, resulting in feelings of nausea and even fainting when I was around such people.

It is ironic that I decided on a career in medicine, where one is constantly exposed to people who are suffering, after starting out as a teenager as a volunteer first-aider at local events. In truth, during those early years I prayed that nobody would ever get sick on my watch. This option was not available to me after I became a doctor, and since fainting is frowned upon in the midst of a busy emergency room, I soon learned to detach from the emotions of the patient and become strictly "professional."

This worked for almost twenty years of working within both the complementary and the allopathic medical fields, until I realized that the barriers I had placed around myself as protection were causing me to become less psychically sensitive, a gift I deeply valued. It was then that I decided to close my practice and concentrate on teaching and writing about the wisdom and insights I had received as a child but had buried when I entered medical school.

It has been during the past decade that I have found my thoughts turning increasingly toward the Great Mother's presence here on earth and the sacred role that women are to play in birthing a new consciousness, beginning in the pivotal year of 2012. This has caused me to look at the female role models in my life, beginning, of course, with my own mother.

Mum was Scottish by birth, brought up in a large family on the outskirts of the ancient city of Edinburgh. Like her mother and her mother before her, she was kind and devoted to her husband and children. I could guarantee that if I called her on the telephone or arrived on her doorstep unannounced, she would drop everything she was doing to give me her full attention. I can still taste the scones spread with homemade jam that would mysteriously appear, freshly baked, as if somehow she just knew I would be popping in for a visit.

My mum enjoyed any opportunity to interact with people, whether it was serving tea at a local village fete, working in a friend's shop, or going on one of our many travels together. Both my grandmother and great-grandmother had been recognized as the wise women of their communities. My great-grandmother was the sacred woman called to all the deaths and births in the village, for she had an understanding of the mysteries of life. My grandmother's kitchen table was frequented by leading members of the community, who sought her wisdom and advice because she was known to be "fey," a visionary with the gift of seeing beyond the veil. My mother followed in this talent, and she, too, was sought after for her insights and opinions.

My mother adored clothes, not necessarily the most expensive, but clothes that made her look and feel feminine. As every photo of her attests, at five-foot nothing, she was an attractive and vivacious woman who knew how to carry every one of her assets with pride. She married the love of her life, my gentle and fun-filled father, and they provided for my sister, brother, and me a home that was filled with respect, compassion, and humor. My parents' time together was cut short after twenty-five years of marriage by my father's early death. Yet even though Mum was only fifty-two at the time, still vibrant and sensual, she never remarried, remaining faithful to her dear love's memory until her own passing twenty-eight years later.

My parents showed their affection for each other not only in the sentimental notes they wrote to each other but also through their unwavering respect and encouragement for each other. Despite their marvelous example of mutual, loving supportiveness, my own journey on the path of intimate personal relationship has been less smooth, but nevertheless rich with wisdom and insights and even a certain type of humor. I've known great love and great sadness, sometimes side by side, and I now recognize, in retrospect, the rewards of each. When I first met my beloved Leland eight years ago, I decided to get some things clear right at the start. Upon our first meeting, I stated clearly, "What I need from a relationship is honor, respect, and support; can you do that?" Unaware that we were in that moment embarking on a relationship, he thought for a moment and then said, "That's easy. So I take it that you're up for a second date?"

From that moment on, our courtship moved forward rapidly—at times, too quickly. I often felt like a bird whose freedom was slowly diminishing, trapped by my own perceptions of what I thought were his expectations. I would find myself making up all sorts of excuses why this relationship wouldn't work, finding fault in silly and irrelevant ways. One day, I had the courage to let Leland know what was happening. My wise partner once again became quiet, and then, drawing from the wisdom in his heart, he said: "I will never trap your beautiful inner bird because I love your curiosity and enthusiasm. But I will hold out a finger, and you can land there anytime you want." That was all I needed to hear. Within forty days of meeting we were engaged, and we married soon after that. Now, with my wise, funny, and affectionate beloved by my side, I feel blessed to be experiencing the same tenderness my parents and grandparents felt for each other.

My other early female role models came mainly through my schooling. I went to an all-girls high school and was surrounded by strong and well-educated female teachers who were not easily intimidated. From there I entered the Royal Free Medical School in London, which was founded in 1828 exclusively for female students, as women were not allowed admission into the other male-dominated medical schools. Here, once again, I met professors and consultants who had worked their way to the top of their professions through hard work and determination. During my medical training it was not uncommon to find myself in an operating theater where the entire staff was female. Surrounded at home and at work by women who were confident in their abilities, I personally never encountered any sexual discrimination until I arrived in the United States in 2001.

The first time a man talked down to me took me by surprise, as I had always been treated with respect by men, especially within my own profession. The surgeon I was consulting for a minor problem insisted in speaking over me to his nurse, until I decided to ask a question. In a dismissive manner, he replied, "You don't have to worry about that, dear." I can still see the shocked look on his face, as well as the faces of his staff, when I calmly but clearly demanded respect—and got it! Since then I have met other men who have tried to bully me into accepting their point of view by shouting at me or attempting to humiliate me, but I am my mother's daughter and will not stand for such behavior in my presence. Since then I have also heard from colleagues many stories about sexual discrimination in both their homes and their professional lives, which always surprises me considering the emphasis America places on democracy and equality.

But despite the confidence I have in my professional abilities and the encouragement of many strong female role models, I admit that in the past I was far less self-assured when it came to certain friends and acquaintances, especially when they called for me to step beyond my masculine attributes. In my experience it has been appropriate for me to show certain acceptable feminine qualities, such as kindness, caring, and sensitivity, but it's not okay to show my deep dragon power, which burns and destroys, or my sharp, owl-like insightfulness, which pierces through any pretense, or my deep capacity to love, which seems to threaten so many people who have forgotten that they are unconditionally lovable.

"THE PERFECT WOMAN" MYTH

I'm not the only woman who has presented a certain socially acceptable facade while keeping other aspects of my persona well hidden. This tendency is reinforced by media messages constantly telling us how to look and behave in a male-dominated culture. In addition, there is a dearth of modern-day role models—many of our cultural, religious, and political female leaders have to present their masculine persona to be respected in the world they inhabit. Many women like me have had to abandon the full spectrum of their feminine expressiveness in order to be treated as an equal in a man's world, little realizing that it is only by embodying *all* the qualities of the Great Mother that true equality and power can be found.

Take, for instance, sex. In Europe and the United States, 13 percent of teens have had intercourse by the age of fifteen, and 65 percent by their nineteenth birthday.[2] At least 55 percent of young people between the ages of fifteen and nineteen reported having had oral sex with someone of the opposite sex.[3] These statistics imply that a lot of sex is going on among young people—as it probably always has—but we need to ask whether sex education beyond just teaching the mechanics of the act and instruction in "safe sex" is occurring. Are mothers teaching their daughters that sex is the coming together of two people to experience the intimacy of eternal oneness? Do mothers explain that tenderness and respect enhance the satisfaction and enjoyment of lovemaking? Do daughters know that it is the woman who should be directing the rhythm of sex using the contractions of the vaginal muscles, rather than allowing the man to dictate the pace through the thrusts of his penis? And how many young women know that there is a difference between having sex with a man who is circumcised and one who is not, with the latter group experiencing far greater sensitivity around the penile head, changing the level of sexual intimacy for both partners?

Sex is a sacred and healing act. In ancient times, certain women were trained as priestesses to raise their sexual or kundalini energy and thereby achieve a state of oneness. They were also taught how to carry a man along this serpentine ladder so that he too could experience this perfected state. When men decided they no longer needed to turn to women for enlightenment, the sacred sexual priestesses were cast out and denigrated as prostitutes and whores. Whereas many women today claim they experience a satisfactory and enjoyable sex life, I would venture to suggest we are still a long way from the sacred priestesses whose connection to the Great Mother allowed them to take the lead in what can truly be a spiritually as well as physically transcendent experience.

VIOLENCE AGAINST WOMEN

The disconnection from sacred sexuality and sacred femininity can be seen in the prevalence of sexual violence against women in the world's cultures today. Around the world, a whole range of abuses are taking place: domestic rape, the use of rape as a weapon against populations in times of war, the trafficking of young people as sex slaves, female genital mutilation, dowry and honor killings, and sexual harassment of all kinds. In 2003, the United Nations estimated that one out of every three women is beaten, raped, or otherwise abused during her lifetime, with the abuser most often coming from her own family.[4] In parts of southern and eastern Asia, notably China and India, abortion based on prenatal sex selection, and female infanticide, are regularly carried out, showing the low value placed on girls and women in these countries.[5]

Rape is just as prevalent in the first world as in the third. In the United States, 17.6 percent of women have survived an attempted or completed rape, with 21.6 percent of these women being under the age of twelve and 50 percent under the age of eighteen.[6] By comparison, approximately 3 percent of American males have been raped, 71 percent before their eighteenth birthday.[7] Between 20 and 25 percent of all female students in the United States report having been raped or threatened with rape during their college years, and it is estimated that many more cases of sexual assault go unreported.[8]

It is estimated that between 10 and 50 percent of women all over the world have been victims of domestic assault, with 3 to 50 percent* reporting violence in the previous year; 25 percent of those questioned had also been raped, while 26 percent had received verbal abuse or threats.[9] In the United States, a woman is beaten every eighteen minutes, with 1.3 million women affected annually.[10]

The incidence and type of assault vary depending on the country,

*This wide statistical range can be attributed to the fact that the highest levels are found in developing countries. Those in industrialized countries have greater access to support services and hence increased opportunities to escape abusive relationships.

culture, and ethnicity. For example, a Native American woman is twice as likely to be a victim of sexual assault as a woman from any other racial background. African American women, on the other hand, are much more susceptible to deadly violence from a member of their own family. On many occasions domestic violence is accompanied by emotional abuse, which includes prohibiting a woman from seeing her family and friends, ongoing humiliation or intimidation, economic restrictions such as preventing a woman from working or confiscating her earnings, and other controlling behaviors. In fact, demographic surveys from a variety of countries show that gender-based violence is often considered normal, with both men and women assuming that a husband has the right to punish his wife if she neglects the children, answers him back, refuses sex, or burns the food. In many Asian countries, honor killing, in which a male member of a family kills a female relative for tarnishing the family image, is still considered acceptable, while female circumcision and genital mutilation affect over 140 million women worldwide.[11]

Trafficking, defined as the recruitment of persons, whether by coercion, deception, or outright abduction, places people in economic and sexual bondage worldwide. The United Nations estimates that 75 percent of trafficked persons are women, and 20 percent are children, and that nearly 2.5 million people from 127 countries are being trafficked around the world at any given time, making this a multibillion-dollar industry.[12]

Many organizations, such as the Global Alliance against Traffic in Women (GAATW), Amnesty International, and the United Nations, have created worldwide platforms for advocacy and action, like the U.N.'s "Say No: Unite to End Violence against Women" campaign. But although eighty-nine countries have passed tougher legislation against domestic violence, many crimes against women go unreported and unpunished, and 102 countries are still without laws against domestic violence.[13] There are many outstanding, courageous women all over the world actively working to expose and reduce these atrocities against women. Yet they need our support, as the issues affect not one country, race, or religion but every single woman.

Looking at these figures, it is easy to feel overwhelmed, especially when we realize that people suffer emotional abuse every day from so-called friends and family, without believing they have a right to question the morality and ethics of such abuse. For many women, some of the most emotionally painful episodes of disrespect and humiliation have occurred at the hands of not men but other women, whether due to their words or their actions. In my experience, the abused child often carries feelings of anger toward the female figures in the family, especially the mother, not always because of what they did, but because of what they didn't do to prevent the abuse. Women have an innate belief in the power of community support, which has protected and ensured the tribe's survival, whatever the crisis, over thousands of years. When this is not present, the wounds of isolation, insecurity, unworthiness, and betrayal easily rise to the surface, affecting a woman's life right down to the core of her being.

Change will come, but it begins with each individual woman; we need to step back from the big picture and instead find ways to restore self-love and self-respect, one woman at a time. Only then can we hope to create the longed-for dynamic shift of consciousness that will lead to the eventual end of violence and abuse against women. For this to happen, every single woman must begin to honor and respect her essential and sacred purpose here on earth, which, as we shall see, goes far, far beyond mere procreation.

Men, as well as women, carry deep wounds as a result of thousands of years of imbalance between the genders. These hurts cannot be healed if, fueled by anger and blame, they are used to create further division between the sexes. The greatest gift we can leave future generations is to ensure that from this moment on, our words and deeds are motivated not by wounds from the past, but by our vision for the future.

The archetypal identity of womanhood is not lost but sleeps deep within our collective unconscious. It is to be found in our history, mythology, and most of all the one thing that hasn't changed for millions of years: the form and function of a woman's body. Our collective identity awaits the day when women like myself and like you, dear reader, wake up and allow the yearnings of the heart, breasts, womb, and soul to lead us. As the sleeping goddess reawakens and we fully embody the true nature of what it is to be a woman, our inner and outer environments will transform, making the world a very different place to live.

2

MEETING OUR ANCESTRAL
GRANDMOTHERS

We are not makers of history. We are made by history.
                              MARTIN LUTHER KING JR.

A wise kahuna from the Hawaiian Islands once said to me, "If you want to know where you're going, you first have to know where you've come from."

So it is for women: if we want to recover our feminine identity, we must first travel back in time and meet our ancient grandmothers. I have confined my search to those civilizations that existed more than 3,500 years ago, after which time, as I suggest in chapter 1, the principles of patriarchy took hold and became increasingly dominant in the world. Other fine writers have documented the story of women during the past few millennia, highlighting their struggle to find, and maintain, a respectful and equal position in society; my search goes back much farther.

Most of the early archeological evidence of the role women played in societies prior to 3400 BCE is not found in any kind of recognizable written form; it has rather been preserved in drawings, carvings, and mythological tales. We are dependent on the skills and hypotheses of archaeologists and scholars who have pieced together their conclusions based on findings such as shards of pottery, faint images painted on walls, and age-worn statuettes. Yet we should never underestimate the desire of the collective unconscious to be heard, subtly stirring the imagination of researchers in such a way that the true story is revealed. Or, as American poet Stanley Kunitz said, "Old myths, old gods, old heroes have never died. They are only sleeping at the bottom of our mind, waiting for our call. We have need for them. They represent the wisdom of our race."

As we attempt to lift the veil that shrouds the sacred purpose of womanhood, we need to rely on those who have had the courage and curiosity to look beyond what has been written in standard textbooks to ask the difficult questions. Such a pioneer was the late Marija Gimbutas, who was a fellow of Harvard's Peabody Museum and a professor of European archaeology at the University of California in Los Angeles. She upset many of her colleagues by claiming that prior to the invasion by the Indo-European patriarchal culture around 2500 BCE, there was a culture known as Old Europe, a matriarchal society with strong evidence of goddess worship.[1] She backed up her findings with prolific writings, including *The Goddesses and Gods of Old Europe* (1982) and the *The Language of the Goddess* (1989).

Gimbutas's conclusions were criticized by her contemporaries, both male and female, for being biased as a result of her 1970s feminist leanings, although her findings did not exclude the the role of men within these ancient societies. More recent explorations carried out in the same area of the world—in particular Anatolia or western and central Turkey—have refined her original research, leading to the conclusion that both gods and goddesses were revered during the era from 6500 to 2500 BCE. However, the discovery of Old Europe by Professor Gimbutas opened our eyes to the fact that well-organized, civilized societies existed at a time when most conventional historians and archaeologists have assumed that we were still living in caves and wearing only animal skins as clothing. More importantly, Gimbutas revealed that within these cultures, contrary to the present day, women held high positions, positions of power, and were greatly revered throughout society.

But archaeological evidence about our ancestral grandmothers stretches even further back in time, requiring us to enter bygone planetary eras that are almost beyond our imagination.

PALEOLITHIC WOMAN

The Paleolithic era began approximately 2.5 million years ago and lasted up to around 10,000 BCE. This immense stretch of time, also known as the prehistoric, or Old Stone Age, was characterized by the use of stone tools, the development of small societies, and the emergence of the anatomically modern human, *Homo sapiens.* This newcomer gradually marginalized the older, archaic varieties of human beings, until their extinction about 30,000 years ago.

Any evidence of the presence of the feminine during this era is relatively scant due to the obvious effects of the aging process on organic materials. Yet carved stones and bones, as well as paintings, have survived from this period. The earliest stones to depict a human form, thought to date from between 300,000 to 500,000 years ago, are known as the Venus of Tan-Tan and the Venus of Berekhat Ram.* There is evidence that these stones were carved by human hand and adorned with red ocher; nevertheless, some archaeologists are not convinced of the authenticity of these objects and believe they are just stones or pebbles that were fashioned by natural forces.[2] Time will tell.

Paintings of the Blood of Life and Death

As we move forward chronologically, to the time 40,000 to 30,000 years ago, we encounter the first evidence of abstract thinking by modern humans with the appearance of cave paintings in various parts of the world, including southwest Europe, South America, Siberia, Africa, Australia, and India. For these cavemen and cavewomen, the ability to think in an abstract manner transformed them from the stereotypical

---

*Though called Venus, the gender of these figurines is indeterminate. The word Venus is usually applied to artifacts that are more modern, as will be described shortly.

image of "see food, kill food, eat food" to a culture that perceived its reality as consisting of relationships and patterns enveloping both the immediate environment as well as the supernatural world. Most of the cave paintings of this period are of large animals such as bison, woolly mammoths, horses, and deer, which are all thought to have roamed the lands during this period.

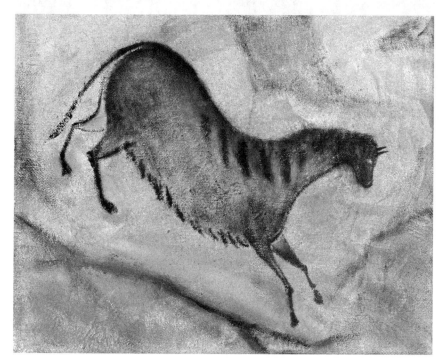

Ancient cave painting

Prehistoric graffiti is also present, often of an explicit sexual nature—revealing marked similarities to graffiti found on the walls of many of our cities today. There are also many examples of traced handprints believed to have belonged to the artists; the size and shape of these prints suggest that at least a quarter of the wall paintings were produced by women.

These prehistoric artists used red ocher to add color to their depictions. This naturally occurring clay contains mainly iron oxides, suggesting a strong association with blood, in particular, iron-bearing

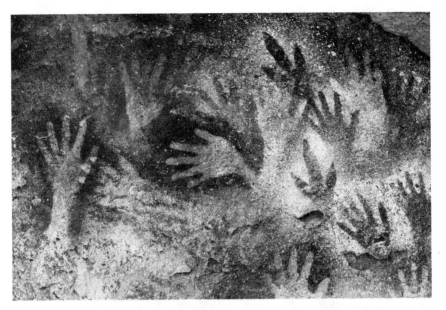

Feminine handprints from our prehistoric ancestors?

hemoglobin. Because so many of the prehistoric feminine images are daubed with red ocher, especially around the vulva and vagina area, it was thought at first that the artists were attempting to emphasize the passion of sexuality. However, further excavations revealed that red ocher was commonly used to paint the bodies of the dead, while vulva-shaped cowrie shells were also painted red and carefully placed around the corpse. This has led archaeologists to conclude that in prehistoric times the feminine was seen as having not only the power to give life but also the ability to intercede with the supernatural world and in fact to bring about resurrection.[3] Symbolically, this continuous flow between the worlds of life and death is expressed through the menstrual cycle, with the blood of menses being seen as mystically endowed with the power of purification and death, as well as rebirth and renewal.

One particular set of caves, known as Pech Merle, in southwest France, has caught the imagination of many explorers, as it contains some of the finest examples of prehistoric cave art to be found anywhere. Pech Merle is an underground limestone labyrinth of chambers and passageways covering over four kilometers, naturally carved out millions of years ago by a now-extinct river. Occupied by humans for 15,000 years, from approximately 25,000 BCE, the labyrinth once had an entrance that eventually closed because of a landslide, and the cave complex was not rediscovered until 1922. Inside the caves, alongside depictions of wild animals, can be found much stranger images showing animals with very small heads on normal-size bodies, or beings that are half man and half animal.[4] The creation of this art did not occur over just a few years' time but covered an extraordinary length of time, emphasizing its importance to the growth of consciousness over multiple generations. Much of the art is found in extremely narrow spaces, suggesting that the artists worked in cramped and relatively uncomfortable conditions. Clearly, these particular caverns were not used for habitation because of the inadequate space, fresh air, and light; and so this leaves us with three questions: Who were the artists? Why did they work under such conditions? And what did the paintings mean to them?

Many interpretations have been put forward to answer these questions, with the most intriguing coming from British writer and journalist Graham Hancock, in his book *Supernatural*. Hancock, who has made a successful literary career out of questioning the unquestioned orthodox views put forth by the educational system, the media, and society at large, believes that these drawings represent the visions of ancient shamans who, having consumed a consciousness-altering plant, entered the world of the supernatural, where they met these obscure and unworldly figures. It is understood that the purpose of such a shamanic journey—like any shamanic journey—would be to escape the confines of this three-dimensional world to explore multidimensional spiritual realities, often to acquire insight into earth-related issues. That these shamanic journeys took place over a period of thousands of years suggests that this process was successful: it not only provided answers, but it renewed the energy of the soul, much as sleep allows the body to recuperate. The darkness, isolation, and sensory deprivation that the caves offered the prehistoric shaman obviously increased the effectiveness of interdimensional travel; otherwise, why crawl into such inconvenient, cramped space? So the next question is: Is such discomfort always necessary for communication with the supernatural world?

I don't think so. I believe that women have a lifetime permit that allows them to access the spiritual realms at will, without the need for mind-altering drugs, especially at certain times in their lives: the moon time, at the time of childbirth, and after menopause. At these junctures in a woman's life there is no need for her to go outside and find a physical cave, for she carries her cave with her constantly; it is the sacral chakra and its physical powerhouse, the uterus. Whatever a woman's age or whether or not she still possesses her uterus, the energy of the cave is always present and can be used to purify her of old, unwanted emotions so that she can reconnect to the heart of the Great Mother and give birth to creative ideas and inspirations.

The Venus Figurines

During the same time frame as the Pech Merle cave paintings, between approximately 32,000 and 20,000 BCE, other prehistoric artists were crafting exquisite, undeniably female sculptures throughout the lands that stretch from present-day France to Siberia. Many researchers believe these artifacts were archetypal representations of the Great Mother, sometimes called the Great Goddess, the Creatrix, and the Life Giver. The archaeologists named all of these small statuettes after Venus—the Roman goddess of love—followed by the place name of the location they were found.

These figurines were carved from a variety of materials, including soft stone (steatite, calcite, or limestone), bone, ivory, wood, and ceramic clays, with most measuring between two and eight inches in height. Since the appearance of the first Venus figurine in 1894, hundreds have been located, with one of the oldest, a statue made from mammoth tusk, believed to be 35,000 years old. It was found in Germany's Hohle Fels cave in 2008.

There can be few women who don't feel a deep rapport with these female images, which display an ease and comfort with abundant female

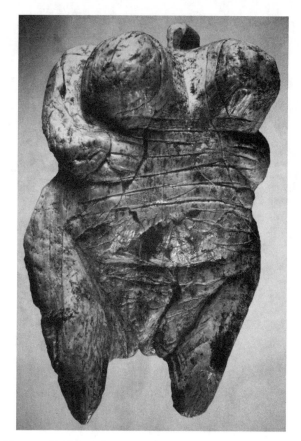

Venus of Hohle Fels, near Ulm, Germany, 33,000 BCE

curves and beautiful nakedness. The characteristics of all these statuettes are markedly similar: an emphasized pubic triangle, a vulvar slit, and exaggerated belly, breasts, thighs, and hips. The large proportions, especially around the buttocks, are thought to signify fecundity in all forms. There are usually no hands or feet, and the facial features are indistinct.

Whether paintings or carved figures, these icons are believed by archaeologists to represent fertility goddesses who were called on to ensure the continuity of a family or tribe. However, this is a modern viewpoint, one that neglects the fact that these prehistoric humans were deeply immersed in an appreciation of the supernatural world. It is highly probable that fertility meant more than mere procreation and physical survival to these people. Could it have described spiritual

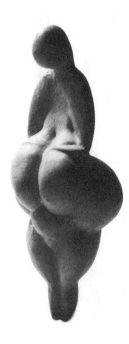

*Replica of the Venus of Lespugue,
France, 23,000 BCE*

fruitfulness and the growth of humanity's consciousness, wherein the female body becomes the essential vessel?

With this in mind, I propose that these artifacts exemplify three different levels of fertility:

- The first area, represented by the buttocks, includes the sacral chakra, uterus, ovaries, and the cave, symbolizing cycles of birth, nurturing, and death.
- The second area, represented by the breasts, includes the heart chakra and reflects bonding, connection, and transformation.
- The third area, represented by the head, includes the crown chakra and the pineal gland and is symbolic of merging with the collective oneness and receiving creative inspiration.

As with the cave paintings, some figurines are painted with red ocher, especially around the vulva and breasts. This is certainly true of the figurine known as the Venus of Laussel, which dates from around 23,000 BCE and still shows signs of this distinctive red paint. She carries in her hand a bison horn, which is said to represent a cornucopia, or horn of plenty, an ancient symbol of the abundance and fertility of the Great Mother. The horn is carved with thirteen notches, which are thought to represent the thirteen lunar cycles that have comprised the lunar (female) calendar of indigenous peoples since time immemorial.

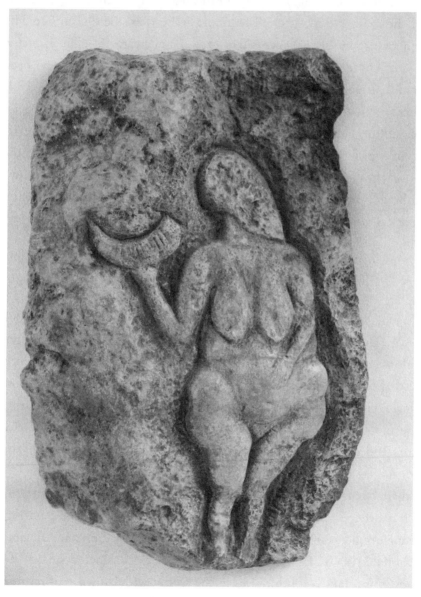

Venus of Laussel, France, 23,000 BCE

Among the best known of these figurines is the Venus of Willendorf, which was found in 1908 close to the Danube River and now resides in Vienna's Natural History Museum. Five inches tall, she was carved from limestone and has been dated from between 24,000 and 22,000 BCE. She has many fascinating features that I believe sets her apart from many of the other Venus figurines, and in this regard she opens our eyes to one of the most important of all feminine archetypes, the Queen Bee. Her inheritance and significance will be explored in greater detail in chapter 9.

It is noteworthy that although some 200 Venus statuettes have been found around the world, male figurines are surprisingly absent; while there are many examples of phallic artifacts and paintings that depict masculine characteristics, there are no comparable male statuettes from this period. One modern British archaeologist has promoted the novel theory that the female figures are a kind of prehistoric sex toy,[5] although in my opinion this should be taken as a product of a twenty-first-century (male) imagination.

NEOLITHIC WOMAN

The Neolithic period began around 10,000 BCE and lasted until 3000 BCE. This rich era of human evolution saw the development of agriculture, the domestication of animals, and the creation of permanently settled communities. The timing of such innovations varied across the world, largely depending on the climate and the melting of ice from the most recent ice age. In northeast Africa, domestication of animals and cultivation of grains began as far back as 10,000 BCE and continued until around 5000 BCE, when the desertification of the Sahara occurred, causing communities to move in search of water. In China, there is evidence of early farming practices and cave paintings from around 7000 BCE, although the first dynasty didn't appear until around 2100 BCE. Mehrgarh, in Pakistan, is considered one of the most important Neolithic sites in the world, with evidence of farming settlements dating back to between 7000 and 5000 BCE.

Many historians and archaeologists believe that it is precisely in these Neolithic settlements in the area of what is now called the Near East that we find evidence of the source of many Western civilizations. This is the area that once encompassed the ancient regions of Mesopotamia (now Iraq, parts of Syria, Turkey, and Iran), Canaan (now Palestine), and Egypt. Because of a temperate climate and a rich source of water, the land in this region was fertile, and by 10,000 BCE the people here were producing wheat and barley on a large scale. By 9000 BCE sheep farming was popular, and by 6000 BCE pigs, dogs, and cattle had been domesticated. During this period, people lived in villages and townships, with the settlements often positioned on hills to provide natural protection. From evidence dated to around 6500 BCE, it is clear that the plow and the wheel were in widespread use, and people had progressed to being able to combine copper and tin to produce a highly durable bronze.[6]

There is little archaeological evidence of social stratification in these Neolithic societies, with most exhibiting egalitarian and polytheistic principles, whereby all people were considered socially equal and numerous expressions of divine inspiration were allowed. This has confounded many modern historians who come from the perspective of modern society, which is hierarchal; they tend to think that all previous cultures must have also been hierarchal, with social stratification much like what we have become accustomed to. Based on this fallacy, there is a propensity to look for evidence of a power structure whereby the leader is deified, i.e., raised above the status of the common man. Similarly, as soon as there is a suggestion that a particular artifact exhibits superhuman characteristics, it is referred to as a god or goddess and there is a concurrent belief that this archetype must have been worshipped and placed on a pedestal. Very likely, however, everything was honored equally in Neolithic society—the sacred was seen in all things.

One of the best-preserved Neolithic sites is Çatalhöyük, in southern Anatolia, Turkey, which is dated from between 7500 and 5700

BCE. When James Mellaart, the archaeologist who first excavated the site in 1958, found beautiful feminine statuettes that are evidence of goddess worship, he declared that the society must have been matriarchal.[7] However, in more recent years, researchers under the direction of Ian Hodder, professor of archaeology at Stanford University, have unearthed evidence that suggests that both men and women were equally honored.

Çatalhöyük reveals many significant findings in our search for the female archetype. One of the most powerful images, dated to around 6000 BCE, is a terra-cotta figure of a seated woman with large breasts and buttocks. The head of an infant appears between her ample thighs. She is flanked by two felines, probably leopards, which were often associated with feminine strength as far back as the Paleolithic era. This image clearly represents fertility, so we need to go back 8,000 years and investigate the significance of giving birth, and especially the right to inherit, before we can truly understand the importance of this statue.

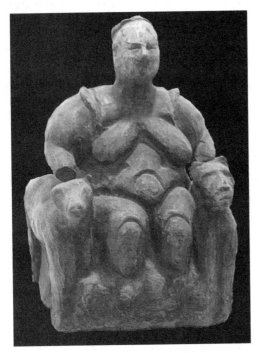

Great Mother figure found at the archaeological site of Çatalhöyük

Matrilineality

Today, almost any child beyond the age of innocence knows where babies come from. Yet this was not always the case, as historically pregnancy and birth have been shrouded in mystery. In her groundbreaking book *When God Was a Woman,* Merlin Stone describes the findings of several anthropologists regarding the subject of fertility. They concluded that, unbelievable as it may sound, in many prehistoric cultures no connection was made between the act of coitus between a man and a woman and the birth of a baby nine months later. This, anthropologists believe, led to women being revered as life givers, while the role of the male in conception went unacknowledged.[8] Whether the women of this era knew of his part in the process—as seems likely—and chose to keep the information to themselves for whatever reason we will never know.

Anthropologists believe it is for this reason that so many images and statuettes of pregnant women and women giving birth—which honor woman's mystical fertility and her ability to ensure the survival of the tribe or clan—have been found at ancient sites. It is also suggested that it was this perception of a woman's supernatural powers in birth that fostered matrilineality, in which the maternal name and property are transferred from one generation to the next, allowing women to amass substantial wealth and privilege within society. This also led to the practice in the earlier dynasties of Egypt whereby a princess commonly married her brother in order to keep the wealth in the ruling family.

From accounts describing life in Egypt between 3000 and 1500 BCE, we learn that because of the veneration of the Great Mother and matrilineal inheritance, women were highly involved in matters of state and finance, while their husbands remained at home. Similar reports have emerged from other parts of Africa, where, much like the Amazons, a nation of all-female warriors in Greek mythology and classical antiquity, it was the women who formed the armies while the men stayed at home to look after the children.[9] Because of a woman's esteemed status, it was she who chose her husband, as well as making the decision to separate when she considered the marriage was over.

Despite the authority given to women during these times, anthropologists are not convinced that these societies exhibited matriarchal domination. In other words, although inheritance was passed down through the mother's lineage, there was no evidence of an unequal distribution of power and governance between men and women. Such matrilineal societies are believed to have been in existence from 30,000 BCE until approximately 1200 BCE, when a change occurred and the system converted to patrilineality. I believe the most likely cause of this shift was also the motivation for the medieval witch hunts and is still active in our world today: *avarice,* a desire to own something that doesn't belong to you, commonly advanced by spreading false information and generating fear. Slowly, the land, property, and prestige were removed from the women and became the possession of men. However, these were merely outer trappings to the real prize, the power of fertility, which could only ever be owned by women.

Even though most of the Western world follows the patrilineal pattern of inheritance today, there are still some isolated peoples in Africa, India, China, Sumatra, and Indonesia that continue the matrilineal system. The Cherokee, Choctaw, Hopi, Navajo (Diné), and Tlingit peoples of North America were also all matrilineal societies, as were the Hawaiians and Polynesians, up until the time the Christian missionaries arrived, beginning in the early 1800s.

The Iroquois nation, whose oral constitution, known as the Gayanashagowa, or the Great Law of Peace, was the basis for the constitution of the United States, was a matrilineal society. Women were considered the keepers of the culture, responsible for deciding political, social, spiritual, and economic policies for the tribe. It was a man known as the Great Peacemaker, Deganawidah, who brought together the original clan mothers, because he believed that only women could decide what was best for the good of all the people. He also understood that women alone knew the pain of burying a child they had suckled at their breast, and therefore only women had the wisdom to decide whether a battle or war was worth the potential loss of life.

It was the clan mothers who were inspired with the ideals and visions that would benefit the Iroquois nation, while the men were entrusted to carry out the policies as established by the women. Although outwardly the leaders appeared to be the men, it was the clan mothers who nominated and elected them and who removed them from their positions of authority if they failed to live up to their responsibilities. Yet it is important to understand that in societies such as the Iroquois, both genders were honored for the roles they played in the community, receiving equal respect for their contributions.[10] One can only imagine the social and political landscape today if such a system were in place! How different our world would be if men cherished and appreciated the intuitive visions and insights of women, while women valued and celebrated the achievements of men.

Mitochondrial Eve

It could be hypothesized that matrilineal descent was based not merely on a perception about what it takes to make a baby, but on the awareness that some family lines survive better than others. Scientifically, we now know that one's physical endurance is determined by tiny intracellular particles known as mitochondria, the genes of which are exclusively those of our mother. Mitochondria are stored outside the cell nucleus, in the cytoplasm. The cytoplasm of a human egg is packed with a quarter of a million mitochondria, while the sperm contains very few mitochondria—just enough to provide the energy to swim to the egg. When the sperm has delivered its nuclear DNA, the mitochondrial DNA of the father plus the tail of the sperm are jettisoned.[11]

Mitochondria are the power generators of the cell, converting oxygen and nutrients from food into adenosine triphosphate (ATP), which the cell uses as an energy source. When there are mutations within the mitochondrial DNA, energy production is much slower, leading to malfunction within the organs that rely on quick sources of vitality, such as the heart, the muscles, and the brain; this ultimately accelerates the aging process.[12] Research has also shown that in illnesses such as fibromyalgia and chronic fatigue syndrome, there is mitochondrial dysfunction that leads to a decrease in available energy.[13]

Because of this unique feature of maternal mitochondrial DNA being passed down through the generations, researchers have been able to look back in history at the origins of our species. Bryan Sykes, professor of human genetics at Oxford University, has concluded that all races can be traced back to a common maternal ancestry. He cites the existence of four such women among the Native Americans, nine in the Japanese culture, and just seven women for 97 percent of native Europeans; all of these mitochondrial ancestors of ours lived sometime between 10,000 and 45,000 years ago.[14]

Going back even farther in time, statistical analysis has revealed the presence of a gene pattern that first appeared 200,000 years ago, the legacy of an ancient ancestor called Mitochondrial Eve. However, it's important to point out that Mitochondrial Eve was probably not the first woman to appear on Earth, nor was she the only woman alive 200,000 years ago, but her genetic lineage was the first to survive to this day. If a woman gives birth to only male offspring, then her mitochondrial DNA will be lost. In other words, in ancient times parents would rejoice when a daughter was born, for it was through her that a strong maternal line was preserved.

In summary, matrilineal inheritance and the reverence shown to women as the progenitors of life are probably attributable to a number of factors, one of which is very practical: survival of the fittest. Even today, some children fare better than others because of the mitochondrial genes gifted to them by their mother.

The Primordial Waters

As we continue our exploration of Neolithic women, it is important to examine the key spiritual beliefs that shaped their daily routines. To do this, we need to set aside for a moment any Creation narratives wherein the singular creative force is masculine, and instead we must imagine a life born from primordial waters, or chaos. The Greeks coined the word *chaos* to describe the dark void from which all life emerged. According to Greek mythology, chaos gave birth first to Gaia, the Earth Mother, and then to Eros, the god of love. In this chaotic form, the primordial waters are often described as possessing deep, mysterious, destructive powers; they are symbolized by fiery dragons and cunning serpents.

Cultures that existed prior to 500 BCE, including those of Sumer, Babylonia, and Egypt, also honored the primordial waters as the source of all life. To the Egyptians, this creative energy was known as the masculine Nu, or Nun, but also manifested in goddesses such as Maat, Ua Zit, and Hat-Hor, all of whom took the form of the primeval serpent or cobra. The Sumerians and Babylonians believed that the primordial waters were feminine, calling them Nammu and Tiamat. The ancient Maya of Central America believed that the source of life was the watery serpent in the sky, the Milky Way, also regarded as the Mother from whose white belly of stars we emerged.[15] In Hinduism, the primordial goddess mentioned in Vedic scriptures is called Danu, while the ancient Persians called the goddess Anahita. Even the Bible, in Genesis 1:2, describes the primordial waters: "And the Earth was without form, and void and darkness was upon the face of the deep. And the Spirit of God moved upon the face of the waters."

The flow of the primordial waters is closely aligned to the cycles of the moon, which also express phases of birth and death. The waters should not be seen as mere H_2O, for they contain all the vital ingredients required for life on Earth, just as a mother's blood and amniotic fluid provide all the needs of the unborn baby. The waters pulsate with the potential of creative energy, often described as possessing the vibration of primordial sounds that give life to all forms. According to the myths of these civilizations, our existence consists of cycles of birth and death. All beings emerge originally from the primordial waters and are bound to return there at the end of life. This is not so difficult to envisage when we remember that each one of us emerged from the amniotic fluid of our mother, and at death our tissues liquefy under the influence of enzymes, until all that is left are dry bones.

Other names for the primordial waters include the ocean of possibilities, the void, the ocean of milk, the abyss, the Great Mother, and the collective unconscious, where everything exists as an energized potential awaiting focused attention to bring the dream into reality. Depending on the culture, the agents of actualization have been described as a seed, sperm, Spirit of God, thunderbolt, breath, and sun fire. When the sacred union takes place between these energized waters of feminine potential and focused masculine attention, new life is born within the world of matter.

As patriarchal domination increased some 3,000 years ago, any veneration given to the inherent power of the primordial waters diminished, with more value being placed on the actualizing agent than on the source of the creation force. During that time, a number of mythical tales emerged about heroes controlling or destroying the fearful serpentine monster that inhabited the chaotic waters.[16] These include the Babylonian Marduk, who killed the monster Tiamat; the Hindu sky god Indra, who used thunderbolts to slay Vritra, the demonic serpent child of Danu; the Greek god Apollo, who slayed the monstrous serpent Python at Delphi; and Hercules, who killed the serpent Ladon, which was wrapped around Hera's golden apple tree, the tree of immortality.

Why did the slaughter happen? From an esoteric perspective, the primordial waters, or collective unconscious, represent a mysterious and

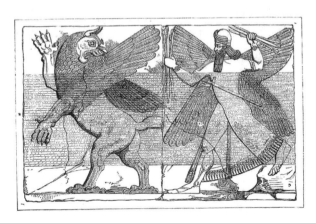

Marduk killing the monster Tiamat

powerful force that influences and penetrates every thought, word, and action. Associated with the death of the old and the birth of the new, this mysterious force often appears to strike without warning, leaving carnage and chaos in its wake. There came a time during the rise of the patriarchy when the male leaders were no longer willing to relinquish their power to an energy they couldn't control. Similar to the way that people deal with unpleasant emotions or memories, the priesthood of the second millennium BCE attempted to take control of their lives by creating doctrines and laws that "made sense" of illogical and unthinkable occurrences, or the mystery of life. With this decision the priesthood effectively banished any mention or worship of this unwelcome guest, the feminine primordial chaos, making them believe that man was more powerful than the source of his creation.

Yet as any parent knows, simply refusing to mention a subject does not mean that a child's curiosity is satisfied. Therefore, the priests had to come up with a new set of rules to rationalize the mysteries of life, especially those that occurred out of the blue, such as death and natural phenomena. They evoked the power of a sky deity, Yahweh, who was out of reach of the people and whose decisions should therefore not be questioned for fear of punishment or being accused of blasphemy. In this way the leaders gained control and power. However, if you have ever tried this approach, you probably know that the more you move away from the truth, the greater the web of deception you weave, building stories upon stories until you can't remember where it all started. I am not suggesting that religious doctrines are false; however, it is appropriate to say that certain omissions or distortions of the truth have perhaps led to more confusion, especially since the original reason for the deception—subduing the primordial waters—has never been possible, and these waters, this collective unconscious, continue to hold sway over our lives.

Fast-forward to today and we find ourselves enmeshed in a complex web of thought patterns that we ourselves have created in the belief that we can control and defy the continual presence of chaos and death. In countries like the United States, a vast array of products are continually marketed to a population that places great value on long life and preventing the aging process. However, the primordial energy cannot be eradicated or evaded, for it is the very power that maintains our existence, and as the caterpillar knows, without death there is no birth.

What if we were to stop running from this energy and just accept it, or even embrace it? If we were to do this, our little self, the ego, would have to admit that it is not an isolated, self-contained island, but rather a part of the mighty ocean that surrounds it. The ocean gave birth to the island but can just as quickly take it back, until there is no trace left of it. I suspect that if we were to allow ourselves to blend with the larger encompassing field of consciousness, any feelings we have of being unloved, abandoned, and rejected—emotions so commonly expressed by my clients—would disappear. Perhaps it is time to appreciate that despair, confusion, and chaos, factors often associated with illness, are merely the means by which we are being encouraged to release our hold on life patterns that don't work for us and reconnect to something deeper and more meaningful.

I suggest that there is a practical and urgent need for humanity, whatever the religious persuasion, to reconnect with this primordial energy. If this does not happen, we will fail to receive the vitalizing and renewing force that exists within these waters, and our lives as well as the earth will become unproductive and barren.

How can we reestablish this connection? By immersing ourselves in water—whether literally or metaphorically—so that we can return to the place of oneness we experienced in the womb. As we relax into the pure liquid energy, all walls and boundaries between ourselves and the Great Mother are washed away. We find ourselves surrendering to a loving consciousness that knows who we are and accepts us unconditionally, and we know all is well.

With the patriarchy's banishment of the primordial waters to the deepest recesses of the human mind, other feminine attributes that involve chaos and death, such as menstruation and sexuality, were also demon-ized. Yet, despite attempts to dam the wild and untamable waters, the body of every woman carries the memory of such essential mysteries of life. This relationship between a woman and the cyclical powers of death and birth was expressed by archaeologist Ian Hodder upon his discovery of a particular statuette in the Çatalhöyük complex:

> Another important object . . . that upset our long-held views was a clay figurine discovered by the Istanbul team in the burnt fill of a house. Immediately on finding the figurine we were all taken aback by its very strange and unusual imagery. The front of the figurine looks very much like the small, squat, so-called mother goddess figu-rines that are so well known (though rare) from Çatalhöyük. There are full breasts on which the hands rest, and the stomach is extended in the central part. There is a hole in the top for the head which is missing. As one turns the figurine around one notices that the arms are very thin, and then on the back of the figurine one sees a depic-tion of either a skeleton or the bones of a very thin and depleted human. The ribs and vertebrae are clear, as are the scapulae and the main pelvic bones. The figurine can be interpreted in a number of ways—as a woman turning into an ancestor, as a woman associated with death, or as death and life conjoined. It is possible that the lines around the body represent wrapping rather than ribs. Whatever the specific interpretation, this is a unique piece that may force us to change our views of the nature of Çatalhöyük society and imagery. Perhaps the importance of female imagery was related to some spe-cial role of the female in relation to death as much as to the roles of mother and nurturer.[17]

The Minoan Culture

Around 6000 BCE, a civilization began to develop and thrive on the island of Crete that was similar to the cultures of Mesopotamia. While other societies were falling under the control of the patriarchy, reverence for the Goddess continued in this Minoan society. Indeed, not only was the divine feminine respected, with women officiating at most sacred ceremonies, but the culture was flourishing; it was prosperous and there is little evidence of warfare.[18] Even with the appearance of the Mycenaean culture* on the island around the fifteenth century BCE, the Goddess was not displaced. Indeed, her influence was transported back to mainland Greece, where the employment of women priestesses to oversee sacred rites was adopted. The honored position given to the divine feminine in this culture over matters of

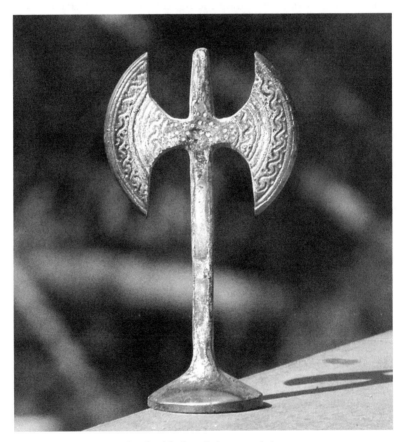

The double-headed ax, or labrys

---

*Quite unlike the Minoans, whose society benefited from trade, the Mycenaeans advanced through conquest. Mycenaean civilization was dominated by a warrior aristocracy.

creativity, fertility, and transformation was symbolized by fascinating images that have intrigued many visitors to Crete.

In the Minoan culture the double-headed ax is believed to have been used during the sacrifice of a bull during religious ceremonies. This tool is always seen in the hands of a priestess, never a priest. The bull was regarded as a sacred animal to the Egyptians and the Minoans, and therefore it was an honored offering to the gods and goddesses in sacred rituals. According to Marija Gimbutas, the ax, in the shape of an *X,* is similar to the contours of a butterfly, both of which represent metamorphosis. The *X* symbol, along with images of serpents and spirals, is often found in sacred locations such as Newgrange, in Ireland, and always signifies a site of spiritual transformation.[19]

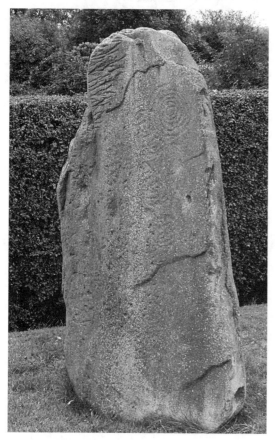

Standing stone at Newgrange showing spiral patterns

The Cretan labyrinth was named after the labrys, or double-headed ax, and was also associated with transformation. The ancient purpose of walking a labyrinth is to leave behind everything that relates to the outer world, until the center of the labyrinth is reached. There the person surrenders completely to the dark and chaotic Goddess—the primordial waters—who instills in the person the gift of new life. The person then leaves the labyrinth with the promise that she will fully manifest her inspiration in the world.

Cretan labyrinth

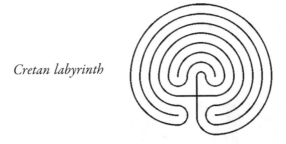

The Serpent

This creature, historically associated with energized potential, is intricately linked to the creative forces that flow through women. In the Minoan civilization, women were trained to have mastery over such powers so they could be used in sacred sexual practices to bring about spiritual evolution. Similar practices were also taught to the priestesses of Isis in Egypt, who wore snake bracelets or serpent tattoos on their arms to reveal their proficiency in such matters. The famous Minoan snake goddess who is seen holding two serpents aloft reveals that she was an initiate of this sacred and pure art.

The Horns

Some of the most intriguing findings in Minoan archaeological sites are the huge stone sculptures that resemble the horns of a cow or bull.

Scholars believe the horns may represent the receptivity of Mother Earth's womb to the sun's rays, especially as many of the huge stones are aligned to the cyclic movement of the sun. Many of the Minoan rituals were carried over from the Egyptian culture, where

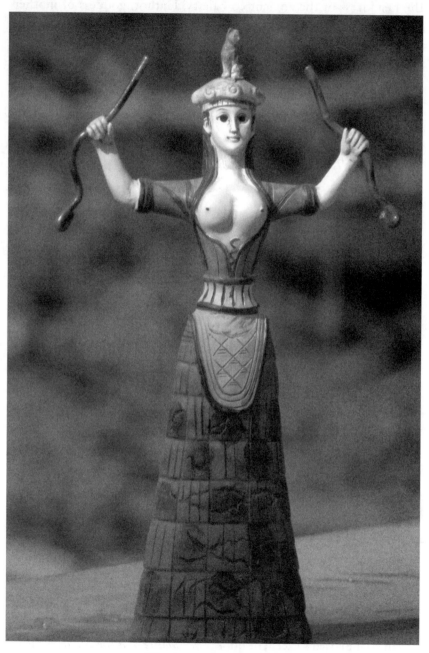

The Cretan snake goddess

the headdress of the ancient cow deity, Hathor, goddess of motherhood, reveals a crescent moon shape, between which sits the sun, or son. Mythology tells us that the Egyptians believed that the Earth gave birth to her son, the rising sun, in the morning, became his consort at noon, and collected his seed into her womb before the sun disappeared from the evening sky. As the goddess Isis came to power, she assimilated the qualities of Hathor and is often seen wearing a similar headdress.

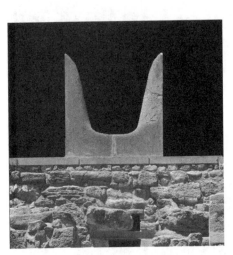

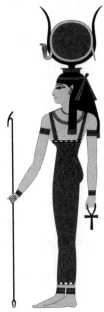

Horns at Knossos, Crete   *The cow goddess Hathor*

If the images of horns found throughout the Minoan culture symbolize the fertility rites that take place daily between the Sun and Earth, then the Minoan sport of bull leaping, wherein young men and women somersaulted through the horns of a cow or bull, could in fact have been replicating this regenerative ritual.

In Riane Eisler's excellent book *The Chalice and the Blade,* we learn that Minoan life was unique, expressing an ardent faith in Goddess nature that led to "a spirit of harmony between men and women, as joyful and equal participants in life." Some of the remarkable features of this society were a high quality of living, whether as king or as peasant, and the absence of statues in honor of the reigning sovereign, indicating that his or her role was not considered any more important than that of any other member of the society.[20]

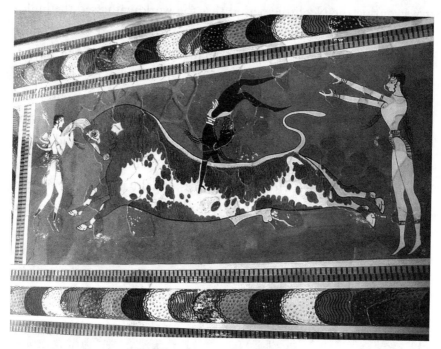

Bull leaping in Minoan culture

Although Minoan weapons have been discovered by archaeologists, it is clear that life was not based on warfare or defense. Everything was designed to be aesthetically pleasing to the eye and in tune with the natural surroundings. Religion was a celebratory affair, closely linked to recreation, especially the bull-leaping game. Some researchers have hypothesized that the Minoans maintained a peaceful and egalitarian society by having a healthy respect for sexuality, with the clothing of both men and women revealing just enough flesh to create a joyful sense of pleasure between the sexes.

Eventually, however, around the eleventh century BCE, paradise was lost to a series of devastating earthquakes and, finally, to invasions by outside conquerors, who callously destroyed the beauty and gracefulness of the civilization that had so much to teach us.

Temples to the Divine Feminine

It was during the Neolithic period that the world witnessed the building of remarkable megalithic temples, many of which are still standing today. It is clear that the ancient architects appreciated the importance of the sacred marriage between the feminine force that inspires, nurtures, and transforms and the masculine strength that focuses and defines. They designed their temples to reenact and celebrate the divine union between Heaven and Earth, in the belief that this would ensure the continued health and prosperity of their culture. To entice the divine feminine to live within the temples, buildings were constructed with curves, imitating the shape of Mother Earth, and especially the female womb.

Such a megalithic site is found at Newgrange, in Ireland, where a circular temple was skillfully designed to capture the rays of the early-morning sun on the 21st of December, the winter solstice. In many cul-

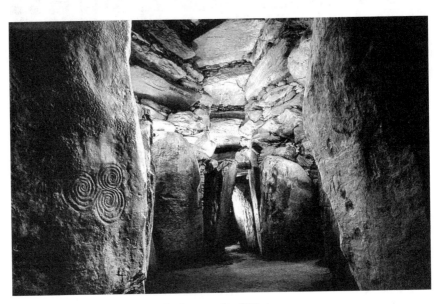

Inside the womb of Newgrange

tures, the winter solstice is regarded as the birth of a new sun, which carries with it a divine intelligence that informs our behavior for the rest of the year. Through a small opening above the entrance of the temple, the sun passes along a passageway—the vagina—before penetrating the cavelike womb of the sanctuary. Here, the masculine intelligence of the sun couples with the wisdom of the earth, and a new child of consciousness is conceived, its energy radiating out from the temple for hundreds of miles.

In the southwest of England we find another beautiful megalithic site, Avebury, with its three stone circles, probably built around 2600 BCE. Linked to several other sacred feminine formations in the area, such as West Kennet Long Barrow and Silbury Hill, the whole complex was dedicated to ceremonies that ensured the fertility of the land and its people.

In still another part of the world, deep in the jungles of the Yucatán, in Mexico, is the temple complex of Uxmal, which was dedicated to training women to become Mayan priestesses. There is evidence that the Mayan culture is tens of thousands of years old, as they often built their newer temples on top of older ones. One of the most imposing structures on this site is known as the Pyramid of the Magician (also known as the Pyramid of the Dwarf). It is perceived as unique because of its rounded sides, considerable height, unusual elliptical base, and the fact that it is made up of three giant steps, three being the number of the Goddess.

A mythical tale tells of a witch who lived in a hut where the temple now stands. Through her wisdom and cunning, her son, a dwarf born from an egg, becomes ruler over the land. I know that it is just a matter of semantics, but I believe the temple should be known as the Pyramid of the Witch, or Female Magician, just to let everybody know that the site is dedicated to the generative powers of the feminine.

Another group of megalithic temples that must be noted as symbols of the embodiment of the feminine force of transformation are

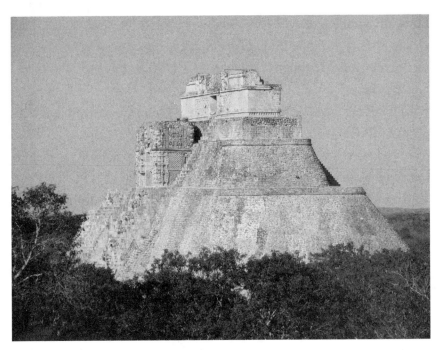

The Pyramid of the Magician at Uxmal, Mexico

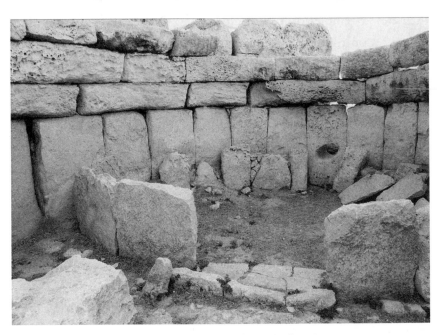

Mnajdra temple on the island of Malta

those found on the tiny islands of Malta and Gozo, in the middle of the Mediterranean Sea, which were erected between 3600 and 2300 BCE. Most of them are aligned with various movements of the celestial bodies, especially the sun, and they thus act as receptacles for the cosmic rays. Nearly all the temples are constructed in the same design, with a central corridor leading through two or more kidney-shaped (ellipsoidal) chambers to reach a small altar apse at the far end. In this way their architecture resembles the curves of a woman.

A deeper explanation of these Mediterranean temples will be provided in chapter 9. There is little doubt that these temples were used for ritual activity, with a strong sense that, once again, women presided over such ceremonies.

SUMERIAN CREATION MYTHOLOGY

Carl Jung said, "We can keep from a child all knowledge of earlier myths, but we cannot take from him the need for mythology." So it is with women.

If women are to understand their true identity, there is one Creation myth that may offer us some valuable clues. This piece of mythology is intricately linked to historical events that have been verified through the translation of hundreds of pieces of Sumerian cuneiform. If there is any truth in the stories found in these ancient texts, beyond mere fantasized ideology, the history books will surely need to be rewritten, not only to correct inaccuracies, but to record the true path of humankind's evolution.

Sumer was a civilization and a historical region in southern Mesopotamia—modern-day Iraq—during the Chalcolithic and Early Bronze ages. Even though this was just a small area of the ancient world, the rapid development of the Sumerian civilization, which took place around 4000 BCE, had enormous implications for humanity. The book of Genesis refers to this era as the birthplace of humankind. Yet as we have already noted, there is strong archaeological evidence that humans existed many thousands of years before this date, before the biblical concept of Adam and Eve.

Perhaps Genesis was never meant to be taken as historical fact, but rather as a synthesis of Creation myths. Given this, and to deepen our exploration, we will start by examining the first book of the Old Testament, which states: "There were nephilim in the earth in those days; and also after that, when the sons of God came in unto the daughters of men, and they bear children to them" (Genesis 6:4). In many modern English translations of the Bible, the word *nephilim* has been changed to *giants*; this, according to writer Laurence Gardner, in his book *Genesis of the Grail Kings*, is not the correct Hebrew translation.[21] The meaning of *nephilim* is "those who came down or descended." Since the Hebrew Bible speaks of the "sons of God" having fallen from grace when they mated with women, it is probable that the nephilim and these sons of God are one and the same.

Returning to Genesis 6, Gardner points out another inaccuracy in the common translation of the original Hebrew, which in fact stems from the advent of monotheism (which itself is a product of patriarchy). The verse refers to God, singular, when in fact the word in the original Hebrew text is Elohim, the plural form of El, meaning god (or goddess). So an accurate interpretation of this line would be: "Sons of gods (and goddesses) came in unto the daughters of men." Now we have a new question; who were these descended gods (and goddesses)? According to Mesopotamian mythology, especially Sumerian and Babylonian, the collective name of the Elohim is Anunnaki, which was translated as "lofty ones, shining ones, or those who from Heaven to Earth came."

Because of the recurrent references to "beings who descended onto Earth," it has been suggested that the Anunnaki were an extraterrestrial race who took an interest in humanity hundreds of thousands of years ago. Whether their intentions were beneficent or malevolent is still debatable. One of the strongest exponents of this theory was the late Zecharia Sitchin, who believed the Anunnaki came from a planet called Nibiru. His findings have been heavily criticized by scientists and academics, although the public obviously resonates with his ideas, as his books, particularly the well-known *Earth Chronicles* series, have sold in the millions worldwide and have been translated into more than twenty-five languages.

According to Gardner, some of the main characters in the assembly of the Anunnaki are:

Nammu, the Dragon Queen and primordial female

Enlil, lord of the air and predecessor to the Canaanite El Elyon and the Hebrew Jehovah

Enki, lord of the earth and the waters, known as The Wise

Nin-khursag, queen of the mountain and wife-sister to both Enki and Enlil

Inanna, Queen of Heaven, also known as Ishtar and Astarte

Eresh-kigal, Queen of the Underworld and sister to Inanna

Lilith, daughter of Eresh-kigal[22]

Gardner states that the first union between the nephilim and women of Earth did not take place around 4000 BCE, the time of the development of the Sumerian civilization, but much earlier, approximately 35,000 years ago. Ancient texts tell of the difficulties encountered by these human prototypes, who were given powers from the nephilim that were often beyond their evolutionary maturity, leading to widespread death and destruction.[23]

Gardner theorizes that eventually the nephilim decided to produce a superior race of Earth leaders who would be created in their image and therefore able to handle their godly powers.* To achieve their goal, they

---

*Ancient texts reveal that the nephilim migrated like birds, although it is not clear where they went and whether they are still influencing the evolution of humanity. Controversial author and speaker David Icke sees the Anunnaki bloodline as a malevolent force that has found its way into many positions of leadership today and is keeping the mass of humanity in slavery. Other researchers believe in the wisdom and love of the successors of Enki and Lilith. Perhaps the way forward is to accept that both forces exist within us all as archetypes, along with many other sources of consciousness that are encoded in our DNA.

took the egg from a woman and inseminated it with the sperm of Enki, placing the fertilized egg in the womb of Nin-khursag so that it was fed with Anunnaki blood. The result was Adama, or Adam, and later came Khawa, the biblical Eve, who was produced in exactly the same manner as her partner, despite the conventional belief that she was created from his rib. According to Gardner, the confusion occurred because of a simple misinterpretation of her title "Lady of Life," because of the fact that the Sumerian word for "life" is almost the same as that for "rib."

Constant disagreements occurred between the brothers Enki and Enlil, with Enki keen to give humanity the same gifts the gods possessed, and Enlil wanting humankind to be, more or less, their slaves. It was probably Enlil who threatened Adam and Eve with death if they ate from the Tree of Knowledge of Good and Evil, while Enki, as the serpent, persuaded Eve to eat the fruit so that her eyes would be opened and she would know herself as immortal. "But of the fruit of the tree which is in the midst of the garden, God hath said, Ye shall not eat of it, neither shall ye touch it, lest ye die. And the serpent said unto the woman, Ye shall not surely die" (Genesis 3:3–4). As one of our most courageous ancestral archetypes, Eve stepped beyond Enlil's threats and, listening to her own inner wisdom— her serpent power—ate the fruit and gifted all women with inner vision and the deep-seated knowledge of our own immortality.

The Legend of Lilith

Within the assembly of the Anunnaki is Lilith, who is described as a wind spirit or the great-winged goddess. In Jewish folklore, from the eighth- through tenth-century Alphabet of Ben Sira onward, Lilith was cast as Adam's first wife. The myth tells of her unwillingness to be subservient and "lie" underneath him and her subsequent departure to the desert. In this Jewish folklore from the Middle Ages, she is commonly regarded as a vengeful, childless goddess who comes at night to steal sleeping children. She is also described as the queen of demons who causes men to have lascivious dreams so that she may steal their seed and create illegitimate children. However, if Lilith was indeed one of the assembly of the Anunnaki,

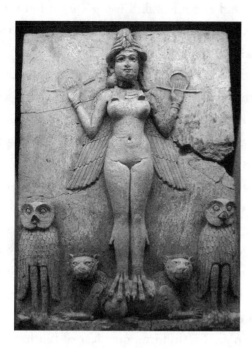

The goddess Lilith

this would probably account for her refusal to be joined in matrimony with Adam, a mere demi-god, let alone to "lie beneath him."

A terra-cotta relief from 2000 BCE shows Lilith as naked and winged, with the feet of an Anzu bird, standing on two lions that rest on a serpent. The Anzu is thought to have been similar to our modern-day owl and was associated with clear vision and insight. The serpent under Lilith's feet represents the creative sexual life force that arises from the earth, also known as dragon power. The lions reveal the power Lilith holds over both the upper and lower worlds. It is her qualities of clear psychic vision and her mastery of sexual energy, as well as her freedom to live in light or darkness, that caused so many to fear her, for she could not be controlled by normal means. She used this unencumbered insight to see a person's spiritual destiny and what obstacles needed to die or be destroyed by her fiery sexual energy in order for a person to reach this potential. She spoke fearlessly from her clear-sighted authority, with her only purpose to ensure spiritual fulfillment, unconcerned by the chaos that might ensue in this transformative process. Like other female archetypes who represent the crone or dark goddess, such as Isis, Kali, and Artemis, Lilith is a powerful force in her own right. She exists in every woman, and it is time that we call her back from the desert and embody her powerful gifts.

As we will see later, there is a time when the serpent and the bird become separated, with the bird of wisdom flying away to later become known as Sophia, or the Holy Spirit, while the serpent power is forced underground. This separation between our wisdom and our powerful creative (sexual) energy is the cause of many of our problems today; it must be healed if humanity is to evolve to a higher state of consciousness and indeed survive at all.

I will never forget the first time I met Lilith. It was at an astrological conference where the female presenter did more than just talk about her subject; she acted out Lilith's main characteristics to a spellbound audience. Portraying the goddess's sensuality and clear insight, the performance triggered extreme reactions from many of the members of the audience who, driven by an archaic and irrational fear of Lilith, became intent on destroying and devaluing the speaker's presentation. It takes a brave and strong woman to take on the persona of a dark goddess.

Nammu, the Dragon Queen who ruled the primordial waters, was Lilith's ancestral grandmother, passing down to her offspring the art of creating expanded consciousness out of death and destruction. It was this legacy that passed down to Mary Magdalen, causing the Christian church to rise up against her teachings and deny her association with Jesus Christ. Whether historical or mythical, Lilith represents the dark goddess within us all, entreating us to enter our own underworld and embody and master the pure dragon energy of sexuality. Only then will we be able to stand in our power with clear vision, wisdom, and inner authority.

BRONZE AGE AND IRON AGE WOMAN IN THE DAWN OF THE PATRIARCHY

From 2400 BCE to 500 CE, the period covering the Bronze and Iron ages, areas such as Iran, Anatolia (ancient Turkey), Egypt, and Greece were invaded by the people from the north who are referred to as Indo-Europeans, Indo-Iranians, Indo-Aryans, or just Aryans.[24] It is clear from archaeological evidence that these invasions occurred over a period of time, however, so it would be probably more appropriate to call them migrations.

Some historians have suggested that the northern people were strictly nomadic warriors who brought carnage to the peaceful matriarchal communities of the southern regions, although evidence suggests that such encounters were far less dramatic and clearly defined. What is known is that the Indo-Aryan tribes brought with them male deities whom they considered far more powerful than the female deities of the indigenous people to the south. The Indo-European male god, unlike the son/lover of the Goddess religion, was portrayed as a storm god who lived high on a mountain, blazing with the light of fire or lightning. To the Hebrews he was known as Yahweh, and later to the Greeks as Jehovah or Zeus, while in Babylonia he was Marduk. Some tales speak of him as a god who destroyed the "evil" Dragon Queen, while others, such as in the story of Zeus and Hera, see the Goddess as the subjugated wife of her all-powerful husband.

The northern people also brought principles of hierarchy to the societies they invaded. They placed their leaders in positions of supreme authority, in contrast to the far more egalitarian principles that had guided Minoan culture. This change brought with it another significant shift in emphasis: the conviction that light, a reference to the fiery male deities, was good, and that dark, a reference to the subterranean goddesses of the lands to the south, was bad or evil. There are some scholars who suggest that this prejudice may have reflected skin coloring as well, as the northern tribes were considerably lighter or fairer of complexion than the native peoples of the south, who had evolved in hotter climates. At the same time, by positioning their distant sky god "up" in the heavens or on top of a mountain, the invaders separated people from their god and instituted priesthoods to speak for the people instead of the people speaking directly to and with the deity.

As the forces of patriarchy turned against the Goddess, terrible injustices were handed down to any woman who disobeyed the new rules. Such decrees proclaimed that women should be virgins when they marry, remain faithful and obedient to their husbands, and adhere to the rules of an omnipotent male deity whose representatives were all men. With increasing loss of prestige within society, women faced a barrage of insults, aimed mainly at sexuality, and specifically at women's powerful moon time. Levite laws laid down between 1000 and 600 BCE were extremely strict, speaking of the right to kill a woman, often by burning or stoning, if she was believed to be adulterous, acted as a "whore" (i.e., a sexual priestess), or "allowed" herself to be raped when betrothed or married.[25] At the same time, men could collect women and create harems; with the husband now in control of the marriage agreement, he could simply rid himself of a wife who did not please him, and by any method he chose.

The various archetypes of the Great Mother/Goddess suffered different fates in the hands of the patriarchal religion. Many of her manifestations were subverted and emerged in the context of patriarchy, while others simply disappeared. All the mythological goddesses of ancient Greece or Rome carried the wounds of submission and humiliation that are still clearly visible in women today.

Sarah and Hagar

The Bible recounts how around 1900 BCE, Sarah, the beautiful wife and half-sister of Abraham, desperate to provide an heir for her husband, agreed that Hagar, her handmaiden and the daughter of an Egyptian pharaoh, should sleep with Abraham. In time, Hagar gave birth to Ishmael, Abraham's firstborn—giving credence to the Islamic belief that it was Ishmael and not Isaac whom God asked Abraham to sacrifice in a show of devotion.

Thirteen years later, at the age of ninety, Sarah gave birth to Isaac and demanded that Hagar and Ishmael should leave her home; hence began their wanderings in the wilderness. It is clear from the Bible that this was Sarah's decision, not Abraham's, as he had to be persuaded by God to listen to Sarah, as noted in Genesis 21:12: "But God said to Abraham, 'Do not be distressed because of the lad and your maid; whatever Sarah tells you, listen to her, for through Isaac your descendants shall be named.'" This suggests that women were still powerful during this time. As Hagar wept over the fate of her child, God made her a promise: that Ishmael would be fruitful and begin a great nation (Genesis 21:18), with his offspring eventually establishing the Islamic faith. It is Hagar's perilous journey to Mecca that underpins the pilgrimage known as the Hajj, which millions of Muslims have undertaken each year for many centuries. Meanwhile, Isaac became one of the patriarchs of the future Jewish religion, inheriting much land, including Egypt (Genesis 15:18).

When we look at today's struggle to find peace between these two religions and two peoples whose founders, Ishmael and Isaac, were brothers, we must understand that the original quarrel was not between the sons, but between their mothers. Sarah's fear that she would not be able to provide Abraham with a son caused her to suggest Hagar as a substitute mother. However, when her own son was born, Sarah rejected her "sister" and banished her from her home. Note that these events took place during the transition from matrilineal to patrilineal inheritance; this, I believe, would account for the insecurity that Sarah must have felt around Hagar, and it probably would not have been an issue in earlier times. It is clear to me that true harmony between these two great religions and magnificent peoples will occur only when the women of both nations make peace between themselves in the name of sisterhood.

Asherah, Consort to Yahweh

As women became increasingly marginalized in patriarchal culture, so were the old female archetypes, the goddesses. Many were married off to one or another male deity and assumed secondary status, and most goddess cults were disbanded and scattered, their temples destroyed. One such Mother goddess was the Semitic Queen of Heaven, Asherah (or Ashtoreth), who was commonly regarded as the consort of Jehovah, or Yahweh. She is identified as the wife or consort to the Sumerian Anu and Ugaritic El, the oldest deities of their pantheons, where she was given similar rank to her male counterparts. In the Ugaritic texts (before 1200 BCE) her name is Athirat and she is known as "she who treads on the sea" as well as the "creatrix of the gods" (the elohim). Her title of Elat (Allat, Ilat) is the female counterpart of El, suggesting that Athirat/ Asherah is a collective name for the consort of gods who evolved from El, including Jehovah and Yahweh.

The idea that the Hebrew God might have had a wife and did not rule alone raises much controversy even today. Yet as William Dever points out in his intriguing book *Did God Have a Wife?* there is plenty of evidence—images, female figurines, and writings—that men and women participated in religious practices in honor of the goddess Asherah within a developing Yahweh cult, which suggests that religious pluralism was initially acceptable.[26] Her many sacred sites of worship typically consisted of pillars and a certain type of tree, which symbolically reassured her followers of the continual, eternal love of the Great Mother.[27]

It was not until around the seventh century BCE that the priesthood finally decided to stamp out evidence of female religion, destroying many of Asherah's altars and assimilating Asherah and Anath (the daughter of Jehovah) into a single entity known as the Shechinah. In Hebrew, this means "a dwelling place," and in Judaism this concept represents the feminine presence of God and divine wisdom. The Shechinah is thought to be present during times of prayer, in music, and in moments of joy; she offers guidance, prophecy, and transformation. A similar feminine energy, Shakinah (or Sakina), is also mentioned in the Qur'an; like the Jewish concept of Shechinah, she represents peace, warmth, reassurance, tranquillity, and strength.

Most likely the tree associated with Asherah was in fact a sycamore fig, which produces large clumps of juicy red fruit. According to Merlin Stone, admiration for this tree was not limited to one culture, as

Cretan pottery and paintings show similar clusters of fruit displayed in honor of the goddess.[28] The Egyptian Mother goddesses Nut, Hathor, and Isis were all associated with the sycamore fig, with ancient images showing Hathor giving fruit to the dead in order to bring them back to life. In Egyptian mythology, the tree represented the eternal presence of the Great Mother here on earth, with the juice representing her blood and the flesh of the fruit her body. When ingested together, they offered eternal life. Sound familiar? Perhaps this is the "forbidden fruit" that Christianity speaks of—which is in fact not a fruit of lust and carnal desire, but the fruit of eternal life, which is free of conditions and dogmas and available to us all today, without the intercession of a priesthood. Rather than an apple tree, perhaps it was a sycamore fig that stood in the Garden of Eden, its fruit an offering from the Great Mother, promising us all a resurrected and immortal life. No wonder the patriarchal god of the day was eager to suppress that knowledge from humanity, for once we attain this wisdom, death loses its sting, and we no longer need anybody to petition on our behalf, for the doors of heaven are open wide to each and every one of us.

Sophia, Keeper of Wisdom

Sophia's name comes from the Greek word for wisdom, giving meaning to the word *philosopher,* "those who love wisdom." She was also known as the Holy Spirit and the feminine face of God, with her wisdom associated with the mind rather than the body.

In the Judeo-Christian tradition, Sophia is the keeper of the knowledge of all things that are righteous and just. In this way she is similar to the Egyptian goddess Ma'at. Her sound wisdom and guidance are sought during times of prayer, as supplicants look to the heavens to receive her answers. This is in sharp contrast to earlier cultures, in which wisdom was perceived to come from deep within the earth, in the calls of animals and birds, in the sound of trees rustling in the wind, and in the sound of the water moving over the surface of the earth.

Venus, Goddess of Eternal Love

There is one aspect of the divine feminine that has been represented throughout time, and this is the goddess of love, who today is known as Venus, but who has also been called Isis, Astarte, Ishtar, Anahita, and Aphrodite. Her name was given to one of the brightest celestial bodies in our sky, the planet Venus, whose cycles have been used by many cultures throughout time to predict the outcome of events.

Venus is known as both the morning and the evening star. This is because there are times when it appears with the first rays of the sun at dawn, while at other times it is seen at twilight, when the sun's rays are fading. Initially, neither the Egyptians nor the Greeks appreciated that the morning and evening stars were the same planet, and therefore they gave them different names. The Greeks called the morning star Phosphoros, "the bringer of light," and the evening star Hesperos, "the star of the evening." Once they realized their mistake—that this was in fact one body—they combined the two names into one: Aphrodite. The Romans translated the names into Latin, with Phosphoros becoming Lucifer, "light bearer," and Hesperos, the evening star, becoming Vesper. These translations give a whole new meaning to the early Christian concept of a fallen angel named Lucifer. Could it be that they were warning us that, like the pathway of Venus, even though we may rise brightly in the morning sky, there will come a time when we will fall into darkness?

Yet it is also possible that the Roman Christians just wanted to make the point that Venus, along with the other Mother goddesses who had preceded her over thousands of years, had now fallen from grace, their beauty dimmed by the brilliance of the masculinized deity. I suspect that Venus represented a much greater fear for the patriarchy, as she is the goddess who fearlessly travels into the darkness before returning sometime later as the morning star. Venus expresses two faces of the Great Mother, the virgin and the crone; she brings inspiration at dawn, and death at dusk. Yet whether descending into darkness or rising into the light, as the goddess of love Venus assures us of one thing: that love is our constant companion.

PATRIARCHAL FORMS OF THE GODDESS

In 392 CE, the Greek emperor Theodosius closed the sanctuary of the goddess Demeter, located in Eleusis, Greece, as well the temple complex in honor of the great goddess Artemis, near Selcuk, in what is now Turkey—the latter often considered to be one of the seven wonders of the ancient world. For 1,500 years, the shrines to Demeter and her daughter Persephone in Eleusis had been the site of initiation ceremonies known as the Eleusinian Mysteries, following the story of Persephone's descent into the underworld, her mother's grief, and Persephone's resurrection as a fully mature woman. These annual events were initially open only to women and later included only certain men. Great secrecy has always surrounded these mysteries, but it is known that participants went through a purification process before descending into the underworld to reconnect to their inherent creative power, inspiration, and rebirth—the mystical essence of a woman's menstrual cycle. Although each participant gained much from the experience, it was the collective expression of the feminine mysteries that influenced the consciousness of the culture, keeping alive the memory of what it is to be a sacred woman for so long, until the sanctuaries were closed by Theodosius's decree.

If you visit these sacred sites today, you will find, as I did, ruins of these ancient temples lying in disrepair, often unvisited by the majority of tourists, who instead flock to sites that glorify gods such as Apollo or Zeus, which have the official imprimatur and have therefore warranted restoration. In fact, it is not uncommon to see sewage-treatment plants or oil refineries built right next to these ancient feminine sanctuaries, or Christian churches built over them.

Despite the suppression of the feminine in the Greek and Roman societies and those that embraced Judeo-Christianity, it was certainly not a global phenomenon, despite the spread of patriarchal ideals around the world. It appears that many cultures and religions are willing to embrace the Goddess, seeing her as an essential part of life, especially in terms of home, family, and fertility. For instance, the Great Mother has always been a part of Hindu and Buddhist traditions. Although an in-depth and complex study of the subject is beyond the scope of this work, here are a few of the best-known faces of the Great Mother in these cultures.

Hindu Goddesses

Hinduism is a religion and a philosophy of life that emerged out of sacred texts known as the Vedas. Written from about 1700 BCE onward, the Vedas honor a pantheon of gods, although the teachings do contain some hymns to the divine feminine, including one to Ushas, the goddess of dawn, and another to Prithivi, the earth goddess. However, it wasn't until the resurgence of Hinduism around 400 CE that the divine feminine was truly revered, appearing as a many-faced goddess whose many aspects include:

Shakti, the feminine face of the divine power, or energy

Sarasvati, one of the oldest goddesses, the patron of music, poetry, and science, and the consort to Brahma

Parvati, the gentle and loving Mother goddess and wife of Shiva

Sita, an earth goddess and wife of Rama, whose exiles and subsequent challenges reflect the trials of all women, offering hope and the power of endurance through true love

Lakshmi, the gentle goddess of wealth, prosperity, and health, and consort to Vishnu

Kali, the dark goddess or face of the crone, associated with death, destruction, and sexuality

Buddhist Goddesses

Buddhism is a leading religion in many countries, including India, Sri Lanka, Tibet, China, and Japan, and its various forms have myriad expressions of the Goddess. Here are just two of the most familiar manifestations:

Tara, the Mother goddess, whose name means "star," and through whose various faces are reflected creation, compassion, enlightenment, and protection

Quan Yin (Kuan Yin or Kannon), goddess of mercy and compassion, whose name means "she who harkens to the needs of the world," for legend tells us that she paused upon entering nirvana when she heard the cries of the world and decided to remain on earth to help sentient beings

Indigenous Cultures

Many indigenous traditions have a pantheon of goddesses, many of whom express the fecundity of Mother Earth. For instance, Pachamama is the fertility goddess of the native peoples of the Andes, who, after the conquest by the Catholic Spaniards, was recast as the Virgin Mary. However, these colonized people never forgot their Great Mother and worshipped Mary knowing she was a cover for the real Pachamama. In the Mayan tradition, Ix Chel was an earth and moon goddess and patroness of weavers and pregnant women. The Hopi refer to the earth as Tuuwaqatsi or "Earth Mother," which is representative of most Native American beliefs. According to the knowledge the Hopi have carefully preserved down the ages, Earth is both our land and our life, which is remembered in their first law: Tutskwa I'qatsi—land and life are one.

The Hawaiians refer to the Earth Mother as Haumea, and she is seen as the Creatrix of the Hawaiian people. It is said that, in preparation for the beginning of civilization, she gave form to the star children, who first walked on the land known as Mu as goddesses and gods. It is believed that she lived as a mortal woman known as La'ila'I and as the cosmic mother known as Uli. Among her children is the dark goddess Pele, whose lives within the volcano on the Big Island of Hawaii and who hair streams out as lava. Her sister is the goddess Hi'iaka, whose presence is evoked through the hula dance.

In New Zealand, images of Maori goddesses such as Hinetuahoanga,

Matuatonga, Horoirangi, and Pani were preserved in stone. However, until a recent resurgence, any interest in their relevance to Maori culture was minimal due to the early European settlers' fixation on the one male God.

In the Shinto tradition of Japan there are many gods and goddesses, commonly associated with the natural world. One of the most famous goddesses is Amaterasu, the goddess of the sun and the universe, and sister of Susanoo, the powerful storm of winter, and of Tsukuyomi, the god of the moon. It is believed that the emperor of Japan is a direct descendant of Amaterasu.

Reverence for the Celtic deities is still widespread even today, despite the influence of Christianity in Britain, Ireland, and other areas of Europe. There are hundreds of gods and goddesses, including Anu (Danu, Don), mother goddess of all gods and patroness of the nourishment that flows from springs and fountains. Brigid (Brigit, Brighid) is seen as a virgin goddess who is guardian of fire, creativity, fertility, and new birth. Two of the dark goddesses are Ceridwen, who possesses a fiery cauldron for transformation, and Morrigan, associated with magic and mystery.

Abrahamic Traditions

Finally, we return to the traditions sired by Abraham. It is not uncommon for these goddesses to express one of three faces of the Great Mother—the Virgin (creator), the Mother (nurturer), or the Crone (destroyer); all three archetypes are essential for the continuation of the creative cycle and the evolution of humanity.

Arabian or Pre-Islamic Goddesses

In Arabic culture, goddess worship was influenced by the religions of Mesopotamia and their strong association with the celestial bodies. Reverence was given to the divine feminine until the rise of Islam in 622 CE, when idolatry was banned, including any association with female deities. However, the Great Goddess of the nomadic people of Arabia was known as Al-Lât, a moon goddess who had three faces. They include:

Qure, the Virgin, or crescent moon, similar to Kore, the virginal face of Persephone in Greek culture

Al'Uzzâ, the fertility goddess who represents the full moon and Mother aspect, also represented as the morning star Venus

Al'Manât (or Menat), the oldest of the trinity, representing the Crone and the waning moon, concerned with fate, prophecy, and divination*

Christian Goddesses

In this tradition, born of the patriarchy, there is only one divine feminine form, which has three faces. Unfortunately, it is not uncommon for only two of her aspects to find expression within officially sanctioned church practices: the Virgin and the Mother. This has caused an imbalance in the energy that emerges from this triple goddess.

The three faces of the Christian Mother goddess are:

The Virgin Mary, seen as an innocent and pure woman who was chosen to give birth to Jesus through divine intervention

Mother Mary, who shows the face of all mothers who love, nurture, and cherish their children unconditionally, joyful in their happiness and weeping when they are in pain

The Crone (i.e., Mary Magdalen), offering enlightenment to all who have the courage to enter into her womb or cauldron of transformation. She was exemplified by Mary Magdelen, who despite often being called a whore or harlot, was in fact a highly evolved soul without whom Jesus could not have fulfilled his mission: to open a doorway for all of humanity to follow, the portal to eternal life. By excluding the Magdalen from its teachings, of

---

*Al'Manât has a well-visited sanctuary, known as Manat, dedicated in her honor. It is located on the seashore between Medina and Mecca.

Christianity prevents its followers from experiencing the fullness of the Great Mother and hence receiving her gift of immortality.

We will meet many more faces of the divine feminine on our journey of reclaiming her true identity and power. Some of these aspects of the archetypal feminine are vibrant and resplendent, while others are hidden, awaiting the call of our hearts to heal their (and our) wounds. It is time for them to take their rightful places within our bodies, minds, and souls, so that we can fully express the totality of the Great Mother here on earth and bring about an evolution in human consciousness.

3

LISTENING TO THE WISDOM OF THE BODY

It is ironic that my decision to write this book was motivated by the remarks of a television interviewer who, in reference to a sports personality, uttered the often-heard remark, "Fancy her getting breast cancer, she's such a nice person." Right then and there I wanted to jump up and shout at the television, "That's the problem—she's *too* nice!"

Now I seem to have joined the ranks of all the "nice" people who get cancer.

In my experience, at least 80 percent of cancer patients are kind people with a chronic tendency to suppress anger and always think of the needs of others before considering themselves. I can still remember the comments of a female patient upon being given a life-threatening prognosis: "I can't tell my family I'm dying, it will only upset them, and they have so many more important matters to worry about." In my own life, I can definitely say I didn't go to medical school, I went to martyr school. I was trained to be "professional" and at my best at all times, however tired, sick, or unhappy I was in the moment. Until relatively recently, I prided myself on being able to bury my own feelings and act as if everything was perfectly well in my world.

Take, for instance, Sally, a long-time patient of mine, who could be described as a chronically nice person—that is, until she was given the diagnosis that she had only two months to live because of an inoperable brain tumor. This is what she told me:

When I was given the prognosis, something inside me snapped, and suddenly I felt waves of anger toward those whom I had allowed to take advantage of me without my ever complaining. I went home and told my twenty-eight-year-old son to leave and take his dirty laundry with him. Then, I ended a five-year relationship that had been dragging on without any real hope of anything deep or meaningful coming out of it. Next, I handed in my notice at work as I thought, Why work when you have only two months to experience the rest of your life? I recorded a message on my answering machine that basically said, "Only leave a message if you have something cheerful to say." At that point I began to live life around my needs, focusing especially on what brought me pleasure.

Two years later, I ran into Sally at a social event; she looked radiant, as if she hadn't a care in the world. She told me her cancer was in remission, and she was working in a new job, which she loved, and was surrounded by friends who honored her wishes as much as their own.

One of the criticisms often leveled at those who practice mind-body medicine is that we are blaming people for their illness. As you may have gathered from the preface to this book, I firmly believe my soul created the cancer I developed, but this has nothing to do with guilt, blame, or shame. Furthermore, I suggest that there is a big difference between giving people the chance to be empowered through knowledge and telling them that their illness has nothing to do with them, that *it's just one of those things,* as many doctors so often tell their patients. I have spoken to many cancer support groups, and each time I meet men and women who say, "Why didn't anybody tell me to treat my illness as a gift rather than leaving me feeling helpless?"

As with the diagnosis of any illness or life-altering experience, cancer gives a person the opportunity to stop and ask, "Where am I not being true to myself?" For me, it was clear that I'd become complacent in my interactions, too busy worrying about the feelings of others to listen to my own emotions. Emboldened by the seriousness of my situation, I am becoming increasingly adept at saying no to anything that either feeds my addiction to martyrdom or merely appeases the emotional needs of another person. It's been quite a process, and I'm still working at it, but I'm getting better all the time at letting go of trying to control how other people feel as I concentrate on my own feelings.

It's strange that some of us seem to need permission to remember we're special so that we can position ourselves at the top of our priority list. I have observed many patients become more self-assured and self-contained because they've stepped out from behind the family agenda and demanded to be seen as someone with unique needs and desires. It's such a shame that we need to get sick to realize it's perfectly okay to be ourselves.

MESSAGES FROM THE SOUL

So let me clearly state: illness is not a mistake, a sign of weakness, or something caused by some outside invader against which we must battle, struggle, or suffer. At least 90 percent of illness is a wake-up call from the soul, the part of us that sees and knows our life plan. Our physical body acts as the soul's most perfect messenger; the body listens more intently to the soul's desires than it does to the desires of the personality or ego. Despite any desire on our egoic self's part to try to block or even shoot the messenger, the body's wisdom will inevitably be heard, as is shown in the following story:

Maria, an actress, had been to see me a couple of times in my homeopathic practice, requesting help with menstrual cramps and severe back pain. She had already been prescribed strong painkillers by her doctor, but she was experiencing side effects, so she was seeking a complementary approach. I suggested that perhaps she needed to take a break from acting just to allow her body to rest, but she was adamant that this was impossible, firmly convinced that "the show must go on." Then one day Maria requested an urgent appointment, as she'd woken up that morning covered with chicken pox, especially all over her face, meaning she couldn't act. It took six weeks before all the spots dried up, allowing her to return to work, during which time her body rested and she was able to come off many of her medications. Three months later she reported that her whole life had been turned around by the humble chicken pox, which had shown her that her life had become an "act" and that there was much more to life than work.

The body never gets the message wrong; you don't get a pain in the neck when you really feel that someone is a pain in the arse! All we need to do is to listen to the message. For example:

Pain in the neck: *Who or what is irritating me even though I suppress my anger?*

Constipation: *What am I holding on to that needs to be released?*

Lower back pain: *Where do I feel unsupported?*

Heart attack: *What am I doing in my life that no longer brings me joy?*

Gallbladder disease: *Where am I frustrated but unable to make a decision to change the situation?*

Fibroid tumors: *Who is there to nurture me?*

Cystitis: *Where am I pissed off but scared to make any changes?*

Unfortunately, with the plethora of modern drugs available to mask the symptoms of almost any condition, there is a far greater tendency to silence the messenger by taking convenient analgesia, in the same way that we may cover a flashing warning light in our car with black tape so we no longer need to see it. Of course, this solution only works for a short time before the car breaks down, and so it is with our body: if we refuse to heed the signs, it will eventually stop us in our tracks.

About twelve years ago, just after my mother died, I decided to leave England and come to the United States. In retrospect, this was a huge move in the midst of a period of grief over the loss of my mother, but intuitively it felt like the right decision, as has since been proved. However, starting a new life in a strange country where I knew very few people was a real challenge. On top of this, at the time I was pre-menopausal, so my hormones and periods were erratic. Within a few months of arriving in the States, I started to develop headaches, aching muscles, exhaustion, and nausea, which became worse when I was under pressure. Nevertheless, ever a martyr to a cause, I did what I had always done since childhood: I ignored my body's messages, engaged my intellect, and powered forward. It's no wonder my upper back and shoulders took the stress, as I used these muscles to push forward with my well-developed willpower.

In retrospect, I can say I had all the symptoms of fibromyalgia or chronic fatigue syndrome. But since there is little medically that can be done for these conditions apart from rest, I kept going. There were times when the pain was so excruciating that any extra stimulus such as touch, smell, or sound would be unbearable; all I wanted to do was lie down and be left alone. Yet, as always, my family work ethic pushed me on. I never let anyone know how I felt during my workday, and I would flop down on the bed for what remained of the rest of the day, which was very little. I truly thought I had gotten away with the deception until the day I started to vomit and my cover was blown. I still remember the scene: I was talking to a client on the telephone and told her, "Excuse me, I'm going to be sick," and she replied, "Don't worry, I'll wait for you to return." There was something very wrong with this conversation!

This incident caused me to see that the headaches were always worse when I wasn't looking after myself and wasn't speaking my truth. I went in search of some healing by asking my inner self to speak to me. I was surprised to meet an angry little girl with pigtails and a hockey stick, who chided me for not listening to her: *I'm trying to keep you away from situations that drain your energy, but you're always overriding my advice. Now I have your attention and I expect some changes!* Slowly, I started to set boundaries and take much more time for myself. In time, the headaches eased, making one little girl very happy.

Listening, not Talking

One of the first questions I ask a new client who presents with an illness is: What was happening in your life when the symptoms first appeared? Over the years, I have been astounded how quickly I am met with the response, "I *know* why I have this disease." I shouldn't be surprised by this, for who better to know what's going on than the patient herself? Yet this question is rarely asked of a patient/client, in my experience.

I remember during my medical training in the 1970s I was expected to make a diagnosis by first listening to the patient's history (80 percent), then conducting an examination (15 percent), and finally testing (5 percent). Today, the whole process has been reversed; on average, a diagnosis relies on tests 80 percent of the time, on examination 10 percent of the time, and on patient history only 10 percent of the time. Unless we listen with open minds and hearts, remembering the uniqueness of the individual patient, our diagnosis can only be based on physical changes, excluding the all-important emotions, beliefs, and dreams of the soul, all of which create the whole human being. As I have found out relatively recently, it is so easy to speak as if we know what someone is going through or to give advice without ever getting to know the person. I had to laugh when someone advised, at the height of my headaches, that I should just "push through the problem." As a self-confessed (and recovering) workaholic, this is 180 degrees from the truth.

Yes, it takes time for a health care practitioner to get to know someone, but it is certainly worth the effort, as I learned when I met Jean.

When Jean came to see me, she had already received chemotherapy and radiotherapy for cancer of the lung and was about to return to work. But it was obvious to me that although her body had been given the all-clear sign, nobody had addressed the turmoil in her mind or the anger she was attempting to control but which was clearly bubbling just beneath the surface. She told me she was the eldest of nine children from a home of alcoholic parents. Everyone in the family came to her with their problems, and she found it very difficult to say no. On top of this, she had four children of her own and worked as a nurse. Jean was literally drowning in a sea of demands that had been placed on her by her family and the nature of her work. She felt impotent to change the situation, as she was bound by a moral duty, she said, to be "of service." She told me that everybody just kept asking her, "When will you be back to your old self?" In other words, "When will you be available to look after me again?" As she spoke, her shoulders sagged and she looked downcast: "I can't do it anymore, I can't be there for other people and deny myself; it's killing me."

It is no wonder Jean developed lung cancer: she was drowning under the weight of responsibility and yet was unable to express her true feelings for fear of attracting disapproval from others. It was so difficult for her to believe that she had a right to develop healthy boundaries and a sense of an autonomous self without the guilt of worrying about family and friends. Our conversation helped her to see that she had choices to free her up and bring more happiness to her life, even though the changes were going create substantial ripples all around her. Yet there was fight in her belly, and slowly but surely she learned to share her feelings with the family members who could hear her, and to those who were too lost in their own worlds to care about what she was feeling and perceiving, she wrote many honest letters that she never sent so that she could release her own feelings. She told me that one of the incentives for her healing was that she didn't want to see her own daughters continue the family pattern of pleasing others while losing their sense of self—with the consequent health effects. Over time, I saw Jean start to develop a good sense of self-respect and self-nurturing, and this in turn boosted her immune system, which is essential for a healthy body. One of the most important aspects of her self-care program was to create sacred time and space in her day that was just for her and, therefore, sacrosanct.

Eventually Jean came to realize that her counseling talents were wasted on her own family, and she went back to school to study to become a *psychotherapist. The last time I saw her, at a seminar, she was glowing with vibrant health. She and her family had moved a healthy distance away from her birth family, and she now had a thriving psychotherapy practice and daughters whose mother had taught them the value of self-love.*

GLOBAL MEDICAL DILEMMA

When I wrote my first book, *Frontiers of Health,* twenty years ago, I intended to offer valuable information about holistic medicine, focusing mainly on the underlying message of disease. I naively assumed then that such an approach would be commonplace in health care by the early twenty-first century. This wasn't merely an ego trip—I was in good company with this viewpoint. Best-selling authors such as Deepak Chopra, Carolyn Myss, and Louise Hay had all reached similar conclusions: that there is a direct correlation between personally held beliefs, a healthy expression of emotions, and health and well-being.

Fast-forward to 2012, and health care seems to have lost its way. Medical costs are skyrocketing to cover expensive drugs and advanced diagnostic technology, and yet despite reductions in the prevalence of certain diseases, illness refuses to go away, and in fact some illnesses have become chronic on a near-epidemic scale. One fascinating statistic from 2005 reveals that despite having less than 5 percent of the world's population, the United States makes up almost 50 percent of the global market for prescription drugs.[1] The figures are increasing every year as doctors prescribe more and more drugs, often driven by public demand following television advertising or to counteract the side effects of the original prescription. When we look a little deeper, we find that women are prescribed more drugs than men, which is believed to be because women consult physicians far more commonly than men. However, in my experience, this isn't necessarily because of any disparity in disease prevalence between the sexes—indeed, women do tend to live longer than men—but because women are generally more interested in their well-being, recognizing that if they are healthy, the family is healthy.

But despite the fact that women are more invested in health, until recently most clinical trials carried out by the pharmaceutical companies to test the safety and efficacy of their drugs commonly excluded women as subjects in the studies.[2] This is because in 1964 the World Medical Association decided to exclude all premenopausal women from the early stages of research because of the potential risk to a fetus if the woman became pregnant during the trial. This of course excluded a huge portion of the female population. In 1995, the U.S. Food and Drug Administration created a new set of standards, acknowledging that women could choose not to become pregnant during the study, although some limitation of participation by such women still exists in the early trial phases.[3] However, is this enough? Women today have a twofold greater risk of experiencing an adverse drug reaction as men.[4] It is clear that more studies are required to ascertain whether this is because of increased prescribing, increased reporting, or the unique nature of female physiology, which synthesizes drugs differently than its male counterpart.

But beyond all the systematic issues confronting our approach to wellness, the present global health care crisis is not necessarily because of a lack of resources, but because of the prevalent belief that illness is a party pooper, an unpleasant interruption to a lifetime of unhealthy choices. The drug companies encourage this delusion: "You don't have to stop anything in your life (however much these habits are destroying your body); just take our drugs." Most people wouldn't treat their car as badly as they treat their body; they have pride in their car and enjoy taking care of it. Well-being is not about restriction, blame, and guilt but enjoyment, pleasure, and a great quality of life—qualities that come from self-love, self-responsibility, and celebration of oneself.

We need to recognize that illness is a call from the soul, urging us to pay attention, to examine our beliefs, and to be honest about our feelings, recognizing that our emotions provide us with powerful clues into what we need to bring about balance in our lives. This is illustrated in a story about the gift that cancer brought to my dear friend from Tokyo, Shin-ichiro Terayama.

Shin, who is known for his large white beard and always-smiling face, radiates happiness. However, this was not always the case. In 1984, Shin was a solid-state physicist working eighteen hours a day when he was diagnosed with cancer of the kidney. Despite the intensive orthodox treatment he received, his cancer progressed until he was just skin and bones and was thought to be in the final stages of his illness. One night he dreamt that he was at his own funeral. As the lid on his coffin was closing, he yelled, "No, I'm still alive!" Shortly after this dream, his sense of smell became so strong that he couldn't sleep in the wards with the constant array of aromas. So one night he took himself up to the roof of the hospital, where the air was fresh and clean. Despite pleas from the nursing staff, Shin refused to come back to the ward. Although his health was fragile, the following day he listened to the signals of his body and discharged himself from the hospital, realizing that now he needed to take responsibility for his own life, and in particular, his illness. Not wanting to take painkillers for the pain in his chest because they dulled his senses, he intuitively was guided to place his own hand on his chest and speak to the cancer: I created you by myself, and I am sorry, but you are still part of my body. It was my mistake and I am sorry, so please forgive me. You are like my baby, so I love you. *As he sent love to his cancer, the pain decreased, and he started to sleep at night. After months of this kind of focused healing, which included changing his diet, meditation, and playing his beloved cello, Shin's cancer went into remission, and he has been cancer-free for many years. He now travels internationally, sharing his story and giving seminars, reminding the audience that the most powerful form of healing is love. Whenever he starts his talk, he taps his chest and says, "I love my cancer!"*

HEAL THE MIND, HEAL THE BODY

Acknowledging that the mind and body are inextricably linked, let us now examine some of the research that underpins this hypothesis. One of the pioneers in this field is Dr. Candace Pert, whose inspirational work spans many decades and was highlighted in the 2004 film and book *What the Bleep Do We Know!?*[5] As a neuroscientist in the 1980s, Pert went in search of receptor sites for natural opiates on the outer membrane of a cell—the so-called bliss molecules—and found them.[6] A receptor can be seen as a lock that, because of its exact specifications, can only be unlocked when the right key is located. When the correct combination does occur, there is a cascade of activity affecting all the cellular components, including the genes, which ultimately changes the way we behave.

Through the research of Dr. Pert and other scientists around the world, we now know that the body secretes hundreds of tiny keys or protein messengers known as neuropeptides, which change our physiology in response to our emotions. Hence, when we hear a young child giggle, through the lock-and-key combination, the happiness we feel inside spreads outward, creating a noticeable relaxation in the body. On the other hand, when a situation causes us to feel angry, the link between the neuropeptides and their receptors leads to a tightening of the muscles of the jaw and upper body and an increase in the heart rate as we prepare to defend our position.

All of this occurs in a split second, and it has now been shown that just thinking about a situation leads to the same neurophysiological response we'd have if we were experiencing the actual event. In other words, the mind-body doesn't know the difference between an imaginary insult and the real thing. Over time, most of us have become hardwired for a wide variety of emotions and reactions; some are healthy, while others are decidedly harmful in the long term. For instance, if as a child we panicked when we were asked to speak in public, we will find that every time we face a similar situation as an adult we will experience the same emotionally stimulated physiological response; this can be attributed to the lock-and-key effect.

However, humans have another mechanism that comes into play to deal with emotional and physical stress. Our mind creates a belief or perception that defuses the situation by offering us a solution that we can control, a known fact. So if, as an adult, we start to panic upon being asked to give a business presentation, not only does our body prepare for survival, but so does our mind. It immediately presents us with a set of beliefs or personal perceptions based on past programming, which lets us know that even though we feel miserable at the thought of having to make a presentation, at least we are dealing with some known facts. For instance, as we panic, our mind provides us with any number of rationales that explain our reaction:

You're no good at your job.
Other people are inconsiderate and mean.
You didn't receive love and encouragement from your parents.
The world is not ready for what you have to say.

Now, with these "facts," the emotional body can take a rest as the mental body allows us to bask in the security and comfort of our own dysfunctional beliefs. Over the years of teaching a seminar I call "The Courage to Change," it has become crystal clear to me that it's not the emotional or the physical body that needs to change in order to create a healthy mind and body; it is the tightly controlled personal beliefs to which we are passionately attached.

CHANGE OUR PERCEPTIONS, CHANGE OUR GENES

Another pioneer in the field of mind-body medicine is cell biologist Dr. Bruce Lipton, whose book *The Biology of Belief* is an international best seller. Through his experiments, he has shown that genes and their DNA do not control our biology. Instead, our genes are controlled by environmental signals received from outside the cell that can be either physical, such as the presence of the hormone estrogen, or energetic, such as our emotions.[7]

Like Pert, Dr. Lipton also recognizes the importance of the receptor sites on the cell membrane, although he takes it one step further by depicting the cell membrane as the "brain" of the cell. He notes that when a specific stimulant—the key—locks into a receptor site, it causes a cascade reaction that eventually leads to a protective protein sleeve around the DNA to peel back to reveal specific genes. The reading of such genes in the nucleus leads to the production of certain proteins that determine such factors as the color of our eyes or the presence of disease.

The body of research that looks at the way our environment controls gene activity is known as epigenetics, and it is one of the fastest-growing areas of scientific study. It describes the fact that even though you may have a gene for an illness, if a particular environmental switch is not present, then the DNA that makes up that gene will remain covered by the sleeve of protein and therefore the disease will not manifest. This is why identical twins who live different lifestyles often present with dramatically different conditions.

Epigenetic mechanisms, or gene markers, have been found to be present in a variety of diseases, including cancer, cardiovascular disease, diabetes, lupus, and even autism. Over the last decade it has been shown that nutrition, stress, and emotions can significantly influence our genes without ever changing the basic genetic structure, with such modifications being passed down to future generations. In my mind this finding confirms that we should describe any disease that is found across the generations as "familial" and not "genetic." In other words, we inherit patterns of familial behavior that have the potential to manifest as physical disease—unless we decide to literally and figurative change our minds!

Dr. Lipton's research comes to the same conclusion as that of Dr. Pert. They both agree that some of the strongest environmental stimulants, or switches, are our emotions, and these are inextricably linked to our perception of reality. In other words, as long as there is a receptor protein for a specific emotionally charged perception, the body will react. However, if there is no receptor protein for a specific stimulant on your cell membrane, there is no reaction. We can see this effect in action when watching a movie with friends. Afterward, it is not uncommon to find that although everyone watched the same film, each person focused on a different character or set of events that typically mirrors the individual's own life experiences and hence his or her perception of the movie. From this we may conclude that if we experience a strong emotional response to a person (or a situation) we are meeting a part of ourselves residing in the shadows, awaiting integration.

Rather than judging or avoiding such a person, I suggest you ask yourself, "What are three qualities within this person that irritate me or make me anxious?" Then ask, "How difficult would it be for me to accept that these qualities may be hidden in me?" For instance, if you are a very responsible person, you may be annoyed by people who are irresponsible, untrustworthy, and lazy, finding yourself spending valuable time trying to change them. However, they are providing you with a mirror, showing you an aspect of yourself—the irresponsible self— that is seeking your attention. Perhaps it's time to relax, letting go of some of the burden of responsibility by asking for help.

Dr. Lipton concluded that if you want to change the function of your body, you must first change your perceptions. As your beliefs change, new receptor sites are created and old ones become inactive, with the potential for such change occurring in just three days. In other words, nothing is ever set in stone—the person who has always stood under the tail of the elephant and thinks that life is shitty has only to make the decision to take one step sideways to start believing that life is not all about manure!

This conclusion correlates with another piece of research that shows the ability of persons with multiple personality disorder to change not only their persona and behavior within hours, but also their state of well-being. For example, in one such case "Joe," one personality, has diabetes that requires insulin injections. However, when "Joe" is replaced by "Fred," the diabetes completely disappears and now the person shows signs of asthma, which requires a steroid inhaler. Yet there is even one more personality, "Stan," who, when he is in control of his body, knows only perfect health, and the injections and inhaler are unnecessary.[8]

Clearly, such a transformation of well-being through the presence of different subpersonalities reinforces Dr. Lipton's message that you are defined not by your genes, but by the environment that influences those genes, in particular, your perception of reality. These perceptions live within the fertile field of the personal unconscious, which is why so many different forms of psychotherapy focus on this area. Yet it is important to remember that our beliefs should not be the sole source of our reality, for they are created by the mind, which will always be limited. Only the soul carries our greater destiny and can see outside the box, speaking to us through the intuitive wisdom of the heart. In reality, there is not a moment we are not being showered with love and inspiration by our soul, and if we still fail to heed its wisdom, it can always call on the body to focus our attention through the manifestation of disease.

ANCIENT MIND-BODY HEALING SYSTEMS

Ancient physicians did not possess modern diagnostic devices but instead developed their own systems of analysis that far predate our medicine. In this brief overview of ancient healing methods, I will confine my comments to three major philosophies, each of which acknowledges the energetic consciousness of the cells and describes a strong link between physical health and the well-being of the mind and spirit.

The Chakras

One of the first non-allopathic sources of information I absorbed after I completed medical school was the ancient Hindu teachings about the chakras, or wheels of energy. Over the years, I have come to rely on my knowledge of these energy centers in my intuitive work with clients, recognizing the chakras as windows into the deeper aspects of a person's psyche, which have the potential to reach the consciousness of the soul.

As many readers probably know, a chakra is a wheel or vortex of energy consisting of several different frequencies of energy that are naturally found within the human aura. Symbolically, a chakra can be seen as a rose with many different layers of petals, the center of which represents the pure consciousness of the soul. Major and minor chakras are found throughout the body and act as doorways between our inner and outer worlds, receiving information and sending out messages. The sensitivity of our chakra system is far more rapid than that of our nervous system, reacting to stimuli long before we have conscious awareness of emotions such as vulnerability, fear, inadequacy, and shame. For example, it is an almost automatic reaction to cross our arms over our stomach to protect the solar plexus—connected to self-esteem—when we feel judged.

There are seven major chakras located along the spine and, as you will see below, at least two other chakras outside the body. Each of the seven chakras is associated with an area of the body, a spiritual essence, specific emotions, and the potential for certain illnesses if the chakra is out of balance. The appendix of this book offers ways to rebalance the energy of each of these centers, including the use of specific sounds and colors. You will notice that the chakras are described in terms of masculine or feminine energy, with the third eye being a balance of the two energies. This book focuses, in particular, on the organs and tissues associated with the feminine chakras. These centers not only align with the unique anatomical features of a woman but are also the chakras that I find are more frequently out of harmony

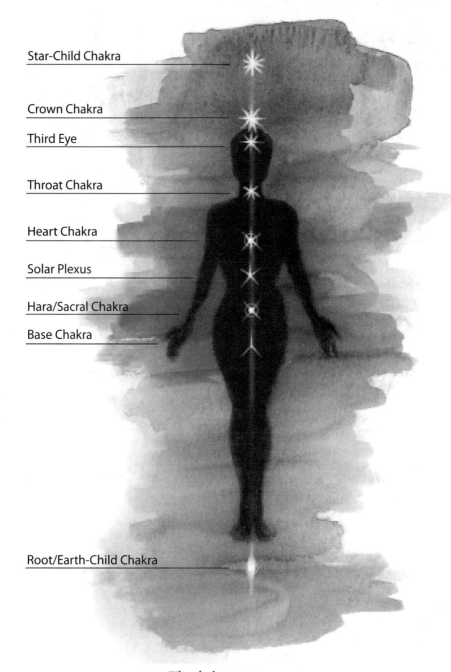

Star-Child Chakra

Crown Chakra

Third Eye

Throat Chakra

Heart Chakra

Solar Plexus

Hara/Sacral Chakra

Base Chakra

Root/Earth-Child Chakra

The chakra system

due to the chronic disconnect from feminine consciousness, not just in women but in men, too.

Base Chakra

Location: base of the spine

Spiritual essence: self-acceptance, security, strength, openness, and sense of belonging to the earth; masculine

Imbalance: fear, anxiety, insecurity, hypervigilance, perfectionism, and need to be in control

Potential disease: illness of the vulva, vagina, kidneys, bladder, rectum, hips, and adrenal glands

Sacral Chakra, or Hara

Location: three fingers below the navel

Spiritual essence: healthy relationships, respect, nurturing, inner power, creativity, and transformation; feminine

Imbalance: shame, disrespect, abuse, inability to receive from others, martyrdom, grief, and lack of creativity

Potential disease: illness of the uterus, ovaries, cervix, prostate, colon, lower back, and testes

Solar Plexus

Location: over the stomach, where the ribs meet

Spiritual essence: self-esteem, confidence, "I'm okay," celebration, and healthy personal boundaries; masculine

Imbalance: guilt, resentment, anger, judgment, hurt, disappointment, and psychic and emotional oversensitivity

Potential disease: illness of the liver, spleen, stomach, small intestine, and pancreas (such as diabetes)

Heart Chakra

Location: center of the chest

Spiritual essence: self-love, joy, compassion, intuition, and connection to eternal consciousness; feminine

Imbalance: self-hatred, loneliness, betrayal, lack of trust, unhappiness, lack of enthusiasm, and depression

Potential disease: illness of the heart, breasts, immune system, and thymus gland

Throat Chakra

Location: over the throat

Spiritual essence: self-expression, willpower, freedom, and accepting the need to change; masculine

Imbalance: stubbornness, fear of change, overanalyzing, excuses, excessive questions, and mind games

Potential disease: illness of the throat, ears, lungs, esophagus, and thyroid gland

Third Eye

Location: between the two eyes

Spiritual essence: self-accountability, wisdom, detachment, clarity, and insight; masculine and feminine

Imbalance: impatience, confusion, and anxiety and worry over trivial matters

Potential disease: illness of the eyes, sinuses, head, and pituitary gland

Crown Chakra

Location: top of the head

Spiritual essence: self-consciousness, spiritual awareness, inspiration, oneness, and bliss; feminine

Imbalance: despair, fatigue, dispiritedness, delusion, and disassociation from the body

Potential disease: illness of the mind, brain, and pineal gland

By now, most practitioners of this ancient science are in agreement that there are five more major chakras, bringing the count to twelve. However, knowledge of the precise locations of these extra energy centers was lost around 1100 CE, when Hindu practitioners decided to work with only those centers along the spine, intensifying the disconnect from the Earth Mother and spiritual Great Mother, which had begun when the patriarchy came into power. However, over the past ten years, I have been intuitively guided to work with two of these chakras outside the body, as the first steps to reconnect humanity to its true origins and power.

The first is a large and powerful chakra located approximately twenty-four inches beneath the soles of our feet, called the root or earth-child chakra, which connects us to pure creative feminine energy, also known as dragon energy. We will look at the importance of this chakra in far more detail in chapter 5. The other chakra is about the same distance, twenty-four inches, above the crown chakra at the top of the head; this is known as the star child. Whereas the root chakra is the portal to the earth's goddess energies, the star-child chakra is a gateway or star gate to the spiritual realms, the home of the Queen Bee, whom we will meet in chapter 9. As we will see, one of the greatest problems at this time is humanity's disconnection from the root and star-child chakras, causing us to lack true spiritual power and inspiration; this, in my opinion, is a major factor when trying to solve issues such as global poverty, infertility, and depression.

Traditional Chinese Medicine

Traditional Chinese medicine considers the human body a microcosm of the universe, with the two inextricably linked; what happens to one immediately affects the other. As Master Nan Lu, a classically trained doctor of traditional Chinese medicine explains, "In order to maintain optimal health, the body must follow not only its internal laws, but the natural laws of the Universe."[9] Such laws encompass the seasons, the foods we eat, and the weather, as well as our emotional status, which naturally changes with the shifting energies of the universe. When we recognize and adapt appropriately to the shifts and challenges that are sent our way, all is well. When we don't, we experience disease.

According to traditional Chinese medicine, the body contains twelve major meridians that network throughout the body; these are linked to the five elements—water, wood, fire, earth, and metal. It is through these energy pathways that *qi* (or *chi*), our internal vital energy, flows, thus providing vitality and balance to every organ and to the surrounding areas. As long as qi remains strong and flows freely, the body's organs work in harmony, and disease and illness cannot manifest.[10]

Below I outline the salient points associated with the major meridians, although for those interested I strongly advise deeper study of this subject, which cannot be adequately covered in a book of this scope.

Kidney and Bladder Meridians

Element: water

Function: to store and supply energy, or qi, essential for the body to function. Ancestral or inborn qi comes from our parents; its quality is dependent on the positive nature of their beliefs and our willingness to be on the earth. Acquired qi comes from food and the wisdom we absorb from life.

Associated emotion: fear. With constant worry, no time to rest, and poor motivational energy from our ancestors, it is easy to experience adrenal burnout.

Organs involved: kidneys, bladder, adrenal glands, teeth, bones, hair, and ears

A healthy kidney requires the ingestion of wholesome foods, restful sleep, and warm conditions, as well as the willingness to value the positive messages we have received and let go of the rest.

Liver and Gallbladder Meridians

Element: wood

Function: to maintain smooth and harmonic movement within the body and, in particular, the flow of blood, emotions, and qi

Associated emotion: anger and frustration. When we feel angry, we need to move, either physically—such as leaving a relationship—

or mentally, by changing our opinion. If anger is allowed to fester through sulking, passive aggression, and bitterness, then eventually the suppressed energy will impact health. The gallbladder controls the ability to make decisions; when we're fearful of making the "right" decision, we won't move, often resulting in gallbladder disease

Organs involved: liver, gallbladder, breasts, uterus, prostate, throat, tendons, nails, and eyes

A healthy liver requires harmony through movement, whether this describes the way we physically move through the world or the way we move our thoughts in order to restore a peaceful state or a sense of easy flow.

Heart and Small Intestine Meridians
Element: fire

Function: when the heart is happy, every other organ is happy; the heart houses *Shen* (spirit), feeding us with creative inspiration.

Associated emotion: joy. When we give voice to our soul's inspiration, our heart sings. When the energy is blocked, we become depressed. The heart needs to act as the queen of our life; otherwise we may experience agitation, insomnia, excessive dreaming, forgetfulness, and even insanity.

Organs involved: heart and small intestine, which filters what is healthy for a person. When imbalanced, indigestion, food sensitivities, and bloating can result.

A healthy heart requires a loving sense of self, the expression of creative ideas, and joyfulness of spirit, which starts with a single smile.

Stomach and Spleen Meridians
Element: earth

Function: to offer security through the generation of energy, whether from physical sources, such as food, or from emotional sources, such as love.

Associated emotion: worry. The ability to nurture ourselves with the energy of food or love is dependent on the bonding with our birth mother and with the spiritual Great Mother. If either are lacking, we develop distrust, obsessive worry, or a compensatory desire to care for others, which can lead to paranoia, difficulties in bonding with others, and issues of separation.

Organs involved: stomach, spleen, breasts, and uterus

A healthy spleen and stomach require healthy bonding with nurturing Mother energy, whether this is achieved by enjoying walks on Mother Earth, receiving loving support from mother figures, or opening one's heart to the eternal love of the Divine Mother.

Lung and Large Intestine Meridians

Element: metal

Function: concerned with the cyclical movement of water and energy, reminding us of the cyclical nature of life through death and rebirth

Associated emotion: grief. When we fail to grieve and release the old, we develop an imbalance in the lung meridian.

Organs involved: lungs, sinuses, skin, and large intestine

Healthy lungs require us to understand that we should fully enjoy the flow of energy that comes with inspiration, or inhalation, and yet we must not forget that exhalation, or death, is inevitable if we are to experience true spiritual growth.

Astrology

The science of astrology goes back at least 3,500 years; in fact, it is from astrology that the sciences of astronomy and psychology later emerged. Having worked with astrology for more than twenty years, running experiential seminars with my husband for the past decade, I want to acknowledge that astrology is a vast and complex science. Every time I look at a person's chart I see not only challenges and strengths but also the soul's unique potential in this life. I believe each of us chose the exact time, date, and place to be born as well as our parents, culture, and religion, all of which appears in the placement of the planets in the sky at the moment of birth. With your first breath, you determined your destiny on earth; all you have to do is manifest your purpose into reality.

Such a manifestation is assisted by the continual movement of the planets through the sky after your birth, leading to times when the energy of an orbiting planet will affect a planet in your natal chart, bringing the energy of that planet alive. For instance, when the planet of Jupiter (associated with expansion) transits your Mercury (associated with talking and intellect), you might find yourself excitedly buying new books, scanning the Internet, or sharing your knowledge with others.

An astrologer can focus on many areas of interest within a chart, including factors that may influence your health and where illness may occur in your body. In ancient times, no doctor would consider practicing medicine without possessing a detailed knowledge of astrology and alchemy. Today, practitioners of medical astrology offer information that, rather than creating alarm and fear, will allow the person to take preventive measures so that illness does not need to manifest. Remember, nothing is set in stone. Below I offer a simplified version of a complex study to allow you to begin to appreciate the link between the celestial bodies and your physical body. Each astrological sign rules a different part of the body. For example, I have several planets in the sign of Gemini, so you will see from the quick reference list below that, because of Gemini's influence, when I find myself "caught up in my head" or overthinking a situation, my shoulders become tight and my nervous system stressed. Regular massages and constant reminders to breathe and relax help me maintain a healthy balance.

If you know only your sun sign, this is a good place to start to begin an exploration into the astrological influences expressed through the mind-body connection. You may also wish to consider consulting with a professional astrologer to gain greater insight into your spiritual potential and the challenges you may face in the future and to explore parts of the self that are still in the shadows.

Aries

Associated traits: ambitious, competitive, forthright, adventurous, great
starter but poor finisher as attention quickly turns to new projects,
impatient, quick temper, lacks direction

Associated parts of the body: head, face, nose, brain, and eyes

Conditions of imbalance: headache, sinus problems, fever, inflammation,
hemorrhage, and burns

Taurus

Associated traits: dependable, kind, practical, generous, sensual, artistic,
loves food and music, enjoys touch and sex, stubborn, need for security,
hates to let go of his or her "stuff," can sabotage his or her own efforts

Associated parts of the body: neck, throat, thyroid gland, lower jaw, ears,
tongue, and vocal cords

Conditions of imbalance: sore throat, stiff neck, hearing problems, and
thyroid gland disorders

Gemini

Associated traits: adaptive; communicative; busy; intellectual; inquisi-
tive; charismatic; loves learning, gathering information, and teaching; restless; easily bored; can be superficial

Associated parts of the body: arms, shoulders, hands, lungs, and nervous
system

Conditions of imbalance: shoulder strain, lung complaints, nervous tension, restlessness, and insomnia

Cancer

Associated traits: caring; sensitive; cries easily; loves home, family, and
being nurtured; avoids conflict, just wants everybody to be happy;
can be moody and whiny if displeased

Associated parts of the body: breasts, breastbone, stomach, alimentary
canal, uterus, and pancreas

Conditions of imbalance: stomach, pancreatic, uterine, and breast disease
and lymphatic disorders

Leo

Associated traits: self-assured, powerful, leader, playful, humorous, enjoys the spotlight, seeks approval, likes to have a following (or "pride"), arrogant, bossy, easily outraged if ignored

Associated parts of the body: heart, chest, spine, and upper back

Conditions of imbalance: hypertension, illness of the heart, and circulation and upper spine disorders

Virgo

Associated traits: analytical, self-contained, love for humanity, aesthetic eye for beauty, introspective, self-critical, hyper-alert, perfectionist, enjoys cleanliness, critical and complaining

Associated parts of the body: digestive system, intestines, spleen, and nervous system

Conditions of imbalance: anxiety, nervous tension, and intestinal and digestive system disorders

Libra

Associated traits: fair, reasonable, diplomatic, mediator, artistic, loves balance and harmony, desires relationship, intellectually indecisive, procrastinator, anxious and fearful

Associated parts of the body: kidneys, skin, lumbar region, and buttocks

Conditions of imbalance: kidney disorders, skin disease, and sciatica

Scorpio

Associated traits: intense, caring, sensitive to deep emotions, transformational, focused, passionate, no fear of death, unforgiving, secretive, holds on too long to things that are dead

Associated parts of the body: sexual organs, bladder, cervix, anus, and prostate gland

Conditions of imbalance: reproductive and excretory disorders

Sagittarius

Associated traits: impulsive, enthusiastic, philosophical, lucky, honest, loves travel and exploration, believes he or she is right and hates being doubted, sarcastic, tactless, can become depressed

Associated parts of the body: liver, hips, thighs, arterial system, sciatic nerve, and pelvis

Conditions of imbalance: liver complaints, hip disorders, arterial disease, and bipolar disorder

Capricorn

Associated traits: loyal; dutiful; responsible; works hard; orderly and practical; loves making plans and lists; structured; can become rigid, over-responsible, pessimistic, and fatalistic

Associated parts of the body: bones, joints, knees, skin, and teeth

Conditions of imbalance: knee complaints, disorders of bones and teeth, skin disease

Aquarius

Associated traits: eccentric; independent; visionary; open-minded; spontaneous; playful; enjoys community and fringe groups; can be emotionally detached, cold, aloof, arrogant, and moody

Associated parts of the body: circulatory system, ankles, calves, and shins

Conditions of imbalance: circulatory problems, varicose veins, and lower leg disorders

Pisces

Associated traits: mystical, romantic, creative, empathic, believes he or she is unlimited, loves nature, one with the Universe, psychic, delusional, addictive, out of touch with reality

Associated parts of the body: feet, toes, adipose tissue (fat), lymphatic system, and mind

Conditions of imbalance: disorders of the feet and lymphatic system, addictions, and schizophrenia

As we continue our exploration of the sacred identity of woman as revealed in the very cells and organs of a woman's body, we will see that knowledge of the chakras, traditional Chinese medicine, and astrology are among those disciplines that can deepen our understanding of how to restore and maintain optimum health. I look forward to the day when these and other ancient healing modalities are considered completely complementary and used in a new form of integrative health care, whereby the body, mind, and spirit are equally considered in the goal of the attainment of well-being.

PART TWO

The Dragon Queen

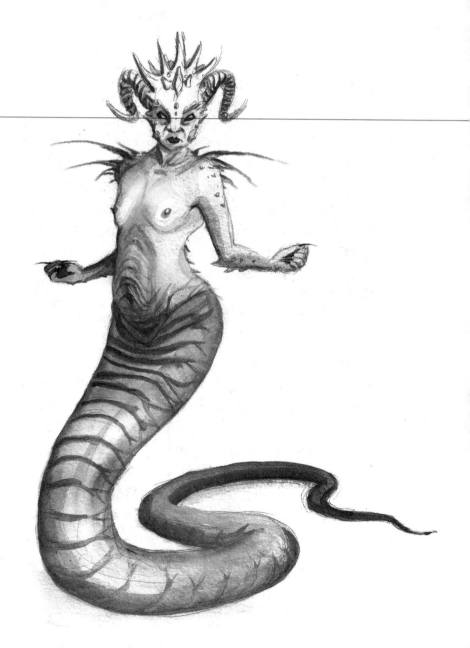

4

VULVA, THE EXOTIC LILY

When woman was made in the image of the Great Mother, no detail was denied. Her curves express the optimal flow of creativity; her softness represents the importance of bonding; and the organs of fertility are carefully protected within the bony pelvis to remind her that these are her sacred jewels. Compare this with the male anatomy and it is easy to see how precious these organs are to the Creator; without them, humanity would not survive. Ancient peoples appreciated this fact, showing great reverence for the female figure by crafting the wonderful Venus statuettes, described in chapter 2, some 20,000 to 30,000 years ago.

Fast-forward to today, where we find that too many curves are definitely *not* in vogue—unless, of course, you're talking about the breasts, which have become a particular object of sexual fascination (more on this subject in chapter 7). When women are complicit in remaking themselves in the image crafted for them by generations of patriarchy, we are surely denying the very things that comprise our sacred identity. Over the centuries, the essential qualities of the female anatomy that have been celebrated and admired—its softness and receptivity—have also been subjected to all manner of abuse, which continues to the present. I suspect the attack on essential femaleness is not because women are inherently powerless; far from it. I suggest that it has been to ensure that women's inherent power remains restrained and under the control of those who fear it. One can only picture the force required to eject an eight-pound baby from the womb to recognize that a woman's power stems from deep within her being, and that once she connects to this core strength—at such times as during childbirth—nothing can stop her from achieving her destiny.

In the following chapters, we will explore the female body, focusing on those parts of her anatomy and physiology that make her unique. This will hopefully encourage each woman to fall in love not only with the shape of her own unique body, but with each precious organ and cell, which hold the memory of what it is to be a sacred woman.

As we begin our journey, I am reminded of the gynecology professor who taught me anatomy in medical school. A quintessential English lady, she would stand in front of the class, her hair neatly gathered in a bun on the top of her head, as she prepared to inspire us with her discourse on the mysteries of the female design. Standing proudly, feet apart, holding a pomegranate in each hand, she would raise her arms shoulder-height as she began: "My body is the uterus, my arms are the fallopian tubes, the fruit are the ovaries, the space between my legs represents the vagina, and my feet are the vulva . . ."

The collection of female organs can be described as the genital,

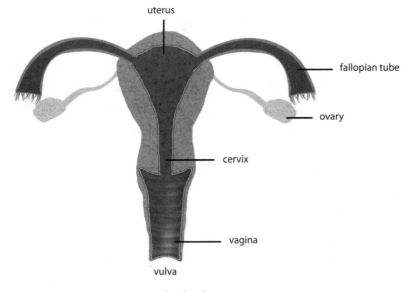

uterus

fallopian tube

ovary

cervix

vagina

vulva

The fertility organs

reproductive, pelvic, and sexual systems, but I prefer the term *fertility organs*. For centuries, these organs have been considered necessary only for procreation and otherwise judged inconvenient, unnecessary, and even at times a "curse." Yet except for the rare occurrence of certain anatomical anomalies, on average every woman's body is naturally programmed to bleed on a monthly basis for about thirty-five years. With the number of children per household currently at an average of 1.2 worldwide, I find it impossible to believe that the only purpose of these approximately 420 hormonal cycles the average woman experiences is reproduction. One explanation that has been used to support the argument that the menstrual cycle is solely for procreation says that in the past, because there was a high infant mortality rate and women died young, there had to be plenty of opportunities for pregnancy to occur within a woman's limited life span. I myself have met women who have been pregnant at least twenty times, and I propose that this old argument does not account for the 400 extra menstrual cycles that a woman's body produces. So let's dig deeper.

According to the ancient Inca, sexual intercourse was never meant to be solely about procreation. The Inca culture regarded intercourse primarily as an act of healing, first for the individual or individuals involved, and then for the planet. The sacred teachings of this ancient culture say that in the past, people in fact lived long lives, so optimal population levels were easy to maintain. Should a soul wish to incarnate into a physical body, this was the decision of the soul and not of the potential parents. The incoming spiritual being would simply choose its parents and then incarnate into the sperm of the man just before it entered the egg.

Perhaps this is not such a farfetched idea for those of us who believe that on a soul level we choose our parents, as well as the time, place, and date of our birth. This brings us to the conclusion that the soul also preselects the outcome of the pregnancy, the method of the incoming being's delivery into physical form, and the level of nurturing it will receive in its formative years. Such a belief would explain why some people are unable to conceive while others become pregnant despite taking every precaution: it is the soul's choice, not the parents'.

In the absence of any deep understanding of the real purpose of a woman's body, it is easy to see how, with the availability of so many different kinds of contraceptives, the sexual act can become divorced from the menstrual cycle. It's as though the sensual arousal of the clitoris and vagina has become disconnected from the deeper workings of the uterus and ovaries. It could be argued that reminding women that lovemaking could result in childbirth maintains that intrinsic perception of the connection between the two functions, but it also hides its deeper truth. As we shall discover, from a sacred perspective, each aspect in the process of sexual arousal prepares a woman to receive healing energy and inspiration, which ultimately affects the fertility and evolution of consciousness on this planet. With this in mind, the status of sex, of lovemaking, needs to be elevated to that of a sacred ritual, and childbirth, menstruation, and menopause should be lifted out of the realm of pathology in which they are now found and back into their exalted positions: as sacred events in the life of a woman.

HEALING THE WOUNDS OF SEXUALITY AND SENSUALITY

Many initiatives to enlighten women and reconnect them to their precious and sacred bodies have occurred over the past fifty years. I want to honor the feminist movement of the seventies, the liberation years of the eighties, and the bold performances in the nineties by people such as Eve Ensler, in her spellbinding theater piece (and subsequent book) *The Vagina Monologues*. All these movements have spoken openly about the true nature of female sexuality. We have been encouraged, with the use of a mirror, to gaze in wonderment at our beautiful lily-shaped vulvas.[1] This is a far cry from the comments I heard from some of my female patients in my early years of practice, who spoke about their problems "down there"; one good Catholic girl nearly fainted from embarrassment when I described the pure pleasure of the clitoris during a lecture.

However, despite the deluge of books, magazine articles, and videos dedicated to a woman's sexual satisfaction, and despite the open manner in which young people today talk about and engage in sex, we should not forget that this area of the body still carries the deep psychological scars of countless generations of women whose sexuality was dishonored and abused. These violations of sacred womanhood go back more than 3,000 years, to the time when sexuality and spirituality became separated and a woman's naked body, especially her genital organs, came to represent a dirty and evil force that had to be tamed at all costs. The consequences of such a longstanding collective desecration of all things feminine are, I believe, major factors in today's epidemic of rape, sexual abuse, sexual harassment, perverse pornography, and female genital mutilation, not to mention the exploitation of Mother Earth herself. When we remind ourselves that in 2012 one in three women around the world will be beaten or sexually abused, and almost one in five women in the United States have survived a rape or attempted rape during their lifetime, we cannot be complacent about the way we view the female genitalia, and ultimately the spiritual sexuality of women.

During my thirty-five-year career, I have listened to thousands of men and women speak of their sexual and physical abuse as children, often at the hands of those they thought they could trust to keep them safe and innocent, such as members of their own family or authority figures such as priests. On many occasions, the child's naturally emerging interest in the sensuality of his or her own body was exploited, leading to additional confusion, shame, and guilt as the child matured into an adult. Many more stories of sexual abuse are probably locked away in the deep recesses of the minds of those who have little or no memory of their childhood, this kind of amnesia being the psyche's safety mechanism when faced with traumatic experiences.

Naively, as a health professional, I always wanted to believe that childhood abuse was a thing of the past, and that modern children were not being subjected to such levels of shame, suffering, pain, and disrespect. However, the facts belie my wishful thinking: in the USA alone, in 2009, 7.5 percent of males and 25.3 percent of females were reported to have experienced sexual abuse before the age of eighteen. However, because of under-reporting and community codes of silence, this continues to be a particularly difficult area for researchers seeking conclusive figures.[2] In 2002 the United Nations estimated that 150 million girls and 73 million boys worldwide under the age of eighteen had experienced some form of coerced sexual intercourse, abuse, or violence.[3]

Faced with such facts, one could easily feel helpless about bringing about change, and yet each of us as adults can make certain decisions that can affect the lives of our children, children around the world, and future generations of children in a positive way. These include:

- Treating our precious body with love, honor, and respect, whatever its size or shape
- Recognizing that the body is programmed for pleasure, and that it is perfectly normal for toddlers, infants, and even fetuses to stimulate their erogenous zones with sheer delight
- Enjoying the sexual response, and appreciating that it can be experienced in many different ways, not all of which need to lead to an ejaculation or an orgasm
- Showing respect toward one another, mindful of how quickly children pick up on subliminal insults, even when we as adults try to make light of them
- Being honest and unashamed when something does not feel comfortable or respectful, especially within a sexual relationship, for in the presence of real love our feelings and needs are always heard

These suggestions may seem superfluous if you watch certain films and television shows that portray sex as a delightful dessert at the end of an enjoyable meal, or read popular women's magazines that lead us to believe every intimate relationship is brimming with discussions about how to bring orgasmic pleasure to each other. Yet 15 percent of women in the United States have never had an orgasm, and approximately 40 percent of women do not orgasm during vaginal intercourse alone. Understandably, an orgasm is not essential for a woman to become pregnant, just as a man can, in certain circumstances, ejaculate without an orgasm. Ninety percent of women who do not experience orgasm are said to have psychological issues—which, if this is true, is not unexpected after such a prolonged period of abuse and wounding of women.[4] These issues, which are not restricted to the bedroom, include poor self-esteem, performance anxiety, a belief that successful intercourse is all about meeting the needs of a partner, fear of asking for what you want, and fear of losing control. Anxiety inhibits the orgasmic release, since reaching an orgasm, physiologically, requires relaxation.

Is it any surprise that 85 percent of men report that their partner experiences orgasm when only 60 percent of women say they do? Men are more likely to orgasm when sex includes vaginal intercourse, but a woman is more likely to orgasm when she engages in a variety of sexual acts, especially when they involve stimulation of such erogenous zones as the clitoris and breasts, which commonly occurs during foreplay.[5] There is no doubt that when a woman's sexual needs are discounted and intercourse is all about relieving a man of his sexual tension, then the length of time spent on foreplay can be extremely limited. I can still hear echoes of a message given to my mother's generation, which was told that sex is not about one's own pleasure, but about the needs of one's husband, and so a woman should "just lie back and think of England!"

THE SACRED YONI

As a doctor I had examined thousands of vulvas before I took the time to really look at my own, with the aid of a mirror. I remember how I cried at the intimacy of the moment, as if I had just been reconnected with a long-lost friend. It was so beautiful, appearing as a delicate and sensual flower. This small area of my anatomy carried so many memories and sensations, even without the gift of having given birth. It reminded me how the ancient people had always revered the vulva, which collectively includes all the external tissue, including the labial lips, pubic triangle, clitoris, and vaginal opening.

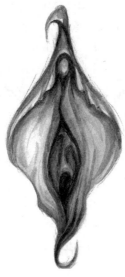

The flowering vulva

The vulva's Sanskrit name is *yoni,* which has several related meanings, including "the origin of life," "a divine passageway," or "being in the presence of the Triple Goddess" (also known as "the One"). To the ancient people, the vulva was sacred, recognized as an opening or portal into another dimension, whether one is emerging from it as a newborn baby or entering into it, as a man does in lovemaking.

The vulvar opening is elliptical or almond-shaped, otherwise known in sacred geometry as a *vesica piscis,* "the bladder of a fish," in Latin. Its outline is formed when the circumference of one circle passes through the center of another, creating between them the two-pointed oval, an interdimensional doorway. As we pass through this opening, whether during our birth or as a man in the act of sex, we are subconsciously being asked to release any previous definition of ourselves and surrender to the loving oneness of the Great Mother so that we can be born anew, on the other side of the doorway. It is only by agreeing to this surrender that we can experience the transformation of our soul. Even those who are born by Caesarean section must pass through a vesica piscis doorway, this being the shape of the uterine incision made by the obstetrician.

During the 3,000 years of feminine repression, the sacred reverence previously shown the vulva diminished, with the external sexual organs, particularly those of a woman, becoming known as the pudendum, from the Latin word *pudere,* meaning "to be ashamed." Indeed, many of the artists of the Greek and Roman civilizations depicted the vulva as a mere longitudinal slit, as if they preferred to imagine the external fertility organs of a woman as innocent and virginal, while the rest of her body was allowed to express sexual maturity.

This was not always the case. Some of the earliest signs of reverence shown toward the primal Goddess and a woman's power of fertility are seen in depictions of the yoni in cave carvings and paintings found throughout the world. In France, 30,000-year-old rock carvings of triangles, circles, and ovals with a central slit are all believed to be expressions of the yoni.

In ancient female initiatory rites, vulvar-shaped rocks were commonly honored, especially where a stone was naturally eroded to reveal two lips and a central hole. If the hole was large enough for a human to pass through, the rock was believed to promote fertility or cure illness. Similar faith in the vulva's power was bestowed on holes in trees, such that children who were weak were passed headfirst into the hole in the belief that it would give them strength. If the object and its hole were smaller, then its presence on your path would be taken as a sign of blessing from the Great Mother.[6] Many other natural objects such as the cowrie shell, apricot, lotus, lily, and rose have all been associated with the Mother, and in particular her yoni.

Even today, all around the world, there are specific places where the Goddess and her yoni are worshipped. One such sacred site is the

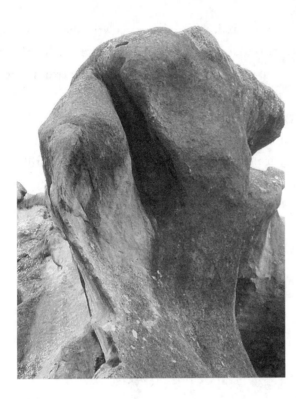

Rock vulva

Yonimandala, in Assam, India. Every year during the monsoon season, red-colored water (pigmented by iron) flows from a natural yoni-shaped rock cleft, believed by local people to represent the menstrual flow of the Goddess. Mythology speaks of the sacred rock being a solidified form of the yoni of the Mother Goddess Shakti (or Sati), which fell to earth as her body was torn apart and spread across the land. As such, the Yonimandala is considered an *axis mundi,* or axis of the world, where both birth and death occur, as symbolized by Shakti's annual bleeding, which represents her promise of continual purification and rebirth for humanity.[7]

Many ancient images of women show that the vulva was viewed with pride, with the size of the labial lips often exaggerated and painted bright red to depict the rich and abundant fertility that emerges from between its folds. It is clear from different portrayals that the yoni was symbolically believed to play an important role at the time of death.

To this end, many red-painted, vulva-shaped cowrie shells have been recovered from ancient burial sites, clearly indicating the belief that the deceased would need to enter a vulva, symbol of an interdimensional gateway, to achieve spiritual transcendence.

As we move forward in time, we find that despite the Romans' negative attitude toward the pudendum, one set of positive female images did emerge during their period of masculine dominance that still causes controversy among researchers. I am referring to the artifacts known as the Sheela-na-gigs, carved between the eleventh and the seventeenth centuries, and found primarily in Ireland, but also in Britain and other European countries.

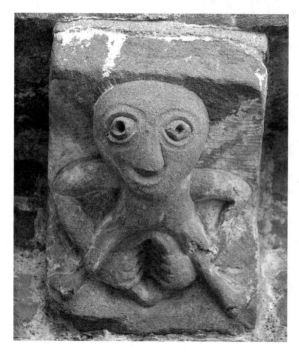

Sheela-na-gig, Kilpeck Church, Hereford, England

These stone carvings, often found over the doorway or windows of a church, depict a naked female with a full belly, posing in such a manner as to display and even emphasize her genitalia. Many of them reveal a woman with her knees apart and with the vulva held open by one or both hands. There are various theories surrounding these images, with different researchers believing that they were created to prevent evil and death from entering a building. This hypothesis is made more credible by the fact that many of the Sheela-na-gigs were located alongside other bizarre images, such as gargoyles, which were commonly used by churches of the eleventh and twelfth centuries to keep wickedness away from their doors, which obviously included the lasciviousness of women. This confirms that the medieval church considered the vulva of a woman to be grotesque and shameful.

There is another, more hopeful theory concerning these feminine artifacts, however. This suggests that the carvings are part of pre-Christian worship of the Mother Goddess, especially as the name Sheela-na-gig is interpreted as "hag woman" or "vulva woman." There is evidence that the images were used as fertility objects, especially by those who wished to become pregnant. The figures closely resemble the yonic statues of the Indian goddess Kali that appear at the doorways of many Hindu temples; these artifacts are still touched today for good luck, and in the hope that the Great Goddess will look kindly on you. The protruding rib cage seen in several of the Irish carvings of Sheela-na-gigs is also prominent in statues of Kalika, the Crone aspect of Kali and the death goddess in Hinduism. Such a female archetype is symbolized in the Irish tradition by Caillech, the Old Woman, who is both the creatrix and the destroyer. In this aspect, Sheela-na-gigs is similar to the clay figurine of the Mother Goddess that was found in Çatalhöyük, which dates from around 7000 BCE and is described by archaeologist Ian Hodder in chapter 2. With the front of this clay carving representing a plump and sensual woman, and the back a skeletal hag, Hodder concluded that "perhaps the importance of female imagery was related to some special role of the female in relation to death as much as to the roles of mother and nurturer."[8]

Many of the more explicit Sheela-na-gigs are still hidden from view, languishing in the dusty vaults of museums. Yet hopefully one day soon they will be restored to their rightful positions, not as talismans to ward off evil spirits, but to welcome visitors to enter the womb of Mother Church. By accepting her invitation to pass through her gaping vulva, we shed our delusional cloaks of separation and become bathed in the unconditional love of the divine feminine. This is not a new concept, for between the twelfth and fifteenth centuries, many of the great Gothic cathedrals of Europe were built with magnificent oval arched doorways, which clearly symbolize the vulva, and which lead to the nave—the womb—of the church.

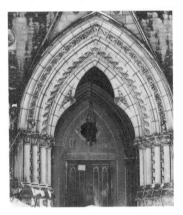

Gothic cathedral entrance

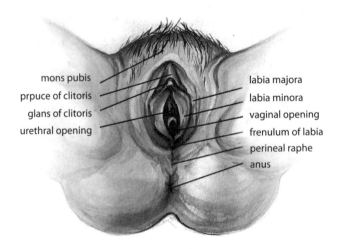

mons pubis

prpuce of clitoris

glans of clitoris

urethral opening

labia majora

labia minora

vaginal opening

frenulum of labia

perineal raphe

anus

The yoni, or vulva

Another symbol commonly used to represent the yoni of the Great Mother is the downward-pointing triangle. Similar in shape to a woman's pubic mound, this is found at the entry point of many sacred sites and is closely associated with the Asian goddess Cunti (also Candra, or Cunda), a female deity in Buddhism who is an emanation of the Buddha Vajrasattva. From this name are derived such words as *county*, *country*, *cunning*, and *cunt*. Unlike modern-day usage, *cunt*, historically, was not a word of derision but one of respect, honoring the embodiment of the Goddess within a woman. The same derivation gives us the word *kin*, or family, leading to the word *kingdom*, which denotes the domain of a king or queen. This confirms the importance of matrilineal inheritance in ancient times, wherein the continuation of a family and its fruitfulness on all levels was seen to be totally dependent on a woman and her link to the Great Mother's energy.

HEAVEN'S DOORWAY

If we think of the yoni, or vulva, as a doorway into another dimension or state of awareness, then it has three important structures: (1) the frame of the doorway, consisting of the mons pubis and the labia; (2) the key to the door, comprised of the sensually excitable tissues such as the clitoris and the G-spot; and (3) the doorway itself, i.e., the vaginal opening.

The Mons Pubis, or Pubic Triangle

Despite the fact that a lover may believe that this mound of fatty tissue is there merely to rest his or her head on, the mons pubis actually protects the delicate joint that connects the anterior halves of the pubic bone. Without this joint and its ligamentous capsule, which loosens during pregnancy, a baby's head would have difficulty passing through the pelvic opening. At puberty, the amount of fat within a girl's pubic mound increases and it becomes covered with pubic hair. The quantity and thickness of this hair varies markedly between cultures and gradually decreases after menopause. The pubic hair, which commonly extends to the groin, perineum, and the uppermost thighs, has led to a number of slang terms for the vulva, including *pussy, fanny, beaver, cooch, kitten, muff,* and *bearded clam.* Pubic hair is coarser and curlier than other hair, growing to its maximum length in a short six months during puberty, and forming a well-recognized triangle.

Nobody is entirely clear why the hair exists. Louis Robinson, a nineteenth-century English physician and evolutionist, hypothesized that the axillary and pubic hairs were remnants of our apelike days, when a baby would cling to these tufts of hair as the adult swung from tree to tree. More recently it has been suggested that the hair prevents dust and other substances from irritating or infecting the sensitive vulvar and vaginal tissues, just as the hairs of the nose and ears filter minute airborne particles.

It has long been the custom of those of the Islamic faith to remove their bodily hair, especially from the armpits and vulva, to maintain cleanliness. This practice is not performed out of shame, but in reverence and the desire to be clean and pure in all actions. Women from other cultures have adopted this practice, but for different reasons, leading to different levels of waxing, up to a Brazilian (also known as a sphinx or Hollywood), in which all the hair is removed from the pelvic area, both front and back. The reasons given for doing this include hygiene, a sense of feeling more attractive, especially when wearing high-cut panties and swimwear, and to give sexual pleasure to one's partner. Whether a lover's desire for hair removal comes from an aesthetic or a hygienic perspective—or because the woman now looks like a prepubescent girl—is not clear. Eve Ensler, in *The Vagina Monologues,* substituting the word *vagina* for *vulva,* sums up her experience this way:

> My first and only husband hated hair. He said it was cluttered and dirty. He made me shave my vagina. It looked puffy and exposed and like a little girl. This excited him. When he made love to me, my vagina felt the way a beard must feel. It felt good to rub it, and painful. Like scratching a mosquito bite. It felt like it was on fire. There were screaming red bumps. I refused to shave it again. Then

my husband had an affair. When we went to marital therapy, he said he screwed around because I wouldn't shave my vagina. The therapist . . . said marriage was a compromise. . . . I needed to jump in.

This time, when we got home, he got to shave my vagina. It was like a therapy bonus prize. He clipped a few times, and there was a little blood in the bathtub. He didn't even notice it, 'cause he was so happy shaving me. Then, later, when my husband was pressing against me, I could feel his spiky sharpness sticking into me, my naked puffy vagina. There was no protection. There was no fluff.

I realized then that hair is there for a reason—it's the leaf around the flower, the lawn around the house. You have to love hair in order to love the vagina. You can't pick the parts you want. And besides, my husband never stopped screwing around.[9]

Labia Majora and Minora

The sides of the vulvar doorway are made up of two pairs of labia, or lips. The outer boundaries are the fatty *labia majora,* which are covered with hair from puberty onward. Creating a link between the inner and outer fertility organs is the ligament that maintains the position of the uterus, known as the round ligament; this stretches from the sides of the uterus and ends in the labia majora.

The inner margins of the doorway are made up of fleshy and hairless folds, known as the *labia minora;* these join together anteriorly to form a hood or prepuce around the clitoris, much as the foreskin covers the glans of the penis. The labia minora remain relatively hidden until after puberty, when they commonly project beyond their fatty counterpart, the degree of protrusion varying between women and cultures.

Although elongated labial lips are considered sexually attractive in some societies, there are women who for aesthetic reasons seek a surgery known as a labiaplasty, to reduce the size of the labia minora. However, this practice, along with other forms of designer surgery, is highly controversial due to the risks that accompany any form of surgery.

The Clitoris

The key that opens the doorway to the abode of the Great Mother is hidden deep within the pelvis. It is no ordinary key, for once touched and stimulated, it unlocks a whole series of responses that ultimately leads to a state of orgasmic oneness. Until recently, the medical fraternity, which had a tendency to take its anatomical information about women from elderly female cadavers, didn't accept that women had any sexual erectile tissue. Fortunately, that misperception has been corrected through the use of modern dynamic exploratory procedures that show that women in fact possess as much erectile tissue as men, if not more.

The clitoris has for too long evoked a certain amount of shame, because until relatively recently a woman's sexual arousal and orgasmic release have been regarded as irrelevant in the greater scheme of things. From a patriarchal standpoint, since a woman can get pregnant without an orgasm, the continuation of the species (and the fortification of a man's self-esteem) must be dependent on the man's impressive ejaculation of sperm. Psychoanalyst Sigmund Freud said that after a girl passes through puberty she should convert to vaginal orgasms, leaving "immature" clitoral stimulation behind. Fortunately, female psychology has advanced somewhat in the past hundred years, although Freud's ruling on the subject still holds sway in the minds of some people, men *and* women.

The meaning of the word *clitoris* is thought to come from the Greek word *kleitoris,* meaning "little hill." However, according to Australian urologist Dr. Helen O'Connell, it would be more appropriate to call it a little mountain, or even a pyramid.[10] Many anatomists speak of the essential similarities between the penis and the clitoris, although they usually infer that the clitoris is far less relevant because of its apparent smaller size. This is because the only aspect of the clitoris that is visible is the pea-size head, or glans. However, when the full length of the clitoris, from the glans to the end of erectile tissue, is assessed, you may be surprised to know that it measures a mighty eight inches. So does size matter now?

It is clear that clitoral stimulation is very important to the orgasmic experience, with the head, or glans, of the clitoris more sexually sensitive

than any other part of a woman's body. Nevertheless, even in these somewhat more enlightened days, for some women clitoral stimulation, and
indeed masturbation itself, is still considered shameful. In addition, even
if a woman is happy to experience this pleasure in solitude, she may be less
keen to ask for clitoral stimulation from her partner, and even less willing
to masturbate in front of him or her.[11] Instead, she may be one of the 40
percent of women who do not orgasm at all during vaginal intercourse
because they are too embarrassed to ask for the specifics of foreplay and
too reticent to demand greater attention to their own sexual needs.

The clitoris is located at the front of the vulva, and its basic structure
is similar to that of the penis. It consists of the visible glans; two con-
joined shafts of erectile tissue, the *corpora cavernosa,* which are roughly
one-half to one inch long; and *crura,* or legs, which are attached to the
lateral bones of the pelvis, the *ischia.*

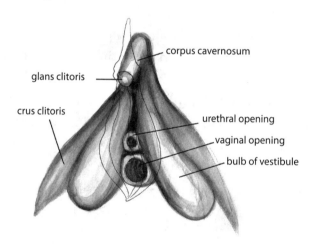

The clitoris

The other important source of erectile tissue in a woman consists
of the bulbs of the vestibule, also known as the clitoral bulbs. These are
analogous to the *corpus spongiosum* of the male, which is a spongy tissue that surrounds the urethra in the penis, ensuring its safety during an
erection. In a woman, the urethra is not at the same level of risk as in
a man, as its exit is separate from the clitoris. Hence the clitoral bulbs

stretch out from the shaft of the clitoris, around the urethra—forming the urethral sponge—and along the sides of the vestibule of the vagina, underneath the labia minora.

In both men and women, the glans contains highly sensitive nerve endings. The clitoral head has a staggering number of such sensory nerve endings—approximately 7,000—more than any other part of the body and, in proportion to its size, four times as many as are found within the glans of the penis.[12] This small and sensual organ, the clitoris, has only one purpose: through touch, stimulation, or pressure, it excites the magnetic field of a woman's body and hence awakens her inner fiery dragon.

Supporting all of these structures are muscles that attach anteriorly to the pubic bone and posteriorly to the coccyx, or tailbone. These muscles bring strength to the pelvic floor as well as causing the whole area to be exquisitely sensitive to touch during sexual arousal, thereby intensifying the sensual experience.

During sexual excitation, contraction of the muscles causes engorgement of the shaft of the clitoris, resulting in an erection similar to a penile erection. At the same time, the clitoral bulbs become full and engorged with blood. Together with the contraction of the muscles, this engorgement causes the vaginal opening to tighten, leading to increased sexual stimulation for the penis. During the orgasmic release that follows, the rhythmic contraction and relaxation of the muscles is felt along their length, from the clitoris to the anal sphincter, resulting eventually in the loss of the clitoral erection.

The G-Spot

Surrounding the urethra is the erectile tissue known as the urethral sponge, which is part of the clitoral or vestibular bulbs. During sexual excitation, the sponge becomes engorged with blood, preventing the release of urine during and, for a while, after orgasm.

The urethral sponge is also associated with the celebrated G-spot, or Grafenberg spot, named for Dr. Ernest Grafenberg, who first described it in a 1950s article in the *International Journal of Sexology* as a highly erogenous zone inside the vagina that gets bigger when directly stimulated. The G-spot is about the size of a fingernail and is located about three inches inside the vagina, on the anterior vaginal wall—which is why intercourse in the missionary position is unlikely to awaken this area. For many women, stimulation of this area creates a more intense orgasm than clitoral stimulation alone. It is extremely sensitive to stroking and vibration and is said to expand to almost the size of a walnut when stimulated.

There has been some debate as to whether this spot actually exists, with some doctors having found little evidence of any difference between this and the surrounding area in terms of an increase in nerve endings or a thickening of the tissues. It is of course possible that the G-spot is actually absent in some women. However, the popularity of a curved, phallic-shaped stimulator known as a G-spot vibrator certainly suggests that adventurous women are not willing to accept that assumption without some personal investigation. The variation in G-spot sensitivity causes concern for some psychologists, who believe that women are being made to feel less than adequate if they cannot locate the spot, leading to an increase in requests for a specific plastic surgery known as a G-spot amplification, a nonsurgical treatment that temporarily augments the G-spot by means of injecting a bioengineered human collagen product directly into the area (a "G-shot"), a procedure whose results last about four months and then wear off.

The Nectar of Youth

In one survey, 45 percent of women questioned acknowledged sensitivity to G-spot stimulation, with 82 percent of these respondents reporting female ejaculation, wherein there is a sudden release of fluid similar to the ejaculatory response of a man.[13] It is believed that the fluid comes from the several paraurethral glands (the largest known as the Skene's glands) that open into the vulvar vestibule close to the urethral opening and probably into the urethra itself. Researchers have discovered that these glands are stimulated during sexual arousal to produce an alkaline fluid very similar to the semen produced by the prostate gland in men, and hence the glands have been called the female prostate. The fluid even contains PSA, an antigen specific to prostatic secretions. The amount can vary from a few drops to a few liquid ounces.

A woman may not recognize her own ejaculation, which can occur independently of any physical arousal of the G-spot. That is because when this fluid gushes, spurts, trickles, or squirts from around the urethral opening, most women, having not been educated in the female ejaculation, think the secretion is urine—which causes many women who experience "the nectar of youth" to instead feel embarrassed and even seek medical intervention. At other times a woman may think that the dampness on the sheets has come from her male partner and doesn't consider that it may be from her own ejaculation.

The female ejaculation has been well documented in the teachings of ancient India, China, and Greece. It appears that it was only in the last two hundred years that the subject slipped from Western medical literature and hence from the minds of the average man and woman— although there are certain pornographic stars who proudly declare that they are "squirters" and "gushers," a proclamation that they are producing an elixir that in fact has been treasured since ancient times. This fluid has been called the divine nectar of the sacred waters and has been linked to other legendary exotic solutions such as liquid gold, the fountain of life, the elixir of immortality, and amrita. In the past, in traditions such as Taoism and Tantra, it was believed that when these white drops of fluid were drunk, the receiver was rewarded with good health, endless youthfulness, and eternal life. In Taoist sexual practice, during cunnilingus, or oral sex, the man uses his tongue, lips, and teeth to bring his woman to orgasmic ecstasy so that he can drink her juices of love, while he himself holds back his ejaculation, ensuring his essential vitality. In certain Tantric rituals, a few drops of these sacred secretions, representing the regenerative juices of Kali, the great Hindu goddess, are mixed with water and wine and then given to a community.[14]

Researchers have shown that the secretions of the Skene's glands contain an enzyme that extends the life of cells; hence female ejaculate has been called the nectar of youth or the enzyme of immortality. It is most probable that this enzyme is telomerase, which decreases the aging of cells.[15] Represented by the lotus or lily, this elixir of life has been linked to the sexual dark goddess Lilith. Like other Crone archetypes such as Isis and Kali, Lilith taught her priestesses how to produce this fountain of youth through sacred sexual practices, so they could confer immortality on those who came into their presence.*

In Hinduism, it is taught that the elixir of life or amrita is also produced by the pineal gland during deep states of meditation that involve raising the serpentine or kundalini energy to the crown chakra. It is said that just a drop of this elixir is enough to conquer death. I believe that despite ancient practices and no doubt the wishful thinking of many men, the mere drinking of the ejaculated fluid of a woman is not enough to confer eternal life. As we will soon see, sexual arousal in a woman causes her magnetic energy body to light up, allowing her to raise her consciousness to the crown chakra as well as carry a partner to that same place. Like it or not, there are no shortcuts when it comes to immortality.

It is only in recent years that urologists have appreciated the immense importance of the urethral sponge to a woman's sexual pleasure, and as a result they are now taking far greater care during surgical procedures. It is not uncommon to find that because of the location of the urethral opening, against the pubic bone, it can become infected or inflamed after intercourse, especially after menopause, when the vaginal tissues start to thin, and this can lead to recurrent bouts of cystitis. Changing positions during intercourse, engaging in regular sexual stimulation, and revitalizing the vaginal tissues can help reduce the occurrence of problems in this area.

---

*It should be noted that the same benefits of immortality have not been mentioned in relation to a man's semen when a woman performs oral sex.

The Entrance to the Goddess's Abode

We have carefully examined heaven's doorway and found the key that opens the door. Now we stand at the threshold of the Goddess's abode. The vaginal opening is the passageway or vestibule to the womb and is located within the vulvar vestibule and behind the urethral opening. Like all secret passageways, the opening and vaginal walls close in on themselves until something is inserted. Just inside the vaginal opening are two tiny glands known as Bartholin's glands or greater vestibular glands; these assist in the lubrication of the vulva and vagina, especially during sexual arousal, although the majority of vaginal lubrication occurs from deep within the vagina. It is now believed that the most important aspect of the secretions from the Bartholin's glands are their pheromone content, which allows interested parties to know of a woman's sexual interest.

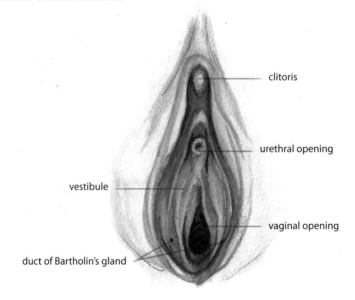

Entrance to the Goddess's abode

From the time of a woman's birth, the opening of the vagina is covered by an incomplete thin layer of tissue known as the hymen, which is usually ruptured during the first sexual experience, through the insertion of tampons, or with vigorous exercise such as horseback riding. In the past, the presence of blood on the matrimonial bedsheets from the rupture of this hymen was considered proof not only that sexual penetration had occurred, but that the newly wedded wife had been still a virgin.

Modifications to the Vulva
Piercing
Apart from the depilation of vulvar hair and cosmetic surgical modifications such as labiaplasty, the practice of piercing, thousands of years old, needs to be considered. Regarded as a status symbol in many cultures around the world, piercing is carried out in various parts of the body, although it most commonly is done in the ears and nose. The piercing of the nipples and labia has been documented in ancient Rome and in India as far back as 350 BCE. Since then, this practice has waxed and waned, over and over again, until its resurgence over the past twenty years.

The reasons for piercing are varied; it can be for religious or spiritual reasons, for sensual enhancement, to boost confidence, as a form of tribalism or peer-group bonding, and as a sign of rebellion. Some people pierce to mark an anniversary or to make a statement about reclaiming their body and their sexual power after sexual abuse.[16] The most common areas of the vulva to be pierced include the labia (minora and majora) and the clitoral hood, with the clitoris included on rare occasions. It is common for studs and rings to be worn, offering both visual and sensual appeal.

Female Genital Cutting (or Mutilation)
Female genital cutting, or mutilation (FGC or FGM), dates back to ancient Egypt and is still practiced on many women today. It is likely that many of the families who insist on this procedure today have forgotten its original meaning and continue the practice because it is a social custom and guarantees that a daughter will not become an outcast in her society.

Before we judge, let's not forget that in the United States, male circumcision is still being carried out routinely, and this too is based on some very spurious reasoning. There is even evidence that gynecologists of the nineteenth century performed clitorectomies to cure female "weaknesses" such as nymphomania, insanity, and masturbation.[17]

The World Health Organization defines FGC as "the partial or total removal of the external female genitalia or other injury to the female genital organs for nonmedical reasons."[18] Those who carry out the practice have demanded that the procedure be known as cutting and not as mutilation, as they resent the stigma attached to something that is considered a ritual. Other terms such as *female circumcision* have also been used, although this is inaccurate, for during circumcision the male foreskin is removed without damage to the underlying structure, unlike the disfiguration that occurs with FGC.

In 2003, the African Union adopted the Maputo Protocol, promoting women's rights and ending female genital cutting. This has certainly led to a decrease in the number of girls undergoing FGC in many countries, although the United Nations estimates that up to three million procedures still take place every year, with up to 140 million women and girls already having undergone the practice. Those most commonly involved include the countries of northeast Africa, the Near East, and Southeast Asia, and some tribes in Australia and South America. Many countries outside those just mentioned have made FGC illegal, even going so far as to prosecute families who send their daughters back to their homeland to receive the treatment; yet the practice continues. Unfortunately, the legislation has caused the procedure to go underground, inciting an even greater risk of complications for a girl, including hemorrhage, infection, and even death.

FGC usually takes place when a girl is between four and eight years old, although it can occur anytime from infancy to adolescence. Depending on the culture, the process is carried out by a doctor or female elder of the tribe, with or without the use of anesthesia and sterile instruments. Apart from the trauma, pain, and risk of infection or hemorrhage during the procedure, many women who have undergone the procedure experience chronic pain, incontinence, and psychological problems for the rest of their lives.

There are different levels of FGC, ranging from partial or total removal of the clitoris to cutting and restructuring the labia majora and minora so that the vaginal opening is closed apart from a hole for urine and menstrual blood to escape. During the first sexual encounter, the opening is made larger to facilitate penetration by the penis. Prior to childbirth, further cutting is required to allow the baby's head to emerge, with the vaginal opening commonly re-sutured after the birth. Although the most extreme procedure is carried out on only about 10 percent of African girls, it is clear that the practice leads to much higher incidences of obstructed labor, Cesarean sections, maternal postpartum hemorrhage, and infant death.[19]

And what are the reasons given for FGC? To prevent a girl from becoming a social outcast and hence to make her suitable for marriage; to reduce a girl's sensuality and her sexual desire, hence maintaining her virginity; to ensure marital fidelity; and to maintain a woman's beauty and purity. But the clitoris is not the only organ to offer sexual pleasure; a 1989 study of Sudanese women who underwent FGC showed that almost 90 percent of them had experienced some level of orgasm during their married lives, although few studies have been done to measure their levels of psychological sexual pleasure.[20]

MASTURBATION: IGNITING THE FIRE OF HEALING

Sex is more than just a few moments of intense pleasure; it is an opportunity for healing and restoration that begins when we turn the excitatory keys and ignite a whole sequence of events that affect the physical body as well as the energetic body, including the chakras. When this occurs, we find ourselves being transported from our humdrum lives into a blissful state, floating in the expansiveness and abundant potential of the Great Mother. For this reason, sexual self-stimulation and foreplay are essential for both genders, with specific areas of the body exquisitely primed to activate the energetic body. There are, of course, other ways for this to happen, especially when the heart opens spontaneously, such as when we're laughing with friends, watching a beautiful sunset, or thinking about someone we love. However this activation of our energy body occurs, without it, it is easy for our lives to become disconnected from the memory that we are spiritual beings having a creative experience within a beautiful and sensual physical body.

The word *masturbate* comes from the Latin *masturbatus,* "to disturb with the hand." It has always offered men and women the chance to activate their energetic bodies and experience sexual satisfaction, with or without a partner. Whether a woman uses her own fingers, a vibrator, a dildo, jets of water, or Ben Wa balls, stimulation is directed toward various erogenous zones, including the nipples, clitoris, G-spot, and anus. She may also apply rhythmic pressure to the clitoris and vulvar region, using a firm object such as a pillow to increase the level of sexual arousal. In the past, there was an attitude that too much of a good thing could be damaging, especially when self-stimulation replaces natural socialization; but many psychologists are coming to the conclusion that masturbation actually improves overall health and well-being.

Statistics from 2010 show that more than half of American women aged eighteen to forty-nine reported masturbating during the previous ninety days; the rates were highest among those aged twenty-five to twenty-nine and progressively lesser in older age groups.[21] Research also shows that 71 percent of British women between the ages of sixteen and forty-four have masturbated in their lifetime, which means 29 percent have never masturbated, mainly for cultural and religious reasons.[22]

Religions that say that masturbation is sinful—the Catholic Church deems it completely impermissible—are a puritanical throwback to earlier times, when the practice was considered "unnatural" and thought to inevitably lead to blindness and stunted growth. Indeed, some popular modern foods were born from the desire to create a bland, meatless diet—especially for men—to reduce the risk of testosterone-driven lust, and hence masturbation. Two such foods include cornflakes, invented by Dr. John Harvey Kellogg, and graham crackers, the brainchild of the Reverend Sylvester Graham, both of whom supported the principles of social conservatism, which advocates puritanical morality and traditional family values and opposes sexual "permissiveness," based on a specific understanding of Abrahamist values.

It was from the same mistaken belief that masturbation leads to insanity that the practice of circumcision—the removal of the foreskin of the penis—was adopted in the United States in the late 1890s. Currently, some 80 percent of U.S.-born males are circumcised, whether for religious reasons (as a sacrifice or rite of passage), for hygienic reasons, or because of the longstanding Victorian belief that this practice reduces the desire to masturbate.[23] Dr. Kellogg, of the aforementioned cornflakes fame, approved of the procedure being carried out without an anesthetic because he believed the pain would be a constant reminder to men of the perils of touching their penis. Even though there is a popular belief that male circumcision prevents infections under the foreskin, especially from sexually transmitted diseases, there is no evidence of this. Nor does it prevent headache, epilepsy, alcoholism, near-sightedness, cancer of the penis, cancer of the cervix, syphilis, or AIDS—all of which have been put forward at one time by the American medical system as rationales for circumcision.[24]

In circumcision, the foreskin of the penis is removed, along with 50 to 80 percent of the penis's erogenous sexual nerves. This means a man loses the pleasure that comes with one of the most natural forms of self-stimulation, when the foreskin slides against the head or glans of the penis during masturbation and intercourse. Studies conducted in 1997 showed that men who are circumcised are more likely to engage in oral and anal sex. This is because the lips of the mouth and the muscles of the anus provide the necessary friction to achieve the kind of sexual arousal that would otherwise have been created by the foreskin. Women who have slept with both circumcised and uncircumcised men definitely notice the difference, with many more reporting a vaginal orgasm with the uncircumcised man. This is thought to be due to the fact that during intercourse the penis of the "natural" man can remain deep within the vagina, as its head, which needs to thrust against another surface to heighten arousal, has its own foreskin to rub against. This means that there is less need for large thrusts by the penis, allowing greater sensual sensitivity to develop between the vagina and the penis.[25]

It is fascinating to learn that at the same time masturbation was being denounced in the late 1800s, it was being used to treat hysteria in women (the word *hysteria* comes from the Greek *hystera,* or uterus), with physicians prescribing an early form of the vibrator, along with various creams to be applied to sensually sensitive areas of the body.[26] Today, popular attitudes toward masturbation have greatly changed from the Victorian era, with many seeing it as a healthy outlet for pent-up energy and stress as well as an aid in bringing relaxation to the body and mind. In the United Kingdom, where there are high levels of teenage pregnancy, many psychologists are sensibly encouraging teachers and parents to recognize masturbation as the means by which young people can have the same pleasures of sex without the unwanted consequences.[27]

Still, most women want more than just a self-pleasuring "quickie" to satisfy their sexual needs. The Goddess within each of us wants her energy field to be ignited through foreplay, which includes wooing, nurturing, caressing, and respect. Any partner who fails to understand this has never had a true sexual experience. Only when a woman's magnetic vessel has been created and her serpentine power aroused can she provide a man with the transformational pathway that leads to transcendence and healing.

When we as women acknowledge the vital role our bodies play in the future of humanity on planet Earth, we will forbid anybody from touching or entering this sanctified space who does not have permission from and reverence for our indwelling Great Goddess. Any sexual practice that fails to arouse the sleeping serpent or that feels degrading to

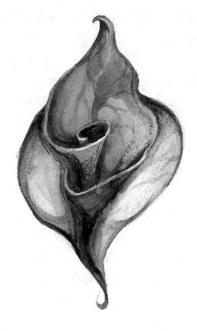

*The transformational
pathway that leads
to transcendence*

the Goddess is obviously unacceptable. At the same time, our partners must agree to take a loving and active interest in our romantic desires as well as our sensitive hot spots. Only then will we experience a sexual interaction as true lovemaking, where both parties feel compassion, first for themselves and then for their partner, leading to the divine and blissful union that we all seek.

THE SEXUAL RESPONSE

What causes us to shift our attention from everyday matters toward something that makes us tingle all over in anticipation? This has been the study of much research over many years. More recently, our knowledge of the process has been enhanced by technology that allows us to see the activity of the brain in real time.

Sexual arousal is a complex process, greatly influenced by our memories, fantasies, emotions, and sensual stimulation. We can be turned on by pleasurable stroking, the memory of an intimate moment, the presence of someone sexy, our own sexual touch, erotic scenes on television or in books, or sexual fantasy, or for some out of plain boredom. Some women are aroused by explicit sexual language, while for others this is a definite turnoff. The more we live outside our body, especially because of a history of sexual abuse, the more we rely on fantasy and less on touch and massage.

Frequently what aids sexual arousal is creating some form of rhythmic motion, whether through stroking, the use of a vibrator, or penile thrusting, although everybody is unique. Some women find using a water jet on the vagina to be highly effective, while ice cream, whipped cream, and melted chocolate provide wonderful incentives for a super-sensual sundae. Whether the experience is solo or involves others, the environment required to create the right atmosphere can be very diverse. For some it involves candles, a bath, and comforting and sweet music; others are turned on by more physical activity or the secretiveness of a situation. Some women can experience an orgasm without even touching their vulvar area. This includes those who are highly sensitive to nipple stimulation and women who can just think themselves into an orgasm.

Whatever the stimulus, when we are sexually aroused our bloodstream is flooded with hormones that provide us with a choice as to whether to follow this path or wait until later. Should we decide to go ahead, the sexual response is delineated into four physiological stages, according to human sexual-response pioneers William Masters and Virginia Johnson:

1. **Excitement or arousal phase.** Increase in heart rate, blood pressure, and respiration. This increase in blood flow leads to many of the following signs:

   - Hardening or erection of the nipples
   - Erection of the clitoris, with the glans appearing from beneath the hood
   - Thickening of the vaginal wall and the labia minora
   - Sexual flush often involving the entire body, and especially the vulva and breasts

- Vaginal lubrication and release of pheromone-laden fluid from Bartholin's glands
- Contraction of various muscles, especially those in the pelvic floor, leading to a heightening of sexual sensitivity in the vulvar and anal regions

2. **Plateau phase.** Intensification of the changes in the excitement phase, including:

- The vagina turning a deep red color
- The vaginal wall lengthening, making it easier for any future sperm to enter the cervix, while also engaging the uterus in the sexual response
- Hypersensitivity of the glans of the clitoris, which may now disappear under the hood to avoid further direct stimulation
- Increased muscle tension, especially of the hands, feet, and legs
- Enlargement of the clitoral bulb and tightening of the vaginal opening
- Swelling of the urethral sponge, with all areas of the vulva hypersensitive and sexually engaged
- Involuntary soundings

3. **Orgasmic phase.** The shortest of all the phases, often lasting only seconds, yet the most euphoric, marked by:

- Sudden release of sexual tension
- Quick cycles of contraction of the vaginal muscles, the clitoris, and the muscles of the pelvic floor, along with release from the paraurethral glands of female ejaculatory fluid
- Spasm of the feet and legs
- Involuntary soundings and movements
- Opioids flooding into the bloodstream

4. **Resolution phase.** Relaxation brings:

- A sense of intimacy, well-being, and bliss, mainly because of the presence of the hormones oxytocin and prolactin from the pituitary gland
- Postcoital sleep (more common in men than in women)
- A return to a normal state of consciousness

On average this entire sequence of events can take approximately four minutes when either a man or a woman is self-pleasuring. When a couple is engaging in intercourse, the orgasmic release in a woman may not come for at least thirty minutes (if at all), compared with ten minutes for the average man. This, according to sex educator and author Claire Hutchins, is because women are less sexually confident in the presence of another person and are therefore less inclined to use fantasy and other aids to intensify their sexual response.[28]

Opponents of the Masters and Johnson model claim that it describes only physiological characteristics of an orgasm and ignores the cognitive or emotional aspects of sexuality. Some of these features are included in another widely accepted model of the human sexual response developed by Dr. Helen Singer Kaplan, a psychiatrist and psychologist and one of the original sex therapists (who trained Dr. Ruth Westheimer). She believed that the process consists of three stages: desire, excitement, and orgasm, the desire phase being, in her opinion, the most difficult to treat when dysfunctional.

S. R. Whalen and D. Roth, researchers in the field of sexuality, created a cognitive model of sexual arousal that outlines a sequence of psychological events:

Perception of a sexual stimulus: *That feels sexy.*
Positive evaluation of the perception: *I like the feeling.*
Physiological arousal
Perception of the arousal: *I feel turned on.*
Positive evaluation of the arousal: *I'm in the mood.*

Sexual behaviors
    Perception of the behaviors: *I'm going all the way.*
    Positive evaluation of the behaviors: *That was bliss!*

Each evaluation acts as a feedback mechanism that increases the level of arousal and sexual behaviors.[29]

The quality of the orgasmic phase varies from person to person and from day to day, depending on an assortment of circumstances. Sometimes the orgasm is an explosive rush of sensations, while on other occasions the effects are far more subtle and milder. The differences in intensity can be attributed to physical factors such as fatigue and length of time since the last orgasm, as well as psychosocial factors, including mood, relationship to the partner, expectations, and self-esteem.

Some Native American tribes teach that once you have mixed fluids with another person, your energies are tied together for the next seven years. This may cause us to reconsider whether that one-night stand was worth it. Even more importantly, the energy that unites us is based on the emotions we felt during the time of coupling. If the experience was pleasurable and enhanced our feelings of self-worth, then the energy bond supports similar relationships. However, if a sexual experience was not based on self-respect and compassion, then unless we want to continue this pattern we need to stop, face the truth, and cut the ties with the past. Only then can we make a promise to our precious body that we will only exchange fluids with those who respect and honor the divine Goddess within and who understand that sex is a beautiful and sacred process.

The Brain and the Sexual Response

It is clear that for both men and women, the orgasmic process is greatly influenced by the brain's activities. Functional magnetic resonance imaging (fMRI) and positron-emission tomography (PET) have shown that at least thirty areas of the brain light up during sexual arousal, whether a woman is self-pleasuring or is being sexually stimulated by a partner. The most dynamic regions involved are those associated with sensation and touch, as well as the areas associated with physical movement.

Researchers have also studied groups of women who are able to think themselves into an orgasm by bringing to mind images that may be erotic, loving, or abstract. These women show the same pattern of physiological changes as women who are sexually aroused through physical stimulation, but they provide a clearer picture of the deeper changes to a woman's psyche when the sensory and motor aspects are removed. The areas of the brain involved include:

Nucleus accumbens: associated with reward, pleasure, and addiction

Paraventricular nucleus of the hypothalamus: controls the release of hormones into the bloodstream, in particular oxytocin and vasopressin, essential for bonding and intimacy

Hippocampus: associated with turning short-term memory into long-term memory

Amygdala: controls our reaction to specific events based on previously stored memories associated with emotional situations

Anterior cingulate cortex: associated with reward anticipation, decision making, empathy, and emotions

Many of these structures are found within the limbic system, whose main job is to guide us toward pleasure and survival and away from pain and death, through the stimulation of emotions and memories. The limbic system also controls our drives and impulses, which include eating, drinking, taking risks, and sex.

In the early stages of sexual arousal, activity in the brain increases in particular in those areas involved in motivation, reward, memory-related imagery, and emotions. It has also been discovered that sexual arousal numbs pain and heightens feelings of pleasure.[30] This response is mediated through the amygdala, which also decreases fear and vigilance, allowing us to feel more trusting and actively seek intimacy—both essential for love-making. This effect is reinforced by the release of oxytocin, known as the love hormone. The activation of the amygdala is less pronounced when the orgasm is thought induced, suggesting that trust is already in place.

When the brain of a man ejaculating was studied by Dutch neuroscientist Gert Holstege and his colleagues, they were surprised to see extraordinary activation of an area of the midbrain associated with reward, the intensity of the response comparable to that induced by heroin. The theory put forward in 2003 was that since impregnation of the female is essential for species survival, it is seen as a rewarding behavior by the brain. But it is clear that the action should not get out of hand; otherwise it becomes pure addiction.[31]

Holstege's team then turned their attention to women. They asked them to receive clitoral stimulation from their partner while a PET scan recorded brain activity. Once again, the team was surprised by the results, which showed that when a woman reached orgasm her brain went silent, particularly the area of the brain that usually exercises self-control over basic desires, including sex. The decrease in activity obviously allowed for a release of tension and inhibition. A similar dip in excitation was seen in the prefrontal cortex, which is involved in moral reasoning and social judgment, the change implying a suspension of judgment and self-reflection.[32] Since a man can orgasm without an ejaculation, it is probable that in this situation he would experience similar changes.

One notable finding is that during orgasm, in both genders the cerebellum is activated. The cerebellum is at the back of the brain and takes up only 10 percent of the brain's overall space, yet it has more nerve cells than all the rest of the brain put together. Known for its importance in motor functions such as coordination, precision, and fine movements, its excitation during an orgasm is thought to relate to psychological functions because of its strong links to the limbic system. Recent research has suggested that this area of brain is associated with balancing emotions and our ability to shift attention from one focus to the next.[33] However, it is clear that more studies are required to understand the true role of the cerebellum, especially during orgasm.

Hormones and the Sexual Response

Dopamine: The Reward Seeker

The activation of certain parts of the brain while other areas are switched off is a function of certain powerful neurochemicals. The main motivating neuropeptide in sexual arousal is dopamine, which activates the pleasure and reward center of the limbic system, telling us that this is something we must have. Dopamine alone is rarely satisfied and loves to take chances. The more dopamine in our system, the more we want something, unless other hormones are available to inhibit dopamine's lust. But dopamine is not the bad guy, for without it we can easily become depressed, lack ambition, and be sexually disinterested and unable to create healthy bonds with other people.

This is certainly the situation for people taking certain antidepression drugs such as Prozac or other SSRIs (selective serotonin reuptake inhibitors). These drugs increase the levels of the neuropeptide serotonin in an attempt to reduce depression. However, serotonin is dopamine's natural inhibitor, which means that increased levels of serotonin decrease our sexual drive. There are new antidepression drugs on the market that affect a different neuropeptide pathway and hopefully will have less of an effect on the libido.

Oxytocin: The Love Hormone

Increased levels of the neuropeptide known as the love hormone are seen in both men and women at orgasm, whether through self-pleasuring or in coupling. Oxytocin is released both from the posterior pituitary gland and from neurons within the brain in response to stimulation of the nipples and genitalia, especially the vaginal tract. It is suggested that the hormone aids the passage of the sperm and egg through the stimulation of muscular contractions.

However, the main effect of oxytocin is increasingly being seen as psychological, as it appears to nurture our desire to create intimate bonds with one another, otherwise known as positive social bonding. Oxytocin receptors in the human brain are mainly distributed in what is called the social brain, the areas involved being activated when adults view pictures of their partners or when mothers look at their children.[34] Oxytocin evokes feelings of contentment, a reduction in anxiety, increased trust, and feelings of calmness and security.[35] To this end, oxytocin is being used as a nasal spray, intranasally, in studies that aim to reduce some of the symptoms of autism, especially where socialization is affected.

Low levels of oxytocin are associated with an increased risk of post-partum depression and illnesses such as fibromyalgia, suggesting that sexual arousal and cuddling play an important part in maintaining a healthy state of mind and immune system.[36] One study showed that oxytocin levels were elevated after women received a relaxing massage, suggesting that such nurturing increases our feelings of self-love and contentment. Women who experience interpersonal problems, especially associated with lack of trust and invasiveness, are less likely to benefit from massage and have more difficulty maintaining their oxytocin levels at optimal levels in the face of sadness.[37]

Prolactin: The Nesting Hormone

Prolactin is secreted mainly from the anterior pituitary gland and is known to cause postcoital relaxation, which is more marked in men than in women. A woman can have multiple orgasms within one session, while a man who has just orgasmed may need anywhere from twelve hours to two weeks before his prolactin level settles and he is ready to go again. The physiological reason for this effect, found in all mammals, is prolactin's inhibition of dopamine. Physiologically, prolactin ensures that once procreation is complete, the parents focus their attention on preparing the nest and ensuring the survival of their offspring rather than continuing to seek satisfaction for their own desires. In humans, the situation is a little more complicated, especially as intercourse doesn't necessarily result in conception. Thus the opposing effects of dopamine and prolactin can trigger moderate highs and lows in libido in both men and women, and this is not necessarily relieved by more sex.

Notably, the release of prolactin in men and women is four times higher after intercourse than after masturbation, suggesting that it is a measure of sexual satisfaction associated with the intimate bonding with a partner.[38]

Estrogen, Testosterone, and Progesterone: The Cyclical Hormones

There is little evidence to show that the female hormone estrogen has a major effect on the specific features of the sexual response. It is true that women are far more sexually aroused around the time of ovulation, but this is thought to be associated with peak levels of testosterone, which, as in men, influences our libido and sex drive, motivating us to conceive during these important days. Testosterone levels decline after ovulation mainly because of the presence of the hormone progesterone, which is far more interested in nurturing and nesting than in desire and conquest.

It is now clear that the contraceptive known as "the pill," which was marketed to women as a source of sexual freedom, actually inhibits testosterone production, thereby reducing sex drive and vaginal lubrication. A study carried out in 2006 showed that the inhibitory effect continues after the pill is discontinued, although the long-term effects are still unknown.[39]

THE ENERGETIC VULVA

The vulva relates to the base chakra, while the sacred organs tucked away inside the pelvis are linked to the sacral chakra. The base chakra is connected to our perception of belonging, whether to a family, tribe, or this planet, ensuring security and the ability to safely root on this earth. If such security is lacking from birth or during the infant years, then the base chakra is highly sensitive to any signs of loss, rejection, or abandonment. Events such as learning of a husband's unfaithfulness or an imminent job loss can ultimately affect organs linked to this chakra, including the vulva, where feelings of insecurity may exacerbate illnesses such as herpes or vulvar pain. In addition, a shock to the base chakra can lead to the other illnesses, including panic attacks and insomnia, which further weaken the immune system's defenses, resulting in infections like candida (thrush) or cystitis.

The base chakra relates to the kidney meridian and its ability to store and supply energy, or qi, which gives us our essential strength and security. In particular, this meridian is dependent on us receiving healthy supplies of ancestral qi at the time of our birth. If our ancestors lived in fear of loss or poverty, then the stores of this energy will already be depleted when we reach this earth, causing us to believe we need only to survive, not thrive. If, in addition, we experienced any threat or insecurity to our life as a fetus or during infancy, then the stores of our life force, or qi, will also be reduced. Finally, survival mechanisms such as hypervigilance and a tendency to live outside our body will, over time, decrease our ability to acquire qi, leading eventually to exhaustion of the adrenal glands and a further lowering of the immune response, possibly leading to infection, inflammation, and cancer.

Healing of this area takes time and is often helped by receiving reliable therapeutic support. Eventually, when we feel secure enough to send our roots down into the earth, we can feel the love and support of Mother Earth. Her natural kingdoms, including the plants and animals, understand what it feels like to live in a world where there is constant uncertainty because of the seasons, the changes in climate, and the cycles of the moon, yet they have learned not only to survive, but to adapt and thrive.

5

SACRED SEXUALITY

Many years ago I toured the wild and beautiful Camargue, in the south of France, in search of the memory of Mary Magdalen. She is believed to have landed here after her escape from Egypt, carrying in her womb the child of Jesus. One sultry afternoon, a group of us visited a church in the center of a town called Saintes-Maries-de-la-Mer, best known for an annual pilgrimage of gypsies who gather in honor of Saint Sarah, or Sara-la-Kali (Sarah the Black). One of the tales associated with Sarah is that three saints, Mary Magdalen, Mary Salome, and Mary Jacobe, were traveling in a boat with Joseph of Arimathea when the water became rough. Immediately, Sarah, a dark-skinned woman, entered the sea to help them, using either a cloak as a raft or by literally walking on the water. Some accounts say that Sarah was a servant, while others regard her as a tribal chief who had foretold of the coming of these three sacred women and was on the shore to welcome them. There is, however, another story that suggests that Sarah, or Sar'h, was the child of Jesus and Mary Magdalen, and it is through her that their bloodline continues to this day.

According to *The Magdalen Manuscript,* written by Tom Kenyon and Judi Sion, Mary gave birth to Sar'h, and when her daughter was twelve Mary returned to Saintes-Maries-de-la-Mer so that the girl could be initiated into the cult of Isis, as Mary had been at the time of her own first menstrual bleeding.[1] According to these writings,

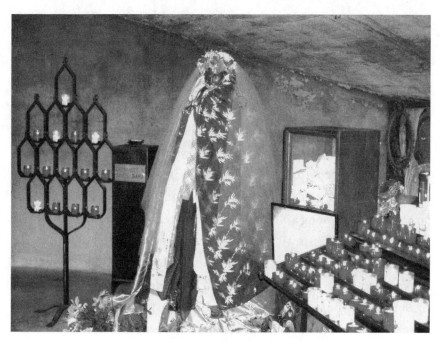

Sar'h in the church of Saintes-Maries-de-la-Mer

the statue of the dark girl that stands in the cool crypt of the church is Sar'h, her dark skin symbolic of both her country of origin and the fact that her mother, Mary Magdalen, is often depicted as the Black Madonna.

As I stood in front of the statue of this slender girl, I became transfixed and was immediately transported back in time to her initiation, where I saw her surrounded by women of all ages, in the center of which stood her proud mother, Mary Magdalen. I watched as the girl's childhood clothes were taken from her and she was laid naked on Mother Earth so she could feel the succulent warmth of moisture begin to stimulate her sensual sensitivity. Then, gently, the women started to massage her body with aromatic oils, leaving no place untouched. I watched as they caressed every one of her sacred sensual spots, including her clitoris, vagina, and nipples. There was no shame, only pure pleasure, as the budding female power and beauty were allowed to burst open with an orgasmic cry, and Sar'h was transformed from a child to a woman.

Her release activated an explosion of energy from deep within my soul, and tears started to run down my face, rising up from my womb. I could feel a profound sadness and regret that I hadn't been raised to see my own body as pleasurable, desirable, and without shame. Because of this, in my younger years I had not always treated it with the respect it deserved. In that moment it became clear that such an initiation was needed in this world today, yet it would work only if the older women were themselves comfortable with the pleasure and sacred purpose of their own bodies. If they carried shame and guilt or a desire to steal power from the young and innocent, then the rite of passage would fail. Children cannot learn without role models and need to be surrounded by women who know how to value and honor their bodies. After millennia of amnesia, it is time to dive into the depths of our psyche and reconnect to the budding seed of consciousness that cherishes and delights in the sensuality and sexuality of the body.

THE ART AND JOY OF SACRED SEX

Despite the fact that each generation thinks that it has invented sex, this alchemical process has been around since the universe formed. It was never meant to be a secretive experience or to be carried out only in the bedroom, for anything that grows, evolves, and transforms, including plants, animals, and galaxies, achieves this through sex, a merging of opposites. Sex is a process of evolution and creativity that comes from our deep and eternal connection to Source, whether it is called God or the Great Mother. Everything we do is in fact sexual, whether we are evoking the magnetic force of attraction, the electrical force of action, or their combined forces of transmutation.

As I researched this subject, I found myself becoming increasingly frustrated as I saw how a perfectly natural and even spiritual practice had been vilified and distorted over thousands of years. Through skillful manipulation by those who have wished to possess the secret of eternal life for themselves, sex has become disconnected from spiritual growth and has been added to the long list of mundane things we do: eat, sleep, shop, watch television, and have sex. Those who do seek further guidance on this subject either have been dissuaded by stories of sin, lustfulness, and vice or have been given a mountain of complicated texts to read and practices to achieve before they may, perhaps, be allowed to practice sacred sex. And, by the way, to be able to practice sacred sex you must receive blessings directly from the godhead or be under the strict tutelage of a guru or master. What an insult to the divine pattern we each carry within us! The natural kingdoms engage in this beautiful process every single day, without ever questioning their divine right to do so.

This deception has been driven for centuries by certain institutions—usually religious—that fear we will come to know ourselves as immortal and therefore will wake up and realize that we no longer need an intermediary to access the divine. These institutions have corrupted a simple and natural act and made it something to be feared—or, conversely, revered. These hierarchal institutions have been able to control the masses by tapping into the most basic human emotions: fear, shame, and desire. You are probably not surprised to learn that most of the judgmental dogmas, rules, and texts created around sexuality were written by men; yet I have sympathy for them, for once they decided to remove the Goddess and all things feminine from their religions and cultures, they lost contact with their intuition and natural instincts and had to rely on their intellect to make sense of the mysteries of the world.

Creativity and fertility are divine qualities associated with the Great Mother, and therefore with all women. Men cannot guide us on this subject, and yet they have been trying to do this for thousands of years, and we have been programmed to follow. When a culture decides to disregard or disconnect from the feminine, productivity cannot be sustained, economies become depressed, infertility levels increase, and the land becomes barren and dry. In the past 2,000 years, many of our ancestors personally experienced the effects of the dismissal of the divine feminine or Mother Goddess from their societies. The rains failed to come, seeds stopped growing, and the people starved.

Like other dying civilizations, the Maya attempted to pacify the gods by sacrificing maidens in the *cenotes,* the natural wells or springs where they believed the rain god and the elementals lived. They refused to accept that water is the medicine of women, and that it will not rain until this element is returned to the Goddess. The Mayan kings and priests also presented blood offerings by piercing their tongue or penis, both seen as sources of creative power, placing the blood on paper before burning it, and sending the ashes to the gods of the sky. But the land continued to die until they, like other tribes, were forced to move to a place where the Goddess was still honored and where the land flowed with milk and honey, so that they could nourish their bodies and souls.

I have no doubt that you understand that we have reached this same tipping point in the world today; unless there is a rebalancing of the masculine and feminine energies, our cultures and civilizations will also be drastically reduced or will die out.

THE EVOLUTIONARY PATHWAY

It is important, I believe, to get an overview of our life here on Earth before we go any further. This will enable you to release any erroneous teachings you might have received that suggest, in effect, that this is a "bad place to be and there's somewhere better to go." Instead, we must understand that especially at this present time, Earth is the *only* place to be; it is here that we find an abundance of creative possibilities for spiritual expansion, beyond our wildest dreams.

In the beginning, there was no personal awareness, for we existed within the unified field of pure consciousness or divine light, known as the Source, the Creator, the Primordial Waters, God, or the Great Mother. Over time, this universal consciousness decided to experience itself in order to expand and evolve. It initially divided itself into two aspects, the sky and the earth, or spirit and matter, with the Great Mother energy becoming known as the Queen of Heavens, offering creative inspiration, and Mother Earth providing nurturing and transformation. Since both contained the consciousness of the Great Mother, they were infused with wisdom and insight and were considered equally important.

Then, like the development of the zygote into a multicelled fetus, the creative energy transformed itself into multiple pieces, each holographic segment containing a reflection of the whole, but from a slightly different angle, making each piece unique. The segment became known as a soul, and it was agreed that this divine aspect would seek to express itself fully on earth while maintaining its connection to Source through an intermediary—the light, etheric, or Ka body. Since the soul was created in the image of its Creator and contained the whole picture, there was never a sense of separation or inferiority. It is only fairly recently in the span of evolutionary time that the mistaken belief developed that we are disconnected from the Source and need to jump through all kinds of hoops to receive the love of the Great Mother. The truth is, she has never stopped loving us, for we are part of her.

The human prototypes were androgynous and existed primarily within their etheric or light bodies, which were continually energized by the eternal life force, much as a baby in the womb is nourished via the umbilical cord. Since the desire was for creative expression, the planet was seeded with a diversity of life-forms, whether a rock, an animal, or the wind, all of which, like humans, reflect an essence of the Source and thus contain consciousness. Since the divine wisdom or creative life force of the Great Mother was now to be found both within the sky and on the earth, it was possible to be enriched by her presence both through prayer and meditation and by the food that is eaten, especially when it is taken fresh from the soil.

As any alchemist knows, the greatest force of creation occurs when there is friction between the different elements of earth, fire, air, and water, because if everything were the same, there would be no growth or new manifestation. It was therefore decided that humankind should also divide into two aspects, male and female, wherein each contains the seed of the other, the anima and animus. At the same time, the soul engaged with the consciousness of Earth, thereby creating an intelligent form—our physical body. This fundamental cooperation between spirit and matter sowed the seeds for the future unification of Heaven and Earth that will be brought about by the creative manifestation of the soul's blueprint.

That decision set the stage for our present-day experience. When two or more entities come together, their energy or light bodies interconnect, and through this sexual process, something new is born that has been directly inspired by this act of communication and connection with the Source. Thus it could be said that every time we engage with anything, be it a person, a tree, a thought, or an idea, we are essentially having sex. This is the true meaning of intercourse, which is formed by the Latin words *inter,* meaning "between," and *course,* meaning "to run," from the verb *currere.* Intercourse thus entails the running of energy between two entities so that together they can reach a state of mutual agreement through the subtle communication that takes place between their energy bodies. Indeed, in many cultures, *intercourse* is interpreted as meaning talking or conversing, while *coitus* is used to describe sexual relations. Notably, the Latin translation of *coitus* also means "to run together," while the word *communion* suggests a mutual sharing.[2] This is the meaning behind Jesus's message, "For where two or three are come together in my name, there am I among them" (Matthew 18:20). This is far more than a mere religious statement; it reflects the fact that when we interact or have intercourse with others, we enter into a state of union with divine consciousness, which nourishes and renews our soul.

Yet for this kind of elevation to happen, whereby revitalization and transformation are available for the benefit of both parties, each one must be consciously present in the process, willing to both give and receive. Otherwise the intercourse can leave the participants tired and drained. It seems clear that if the purpose of all encounters between people is to be inspired and renewed, why wouldn't we choose to be fully present? Perhaps this explains why there is so much chronic fatigue illness and depression in the world today—the value placed on the ability to multitask in our society is in direct conflict with the need to keep our focus aimed consciously in the present. With this in mind, it might be more appropriate to call depression "dispiritedness," as this description better reflects the loss of contact with our spirit, or soul's awareness, which occurs when we are not fully present.

Returning to the early days of our evolution: it wasn't necessary to have physical coitus or intercourse in those times to connect with the Source, as just being in the presence of another person's light body opened the channels to this pure consciousness state. As the energy within our physical and emotional bodies became more static and dense, however, the need for actual physical contact became greater and greater. Yet I am sure that we have each met certain evolved souls in whose presence we feel revitalized because of the strength of their light energy. We can find similar restoration for our soul in nature, as Mother Earth is a pure reflection of the creative Source energy. And while it is possible to revitalize the energy of our etheric bodies on our own, our ancestors might have laughed at such a suggestion: *Why make things so complicated?* they might say, when a more effective and efficient method involves this kind of interconnectedness.

In its purest, essential form, sacred sex is all about the communion of consciousness or light energy between two or more life-forms, whether these forms are people, plants, rocks, or stars. The more present and celebratory we are of the other life-form with which we are connecting, the greater the exchange of energies. If we find ourselves living in our heads or acting from emotions such as judgment, shame, and fear, then we're not present, but merely attempting to control the situation. As humans, we have become distrustful of allowing ourselves to be seen naked, not just physically, but emotionally and mentally. Such a level of trust does not come from the overdeveloped warrior side of our nature, which emerges from the masculine chakras, but from the empowerment of our feminine chakras. Only when there is mutual respect and honor between our inner male and female will we truly be ready to appear naked before another person. This sacred relationship is

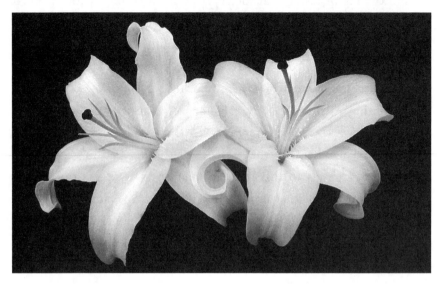

White lilies, representing sacred relationship

under the guardianship of goddesses such as Hera and Juno, who symbolize this kind of love through the exquisite beauty of white lilies.

Since we were born from the divine marriage of opposites, many traditions have incorporated teachings about such a union, describing this in terms of dual yet complementary forces of existence. These pairs are described variously as masculine and feminine, sun and moon, spirit and matter, yang and yin, and Shiva and Shakti. Whatever terms are used, when the two forces communicate, or combine their energies, they create a third force. This combination is often represented as a trinity: father, mother, and child. Yet it would be more appropriate to say that the two create a vessel for the third to exist in, while all are mutually dependent on one another. Such a trinity is expressed by the two ovaries and the uterus, which sits between them. The ovaries are dependent on the womb to provide a safe and nurturing environment for their eggs, while the womb is dependent on the ovaries to produce the hormones that stimulate its cyclical pattern of creativity.

There was never meant to be any enmity between the two opposing forces, but instead an understanding that their uniquely different

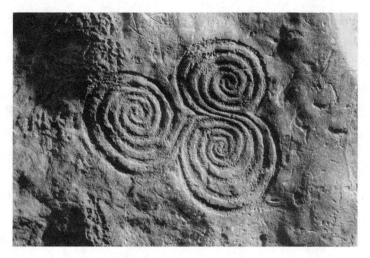

Symbol of the Trinity, from Newgrange, Ireland

yet complementary qualities are essential to the creative process. For example, feminine energy is often described as magnetic, attracting, and negatively polarized, while masculine energy is considered electric, repelling, and positively polarized. Together they create an electromagnetic field that is known to be the force behind the creation and preservation of all life on this planet. Men and women possess both types of energy fields, although a woman's force is mainly magnetic, while a man's is electric.

SACRED SEXUAL PRACTICES: KEEPING THE JUICES FLOWING

Our human ancestors understood that as long as they maintained their conscious connection to the Source, the Great Mother, inspiration and abundance flowed. They developed certain practices to ensure the vitality of their etheric or light bodies, which serve as intermediaries between the worlds. They learned that they could enter their light bodies much more easily when they quieted the mind, spent time in nature or around water, ate simple, life-filled foods, and focused on sacred sounds or shapes. They also discovered that their link to universal consciousness via their light bodies was enhanced at certain times of the year and by specific events, such as during a solar eclipse.

Since the conscious energy of women is primarily magnetic and receptive, our ancestral sisters knew that it was far easier to access their light bodies when external light was dimmed, such as at nighttime and during the period of the waning moon. This explains why, when women come together, their periods are naturally synchronous to this time of the month; it is then, in the darkness of the receding moon, that inspiration and blessings flow directly from the consciousness of the Great Mother. Many women say they find themselves waking around 3 a.m., often roused by insights that have come to them in their dreams. After menopause, the emphasis on earthly creation decreases, and women find themselves spending more time in their light bodies, with their ability to engage with all life-forms within the universe greatly enhanced. From this perspective it could be said that a postmenopausal woman has far more intercourse than her reproductive sisters, with just as much fun, and far less effort!

As women, there are many other ways to enhance the flow of "juice," or energy, through our magnetic fields. Being romanced, laughing with friends, luxuriating in a warm bath, eating good food, walking in nature, enjoying soulful music, and dancing to some sultry Latin American music are all known to increase the energy flow through our bodies. When we add sensual touch that is totally focused on pleasure, we have a winning combination. It is clear that foreplay and masturbation that involve all the erogenous zones lighten up our magnetic field, especially at the levels of the root (earth child), sacral, heart, and crown chakras.

From many archaeological carvings and images it seems clear that our ancient sisters were aware of this kind of knowledge, which is why sexual activities were considered an important part of life, whether they included masturbation or sexual intercourse with a partner. A Neolithic clay figurine that comes from the Tarxien Temples, in Malta, shows a recumbent woman with raised legs, with one hand supporting her head while the other hand touches her swollen vulva. Marija Gimbutas suggests that the figurine represents a woman about to give birth, especially as her back is scored with nine lines, suggestive of the nine months of pregnancy. Yet her belly is only slightly swollen.[3] Could it be that she is merely pleasuring herself? And could the nine lines on her back represent nine chakras and her ability to cause kundalini energy to ascend up her spine through sexual arousal?

There are even older engravings of reclining women dating back to between 13,000 and 10,000 BCE found in the caves of La Magdelaine, France. Once again, we see a woman lying on her back with her knees bent, one hand behind her head and the other arm aiming toward her belly and beyond. Marija Gimbutas believes these are examples of the birthing position of the day, especially as there are images of pregnant bison and mares depicted nearby. Yet, once again, the images certainly resemble the present-day posture of a woman bringing herself to orgasmic bliss.

Such a concept may seem strange, since we are under the illusion that we have just freed masturbation and other sexual pleasures from the interminable dark ages. But thousands of years ago, sexuality does not appear to have been taboo for either men or women. Archaeology tells us that masturbation was a central theme in the Creation myths of ancient Egypt and Mesopotamia, and the art of classical Greece contains images of women using dildos, and they are obviously enjoying themselves.

"SCARLET" WOMEN

Texts and images from Sumer, Babylonia, Canaan, Anatolia, and Greece reveal that sacred sexual practices were considered important for the survival and well-being not only of the people but of the land itself. They reveal that for thousands of years, women lived together in temple complexes. These communities were not merely for worship; they were at the very heart of society, encompassing much of the arable land, with the inhabitants involved in the welfare of domesticated animals and most of the administrative tasks. Women were chosen to oversee such activities, because it was believed that they had the strongest links to the consciousness of Mother Earth and therefore knew what was best for the land and its people.[4]

At certain times of the year, men from the community would enter the temples to pay homage to the Great Mother or Goddess of Creation, known by many names, including Isis, Ishtar, and Inanna, to name a few. There they would be met by priestesses who were representatives of the Goddess, who had been trained in the ways of sexual transformation. It is often written that these priestesses were virgins, suggesting someone sexually inexperienced or uninitiated, although it would be more accurate to apply the real meaning of the word *virgin:* "someone who is complete within themselves, without the need of another to make them whole." In Sumerian legends, sacred sexual customs were considered gifts given by the goddess Inanna to civilize the people. The goddess Lilith, her niece, is described as the young maiden who gathered the lucky men from the streets for their one night of ecstasy with the Goddess of Creation's representative.[5]

Each priestess would choose one of the men and perform a *hieros gamos,* or sacred marriage, making love to him within the sanctity of the temple. The men represented different faces of the godhead, known to the Egyptians as Osiris, to the Akkadians as Tammuz, and to the Sumerians as Dumizid, to name just a few of the appellations. There were at least four special days when this ceremony would occur, each of them representing the changing relationship between the masculine energies of action, focus, and definition and the feminine energies of inspiration, nurturing, and transformation:

- Winter solstice: The seed of the new son, or Sun, carrying the consciousness of the Queen of Heaven, is planted in the womb of Mother Earth, to develop within the darkness.
- Spring equinox: The first sign of his growth appears above the surface of Earth. This is celebrated by the sacred marriage or bond-

ing between the feminine Queen of Heaven and the masculine vegetation deity, ensuring the abundance of crops.

- Summer solstice: The celebration of the fully grown, blooming vegetation god occurs before he prepares to descend once again into Mother Earth, not to be nurtured this time, but to be transformed—to die—in her tomb.
- Autumn equinox: Within the sexual fires of Mother Earth, the god releases his seeds of wisdom back to the Queen of Heavens so that her consciousness may grow and his decomposing body is returned to Mother Earth.

And the cycle begins anew with the winter solstice, in which, once again, the new Sun, enriched by the wisdom of the experience of the previous year, is planted into Mother Earth.

This continuous cycle reveals the magical qualities of the sexual process, whereby both the male and female aspects are essential for the continuation of life. It also shows that the ancient people understood that one of the most transformative and restorative times for a human being is during her or his descent into the tomb of Mother Earth, otherwise known as the underworld. For just as our descent into sleep is essential for wellness of our mind and body, so do we also need times in our lives when we can withdraw and become self-reflective, to ensure wellness of the spirit. As we will discover later, the lack of this kind of sacred time and space for introspection is a definite causative factor in PMS (premenstrual syndrome). Women today have become too focused on the activities of the outer world, with little time left for self-nurturing and harvesting the seeds of wisdom. And this is not merely a problem just for women; all over the globe we are witnessing the results of the imbalance between our inner and outer worlds, with one result being the worldwide financial systems collapse, in which chaos has increased and productivity has stalled. These are signs that the Goddess of the underworld is drawing us into her lair, forcing us to die to our old patterns so that a new world can be born.

According to Merlin Stone, a pioneering author, sculptor, and professor of art and art history, the women who participated in the sexual practices as representatives of the Goddess would live for periods of time within the temple complex, even though they may have been married. It was seen as an honor, not as a taboo, to take place in extramarital sex, with the husband giving his full approval, flattered by his wife's position in society. The women were known as sacred or holy women and were perceived to be pure, undefiled, and spotless—i.e., "virgins." It was only when patriarchal principles took hold that the term *prostitute* came into use.

Laurence Gardner writes that the wombs of women were considered to be the source of a life-giving energy known as star fire. The priestesses who were trained to produce this star fire for ritual purposes were identified as "scarlet" women—in Greek, *hierodulai,* "sacred women," a term translated later from French into English as *harlot*. In the early Germanic tongue, the name was *hores,* which became the English *whore*. Never, at any point, was the name meant to be derogatory, for it literally meant "beloved one."[6]

Any child born from this sacred intercourse was considered legitimate and inherited the name and the social status of the mother. This is thought to be one of the reasons why the practice was later banned by laws created by patriarchal Levite priests, who ruled that a woman should be a virgin—as in the conventional meaning of a sexually uninitiated woman—when she married and should maintain marital fidelity to her husband. The priests were concerned that if a woman made love to more than one man, paternity would always be in question and thus rights could not be accorded any particular man. The patriarchy knew that the only way to seize the land and its considerable wealth from women would be to ban the practice of sacred sex and defile and denigrate the priestesses by calling them whores and prostitutes.

AWAKENING THE SERPENT

Many people today have heard of kundalini energy, described as an inherent serpent power that is coiled up, asleep in the base chakra, at the level of the sacrum. The sacral bone was highly valued in many cultures as the sacred nesting place of the organs of fertility, and therefore it is not surprising that the celebrated serpent rests here. Many traditions see the awakening of this creative energy, often associated with sexual arousal, as essential to reaching self-realization, God consciousness, and enlightenment. Kundalini is generally described as an aspect of the Hindu goddess Shakti, who in turn is perceived as the original spark of life, born from the fertile, primordial waters. As such, Shakti is the creative force responsible for all conception, change, and liberation. Without Shakti, there is no life. It is common to describe Shakti as feminine (with Shiva as her male consort), and all women as embodiments of Shakti, although Shakti resides in men as well. Consequently, the serpent energy, kundalini, is also considered a goddess.

The question that needs to be asked is *why* is she sleeping? We know that over the past three millennia a large part of the female psyche has gone to sleep regarding its true identity. Could the dormant Goddess energy, kundalini, be a reflection of this state of sleep? And why is she stuck in the base chakra, since the base of the spine does not reveal the full range of a person's energy field, with the aura stretching deep into the earth and far above a person's head? One has to question why so many images of the chakras are drawn from the position of a man—and it is commonly a man—sitting cross-legged on the floor, a pose that is a bit unnatural for most human beings.

The concept of there being just seven chakras running along the spine from the base to the crown appears to have evolved from teachings developed in the eleventh century CE; this has become the common way of viewing these energy centers. But prior to this, it is most probable that twelve chakras were used to symbolize the enlightened person, with the earth-child, or root, chakra acting as the portal to powerful energies within Mother Earth. The Christian Church, terri-fied of this arena of feminine chaos that it could not control, designated it as a place to be feared: the underworld, or hell. It persuaded its mem-bers to steer clear of anything beneath their feet, despite the fact that this is exactly where we find our sole and our soul!

This interruption in the free flow of energy between our lower spine and the energy of Mother Earth appears to be a reasonable hypothesis as to why kundalini remains asleep. In other words, any attempts to arouse kundalini are futile if you start in the base chakra, as the energy located there is a mere remnant of its original source of immense power located in the root chakra. This is why it is imperative to enter the dragon's lair and experience the pure fire power of Mother Earth if we are ever to understand the essential nature of sexual and creative energy.

DRAGON POWER

Until the rise of Christianity, the mythology of nearly every culture around the world spoke of dragons. This legendary beast was commonly depicted with a huge crested head, a mouth that breathed fire, the scales and tail of a serpent, and the claws of an eagle. This description led to serpents and dragons becoming interchangeable, both understood to possess wisdom and the power of transformation because of their ability to shed their skins. European dragons, which emerged from the Middle Eastern and Greek traditions, commonly possessed wings, while those

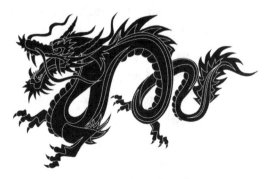

Dragon, the legendary beast

of East Asian origin—in particular, Japan, China, Tibet, and Korea—
are wingless. Dragons are generally believed to live in underground lairs
or caves that are often connected to deep rivers or seas. There, they are
seen to guard vast treasures, including the precious metals of the earth,
especially natural pearls. It is noteworthy that the planet Pluto is named
after the Greek word *plouton,* meaning "wealth," and as the ruler of the
astrological sign of Scorpio it is often described as both a scorpion and
a dragon. In many Asian cultures, a dragon's power is perceived to come
from its ability to control the waters of Earth, and it is thus regarded as
a benevolent or benefitting force.

As a primal force of nature, a dragon is alleged to possess great wisdom and longevity and is believed to have taught humans to talk. In
the earliest schools of mysticism, the symbol for the Word, or Logos, is
a serpent, while the womb is known to give expression or voice to the
Word, as the utterer, or uterus.[7] This clearly suggests that the womb is a
powerful repository and transformer for the dragon's inherent wisdom
or spark of creative energy.

The English word *dragon* denotes a "water snake whose clear sight
can be deadly." Such a portrayal reminds us of Lilith, the daughter of
Eresh-kigal, Sumerian Queen of the Underworld, who with the wings
and feet of a bird and the body of a serpent exhibited clear insight and
a strong sexual force. Lilith's ancestor was Nammu, the Dragon Queen,
out of whose primordial waters, or chaos, all life was conceived. As previously mentioned, this chaotic creative energy greatly troubled mainly
patriarchal institutions, who wanted control and mastery over such a
primal feminine force. The early Christian church solved the problem
by linking the power of the dragon and the serpent to that of Satan, or
the devil.

In the Epic of Gilgamesh, Lilith takes possession of Inanna's favorite
tree, out of which the Sumerian Queen of Heaven had hoped to make her
throne and wedding bed. The bird head of Lilith, at the top of the tree, is
symbolic of the tree's branches that reach for the sky. They also represent
the freedom of our soul to fly through clear insight, wisdom, and the ability

to detach from the world of illusion. In Middle Eastern and Asian cultures, birds and other flying animals signify immortality and are connected to the pineal gland. The serpentine aspect of Lilith, found at the base of the tree and mirrored by the roots, which run deep into the earth, symbolizes the pure power of creative energy, essential for life itself.

Together with the trunk of the tree, the roots and branches represent a lightning rod along which energy continuously flows in both directions, ensuring the connection between Heaven and Earth. Symbolically, the lightning rod represents Inanna's royal scepter, which offers her magical powers over the forces of the universe, similar to a magician's wand. The concept of the Tree of Life is found in many cultures; it symbolizes the passageway between the world of matter and the world of spirit, where both exist simultaneously. It is understood that when energy flows freely and fully through all the chakras, our energy or light body becomes such a lightning rod. With our feet firmly rooted firmly on the earth, our spine vertical and erect, and our arms raised toward the skies, it is easy to see that the human form is perfectly designed for this role: to become god-like, to realize our inherent divine nature and our ability to turn spirit into form and form back into its spiritual essence.

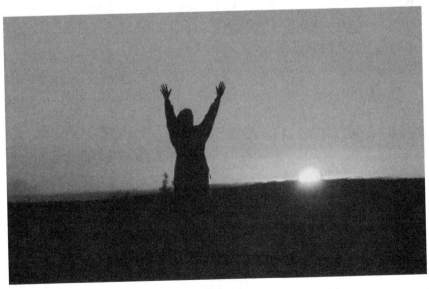

A human lightning rod

In the story, Inanna is fearful of Lilith's presence and asks her brother Gilgamesh to cut down the tree, causing the bird to fly away as a screech owl and the serpent to slither off into the desert. In *Mysteries of the Dark Moon*, Demetra George suggests that Inanna's unexpected reaction to Lilith (since they were related) marked the beginning of the patriarchal influence on the Sumerian civilization, around 2000 BCE.[8] Inanna, like many of the ancient goddesses of those times, was forced to make a decision between her status as queen and her magician's power. Whether by choice or coercion, Inanna agreed to give her lightning rod to the patriarchy by allowing her brother to cut down the tree. This decision led to a violent disconnection of the bird, representing spiritual insight, from the serpent, the creative force, the consequences of which we are still dealing with today in the extreme separation between mind and body on both the individual and collective levels. It is this schism that needs to be healed now if we human beings are ever going to take ownership of our own Goddess-given lightning rods and become the immortal beings we are meant to be. To do this it is essential that we allow the energy of our chakra system—our lightning rod—to flow from the earthly dragon beneath our feet to the spiritual bird above our heads, and not just between the base and crown chakras.

The Dragon Queen

Before this can happen, we must first accept the Dragon Queen, who lives beneath the earth and rules the underworld. Her energy is fluid and fiery, much like volcanic lava that flows much more slowly than water yet is similarly relentless in its passage, destroying anything in its path. The Dragon Queen represents the dark goddess and the Crone, the third face of the Triple Goddess, whose clear insight sees us for what we are, beyond our masks and pretenses. Depictions of her usually show her surrounded by death and chaos, such as in images of Kali the Destroyer, who is seen eating the entrails of her lover. The Dragon Queen is the opposite of the virgin who brings birth and creativity to the world, for the dark goddess represents expiration and death. She carries with her a cauldron of boiling liquid and invites us to enter it so that the meat of our stories can be separated from the bones of our wisdom. She eats the meat as compost for future growth and sends the seeds of wisdom to her sister, the Queen of Heavens.

Yet, lest you are inclined to attempt to shun her, you need to know that she will not be ignored, for she loves you so much that she will not let you be less than who you truly are. Welcome her into your life with an open heart, for otherwise her sudden entrance will wreak chaos and destruction across your life, for she will not be denied what is rightfully hers.

So as we return to the subject of kundalini slumbering in the base chakra, it is clear that she represents just a small piece of the dragon/serpent energy that was abandoned during the brutal disconnection of our consciousness from Mother Earth. The Dragon Queen hides deep within her watery lair, licking her wounds inflicted by the unconscious actions of humankind. This certainly would account for why so many people I work with today feel they don't belong to planet Earth or have profound issues of rejection and abandonment. Without our connection to this powerful restorative energy, it is easy to understand why so many people complain of chronic fatigue, adrenal exhaustion, and persistent anxiety. We need to send our energy down into the earth and allow the healing energies of the Dragon Queen to nourish our roots.

At the same time, when the tree was symbolically cut down by Gilgamesh, the tiny pineal gland linked to the crown chakra became disconnected from the spiritual realms ruled by the Queen of Heavens. It is through the pineal gland that we receive inspiration; not surprisingly, this gland is considered understimulated in most people today. As we will later learn, mythology tells of the archetypal honeybee that acts as the source of germination between the worlds of spirit and matter, and that many thousands of years ago the Queen Bee's wisdom stopped flowing into our pineal glands because she perceived that humanity was misusing her energy; she fell asleep.

It is imperative that we reconnect these energies, for only then can the creative energy ascend from below to above and descend from above to below, creating a vessel for the pure life force to flow once again, between Heaven and Earth. As the alchemical Emerald Tablet states: *As below so above, as above so below.* But remember that if you make that connection, you are also inviting into your life the chaos that the Dragon Queen trails in her wake, for without death there is no enlightenment.

Pearls of Wisdom

The Chinese dragon is often associated with a red or golden luminous pearl, which represents purity, honesty, and spiritual transformation. Similar in size to the pineal gland, a natural pearl is associated with the moon and is created through the hard work of the humble oyster. Representations of the Chinese pearl show it with flaring wings of fire, very similar to the Golden Snitch, the small golden ball about the size of a walnut sought after by Harry Potter in the game of Quidditch— reminding us how often ancient archetypal symbols are portrayed within popular fiction to awaken our consciousness.

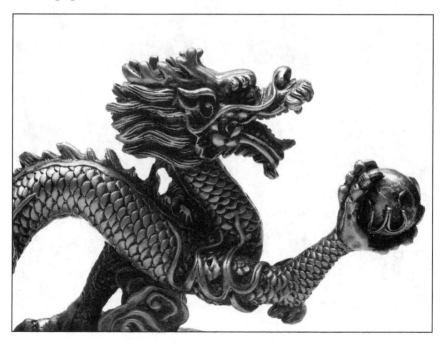

The golden pearl in the hand of the dragon

Other images of the pearl show it being chased by one or two dragons, with the understanding that the pearl represents the treasure we receive when two opposing forces, masculine and feminine, are willing to work together toward a common goal. In the Book of Revelations (21:21), the twelve "pearly gates" of New Jerusalem—i.e., the twelve chakras—are said to be made of twelve pearls, all coming from the one pearl. Later, in the New Testament, in Matthew 7:6, we are warned not to cast our pearls—our precious wisdom—before unappreciative swine.

When we compare this image with that of the caduceus, the alchemical symbol of transmutation, it is easy to see the similarities between the

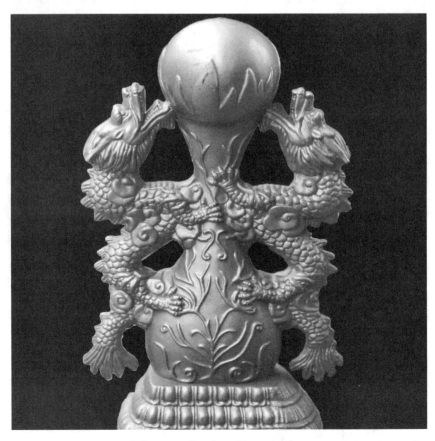

The rewards of working together

Chinese dragons and serpents, both achieving enlightenment through the sacred union of opposites, which ultimately stimulates the pearl or pineal gland to light up and reconnect us to the consciousness of oneness, or Great Mother.

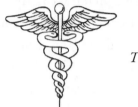

The caduceus

In Hindu texts, the opposing forces that work together for the common good are known as the lunar feminine *ida* and the solar masculine *pingala,* which run alongside either side of the spine. Together they create a third force, the *sushumna,* which is seen as an energy that passes between them and ultimately stimulates the expression of the pineal gland.

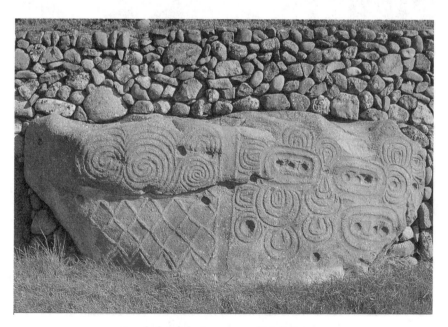

Symbols of the presence of high dragon
energy at Newgrange, Ireland

The Dragon within the Earth

As we descend into the earth in search of the dragon, we come across traditional tales that speak of the serpent or dragon energy that runs beneath the surface, giving rise to ley lines or spirit roads that crisscross the whole planet as low-frequency telluric currents.[9] Ancient peoples like the Druids knew of the strength of the Dragon Queen's energy, which is why they built their sacred sites and temples at the confluence of such lines, often marking such sites with an *X*, a serpent, or a spiral to symbolize the high level of creative power available there.

The temple builders also knew that circulating water focuses and contains the dragon force, so it was not uncommon to build a moat around a sacred site, such as at Stonehenge and Avebury, or to erect buildings near a meandering river, thereby attracting the water energy into the temple.

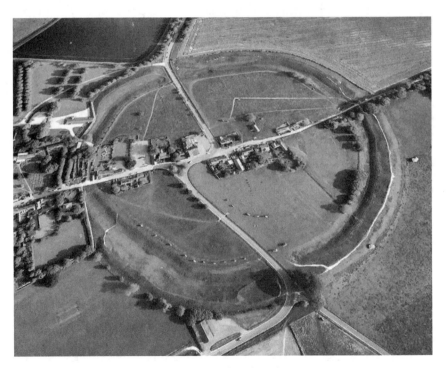

The stone circles of Avebury

Most sacred sites and temples around the world were built to provide a portal or conduit for energy or consciousness to move in both directions, between Heaven and Earth. In many places, such as Egypt and Central America, the temple builders designed the entire temple complex, which often stretched for miles around, to mirror specific star systems, often incorporating a river in imitation of the Milky Way. They believed that such a symbolic representation offered great benefits. Through the enactment of sacred rituals such as *hieros gamos,* divine inspiration flowed to Earth, while at the same time the consciousness of Heaven was enriched.

Dragon energy is synonymous with the Earth Mother's molten core, the fiery cauldron, and is therefore strongly present in areas of high volcanic and seismic activity. Such places include all the countries along the horseshoe-shaped Pacific Ring of Fire, including Chile, Java, Japan, the western coast of the United States, New Zealand, and Canada, as well as the volcanic Hawaiian Islands. I can still remember standing with Makua, a native Hawaiian kahuna from the Big Island of Hawaii, as he pointed to the volcanic mountain Mauna Loa as the sun's first rays fanned her surface and remarked, "Look, the dragon is awakening."

In many sacred sites, trees were seen as the intermediaries between the wisdom of the Dragon Queen and the people. Dodona, located in the mountains of northwest Greece, is one of the oldest sanctuaries devoted to the chthonic oracle, dating back to the second millennium BCE. The shrine is dedicated to Dione, a little-known "mother of all gods" who was described as the daughter of nothingness, born through imagination, capable of controlling the atoms of the universe. She was also known for being able to heal other immortals with just the touch of her hands. Her accompanying animal was the dove, similar to that associated with Sophia, the heavenly source of wisdom in the Judeo-Christian tradition. Dione's priestesses were also known as doves, or *peliades.* She eventually succumbed to the powers of Zeus, who took ownership of her oracular gifts. In the days when the Mother Goddess was still in power, there existed a sacred grove of oak trees in Dodona, in honor of Dione. There, the priestesses, who

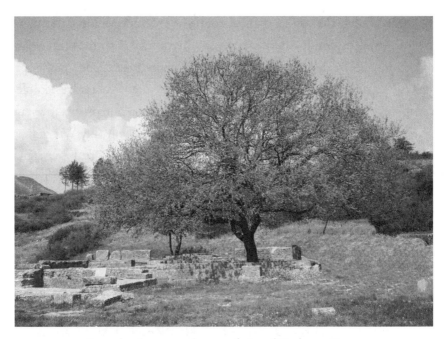

Sacred oak tree at the sacred site of Dodona, Greece

always walked barefoot, would sit on a tripod—a symbol of the yoni—and receive messages from the Dragon Queen below. The messages were transmitted through the clinking of metal vessels hanging in the trees, the call of the birds, and the rustling of oak leaves.

Omphalos, the Navel of the World

Our ancestors saw a strong resemblance between the fertile and transformative strength of the uterus and that of a mountain, believing that both provided a natural lair for the Dragon Queen, who enjoyed curling up deep inside dark places. Indeed, they believed that, like the womb, a mountain is the place where Heaven and Earth unite, giving birth to entire civilizations as its energy radiates out across the land. Over time, certain hills and mountains were designated as axes mundi or omphalos, navels of the world or places of birth. Such mountains include Mount Fuji in Japan, Mount Kun-Lun in China, Mount Kailash in Tibet, and Uluru in the red center of Australia.

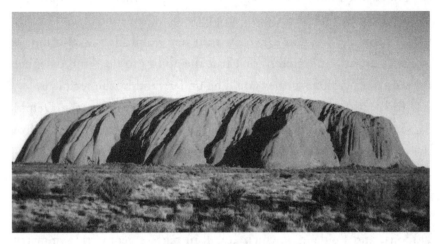

The red stone of Uluru, Australia

The axis mundi or omphalos is seen as a place of both death and birth, with the summit of the sacred mountain believed to be an entry point into the underworld or dragon's lair.

At many of the sites around the world that are designated axes mundi, a round stone can be found that is thought to represent the fertile womb of Earth. These stones often have a dimple on them, denoting the umbilicus on the top of a pregnant belly. Some of these stones also have a hollow passageway, reflecting the portal or umbilical cord that allows energy to flow to and from the dragon's lair.

The best known of these stones was originally located over the lair of the monstrous serpent Python, in what is now known as Delphi, Greece. Mythology tells us that with the arrival of the sky-borne Olympian deities, led by Zeus, the power of such dark, subterranean forces had to be subdued and their allegiance turned toward the sky gods. Thus we learn of Apollo's conquest over Python, the great serpent—although it is noteworthy that Zeus still required a woman, Pythia, to act as a spokesperson or oracle for Python's insights. Seated on a tripod, a symbol of the yoni, Pythia was positioned over a chasm in the earth and gave utterance to the serpent's wisdom. This practice continued for hundreds of years, and I suggest that Zeus required a woman because only she had the strength to gather, control, and master the force of the Dragon Queen within her womb. It was also only a woman's uterus, or "utterer," that had the ability to hear and decipher the words of wisdom so they could be understood by the recipient.

Today, there is a replica of the omphalos stone in the Delphi Museum. The stone is crisscrossed with many lines, which symbolize the energy or spirit lines that radiate out from this axis mundi, influencing the consciousness of the people for hundreds of miles around. The stone acts as a map, with the confluence of the lines on the stone reflecting other sites of ancient Goddess worship, such as Knossos, Dodona, and Epidaurus, which are all in perfect geometric symmetry to one another and are all associated with honoring the Dragon Queen, and especially the process of death and rebirth.[10]

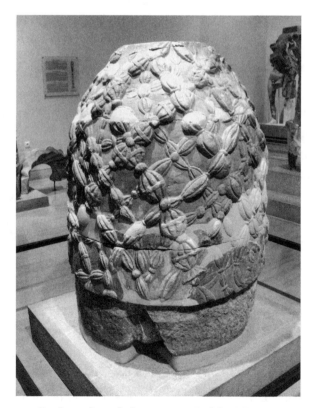

Replica of omphalos stone in Delphi Museum

One other omphalos stone that stands out in my mind is presently leaning against the kitchen wall on the grounds of Glastonbury Abbey, apparently discredited and forgotten. In its center is a dimple, representative of the umbilical opening into the underworld. Since menstruation is a time of heightened sensitivity to the wisdom of the dragon, it is believed that in ancient times a woman would squat on top of the stone and offer her blood to the Dragon Queen before receiving the inspiration she would then share with her family or tribe.

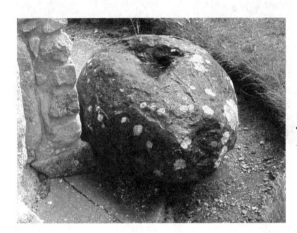

Omphalos stone on the grounds of Glastonbury Abbey

If this is the omphalos stone, where is the actual omphalos in Glastonbury? I believe it is the Tor itself, pierced by a small building, St. Michael's Tower, situated on its summit. Traditionally, the top of the Tor is known as an entry point into the underworld, reached by walking along a serpentine path that describes a three-dimensional labyrinth around the hill. The dragon energy that emerges from the umbilicus at the summit is believed to radiate out in twelve perfectly equal segments, very similar to the energy that radiates out from the center at Delphi.

Whenever I visit the Tor, I am reminded of one of the most powerful experiences of my life. I was in my early forties and troubled at that time by heavy menstrual periods that were very unpredictable. One bright summer's afternoon I joined a group of pilgrims to walk the Tor's labyrinth. As we wound around the hill, my menstrual flow increased. Clear in my own mind that I was meant to complete the pilgrimage, I found

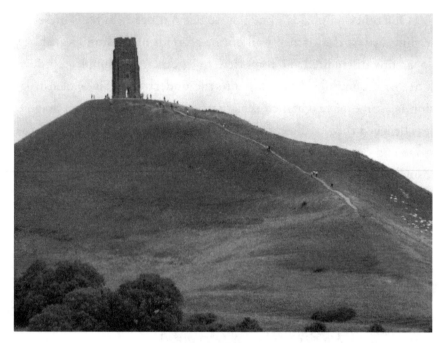

Glastonbury Tor

myself on three occasions squatting down to change my padding, each time spilling a small amount of blood on the ground. Even now, I am amazed that I found privacy on such a busy path and how natural this unexpected ritual felt. Finally, we reached an area on the labyrinth dedicated to the Goddess, where men and women would come to ask for her blessings. As I sat beneath the ancient trees, I knew that through my menstrual bleeding, I had been shedding tears, not only for myself but for humanity. In that moment I was completely embraced by the love of the Great Mother, who gently took from me all the pain and suffering I had been experiencing, until I felt a profound sense of peace wash over me.

There is one other human-made symbol of the fertile and pregnant Mother Earth, found in this same southern corner of England: this is Silbury Hill. Located southwest of the stone circles of Avebury, it is believed to have been built around 2600 BCE under the guidance of a group of beings who predicted that the hill would help humanity at a time when they would be disconnected from the Source. Is that time

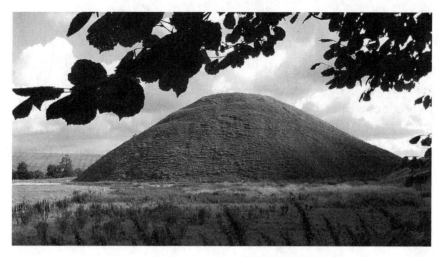

Silbury Hill

now? The meaning of the name Silbury is "enclosure of light." It was built during the phase of the Celtic calendar that symbolizes the harvest or the fullness and abundance of the crops—similar to the very pregnant belly of a woman, which it resembles. It is believed that there is also a vertical shaft in the center of the hill, symbolic of the umbilical cord, which leads down into the domain of the Dragon Queen.

Piercing the Dragon's Skin

In an attempt to focus and harness the dragon's energy for fertility and creative purposes, the ancient people would use a phallic-shaped object such as pillar, obelisk, or standing stone to "pierce" the dragon's skin, inviting the serpent to rise up and curl around the object. Yet, unlike our modern-day obsession with ownership, where we erect a flag, build a church, or raise a multistory office tower to signify conquest over the world of matter, the ancient people understood that when the phallic stone pierced the dragon mountain, an intimate and sexual process was taking place, whereby both would be transformed by the union. For just as the pillar pierces and enters the earth, so does the encircling and spiraling dragon energy begin to devour the stone, drawing it into its lair.

In the same vein, relatively modern teachings about the axes mundi speak of the phallic insemination of Mother Earth by divine intelligence, as if she were merely a passive receptacle for such a blessing. Similarly, the earth's womb is often described as simply providing nourishment for the embedded seed, as if the sperm alone were sufficient to produce a baby. If we arrogantly choose to pierce the earth and suck her dry without ever offering something in return or, more importantly, agreeing to our own transformation, then eventually the Dragon Queen will assert herself and forbid us access to her store of precious treasures.

The Dragon Queen promises that if we agree to surrender our masculine will once we have pierced her surface, then she will curl herself around our rod, our chakra system, and start to climb, until she unites with her sister, the Queen of Heaven. Mythology tells us that we must repeat this process twelve times, each time descending deeper and deeper into the dragon's den, so that our consciousness can rise higher and higher.

It is said that at the start of the thirteenth cycle, we will become free of the cycles of death and birth and will possess a fully functional magician's wand—our lightning rod—and be like the gods and goddesses, immortal. This reminds us that thirteen is the number of self-realization rather than being unlucky, the latter concept found in some religious doctrines to discourage the common human from seeking such a transformational experience. This story of enlightenment is symbolized by the story of Moses, who was called by God to take his rod or shepherd's staff and throw it on ground, whereupon it turned into a serpent. Initially he was afraid, but upon grasping the serpent-rod in his hands, it became his magical wand, with the power to part the waters and quell the storms (Exodus 4:3).

In medieval times, at the beginning of May when animals were sent out into the fields to be fattened up, a pole would be erected in the center of each village that represented the staff or stone that pierces the earth to attract the dragon's attention. During the ritual dances, the villagers, holding different-colored ribbons, would circle the maypole, winding around each other, symbolizing the emergence of the serpentine energy from the winter darkness, bringing purification, abundance, and prosperity.

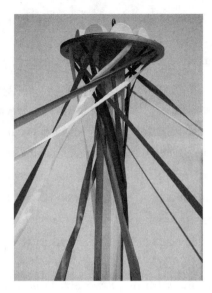

A maypole

The Shaman's Journey

Since ancient times, shamans and mystics have climbed to the tops of mountains to receive inspiration and spiritual attunement. Usually they would drive a staff or stick into the ground in order to focus the dragon earth energies into that place. The shaman would not climb the mountain merely to gain height or to talk to the sky gods; he knew that the mountain is a rich source of dragon wisdom and was therefore willing to descend into the womb of the Dragon Queen so as to be transformed. I suggest that this is one of the reasons why men are often portrayed as sitting cross-legged on the ground in meditation posture, as it allows the non-erect and more submissive penis to metaphorically enter the earth. According to Jean Reddemann, a Native American medicine woman, this is also the reason why priests, judges, and even Scottish warriors wear skirts; the open clothing exposes them, and their masculine energy, to the dragon energy that arises up from within the earth. By accepting and uniting with this female force, they are transformed, their power intensifies, and they are able to reach higher levels of consciousness and authority.

However, since women have a natural affinity with this dragon energy, they don't need to pierce the soil like men do, but rather they can learn how to draw this force up carefully along the vagina and store it in their powerhouse, the uterus, the cave within the mountain. For this to happen, women need to make their vaginas as accessible as possible to this energy, which means that instead of sitting cross-legged, where their vagina is almost horizontal, they should squat or kneel in meditation. At the same time, the wearing of a skirt or dress—with or without underwear—sends out an invitation for the serpent to enter, especially when complemented by a sensual sway of the body, which is much easier when wearing a skirt. Finally, learning how to contract and relax the vaginal muscles, as well as those within the pelvic floor, will naturally tempt the dragon energy to start to wind around women's legs in search of a new home within the womb. This process will be described in more detail in the next chapter.

SEXUAL INTERCOURSE

Let us come full circle and return to discussing sexual intercourse between a man and a woman. When a man's penis enters a woman's vagina, it acts as a piercing stone that focuses her energy to his presence. If sufficient energy has built up in her womb during foreplay, then the presence of the penis should entice her dragon energy out of its dark and damp lair. If he is able to calm his willful drive and be patient, he will feel the serpent start to wrap itself around his penis and draw either his physical seed or the seed of his consciousness through the sacred doorway, the cervix, and into her mound of transformation, the uterus. The more he can surrender, the easier the process. From there, together they will climb the serpentine ladder of consciousness. Like the snake, which moves by successive relaxation and contraction of its muscles, the movement of serpentine energy is achieved through alternating magnetic and electric energy, until a blissful state of oneness is achieved at orgasm.

The sacred art of sex is an inherently natural process that over the past centuries has become increasingly mundane or excessively compli-cated. In simple terms, it allows us to experience the exquisite delight of union, where there is nothing to hide, nothing to learn, and nothing to do except to be as the Great Mother made us, beautiful and perfect in every way.

6

ENTERING THE CAVE OF
TRANSFORMATION

As we pass through the beauty and sensuality of the exotic lily's vulvar doorway, we enter a veiled and darkened passageway that leads to the most sacred of caves, the womb.

When a woman is not pregnant, the uterus is no larger than a small pear, and yet it has the creative power and capacity, within nine months, to be able to accommodate a full-size baby. Not only does it grow exponentially over nine months, but the internal environment of the womb is able to miraculously nurture and transform a few-celled fetus into a multifunctioning human being with ten fingers and ten toes. Then, when the time it is right, the muscles of the uterus are powerful enough to propel an eight-pound baby into the world. No other structure in our body is so gifted with such complex powers of creative transformation. This is clearly the reason why so many of our ancestors revered the pregnant female form, seeing it as the Great Mother at her best.

Yet, as we know, these forces are not exclusively confined to nurturing and birthing a baby: they also serve the all-important expansion of consciousness. Hence, the uterus provides three essential functions that are mirrored in the menstrual cycle: cleansing or purification, gathering the power of creativity to reach the source of inspiration, and the nurturing and expression of our creative ideas. In addition, the womb or uterus of every woman resonates with a much greater chalice or Holy Grail—the womb of Mother Earth.

Around the world are natural and man-made caves where men and women have gathered for thousands of years to cleanse, purify, and receive her wisdom and blessings. Here, in the darkness of Earth's womblike caverns, people surrender their will to her pure love, opening themselves to something more meaningful and more powerful than any other force in the world. According to Padma and Anaiya Aon Prakasha, in their beautiful book *Womb Wisdom,* some of the best-known womb sites are Vaishno Devi in the Indian Himalayas; the Temple of the Sun in Teotihuacan, Mexico; the Isis Pyramid, on the Giza Plateau in Egypt; the Moray Mystery Circles of the Andes, in Peru; the Church of Saint Sulpice in Paris; the Avebury Earth Temple, in England; Rennes-le-Château, in southern France; and an Egyptian birthing site guarded by Anubis, in Australia.[1]

To experience the deep connection to Mother Earth's womb, we must have a respectful relationship with our own womb, the energy of which exists even if we have had a hysterectomy. Unfortunately, as the teachings of the feminine mysteries began to disappear from the awareness of the majority of women thousands of years ago, the rich inheritance of the womb also vanished into the darkness of our collective psyche. The uterus became a place associated with the visibility of pregnancy and the outpourings of menses, the latter often considered more of a curse than a blessing.

Esoterically, the vulva is associated with the base chakra, linked to surviving, doing, competing, risk taking, and assertiveness—all perfectly acceptable in a male-dominated world. As women have become more vocal in their demands for equality in the bedroom, much of that assertion has come from the base chakra, while the sacral chakra, which houses the uterus and ovaries, remains silent.

THE SACRAL CHAKRA

During thirty years of teaching on the subject of the chakras, I have observed that the greatest imbalance in men and women is found within the sacral chakra, often with a compensatory disharmony in its masculine counterpart, the throat chakra. When viewing the energy of the sacral chakra intuitively, I see four distinct patterns:

1. An excess of energy, reflecting an outpouring of nurturing for everybody else, leaving little time or space for self-care.
2. A reduced flow of energy, maintained by walls and metal bars, similar to those found in a tower or prison. It is clear that the barriers were erected by the person to prevent anybody from entering who may abuse or do harm, and yet they also preclude the inflow of love.
3. A desolate and barren land where it feels nobody has visited for a long time. This image is common in those who have developed their masculine persona at the cost of rejecting and abandoning their feminine traits of sensitivity, caring, and interconnectedness.
4. A dark, dense well or cave of energy where painful and shameful feelings have been buried. I sense the person is reluctant to enter this space because this would require her to face and release these emotions, and when she does, she knows that her life would change forever.

The sacral chakra is truly one of the most important seats of the Great Mother, expressing all three of her faces through the qualities of creativity (the Virgin), nurturing (the Mother), and dissolution (the Crone). These facets are beautifully woven into the menstrual cycle, each phase essential for the transformation and expansion of human consciousness. This cyclical pattern continues after menopause, although there is no need for the physical representations because at this point the consciousness of the Great Mother has been fully awakened.

The well-being of the sacral chakra is assured by maintaining a healthy relationship between all three phases of the cycle. If we spend all our time creating new projects and never make time to receive nurturing or enjoy the fruits of our endeavors, then it is probable that we will experience PMS. If we fail to release our hold on things in our life that are finished or complete, then we may experience heavy menstrual bleeding. If our dreams never see the light of day, then our ovaries may become distressed. Just as we need to balance these three phases, so it is important to achieve a balance between our masculine and feminine aspects. Such a harmonious balance is reflected in our ability to give and receive, where we create a truly interdependent relationship, as described in the following story:

> *Once there were two porcupines living in cold conditions. In order to warm each other, they moved close together, but soon felt pain, as the spines of the other pierced each one's skin. They then moved apart and became cold. Eventually, they found the perfect position for their relationship; not so close that they caused each other pain, but close enough to keep each other warm.*

The Hara

The spiritual tradition that emerged from Asia, especially Japan, China, Korea, and Thailand, calls the sacral chakra the *hara*. It is described as the lower of the three *dantians* (or *tan-t'ians*), which are centers of qi, or life-force energy, in various Chinese disciplines such as traditional Chinese medicine, qigong, and tai chi. The other two dantians are situated at the level of the heart (the middle dantian) and at the crown (the upper dantian), with all three regarded as feminine energy centers. In Taoism, the word *dantian* is loosely translated as "elixir field"; the dantians are essential for *neidan,* or inner alchemy, and are accessed through breathing and meditation. The lower dantian, the hara, refines physical matter into essence; the middle dantian, at the heart, refines essence into spirit; while the upper dantian refines spirit into emptiness.[2] In Buddhism and Taoism, it is taught that when we center our awareness within the dantians, our thoughts and emotions become quiet, and we can access the state of *samadhi,* or oneness; here we can see the true nature of reality and release the need for suffering.

The hara is perceived as the door between life and death and the location for both the generation and the storage of qi. The hara is where our physical world meets our inner world. When we focus our mind in the hara and allow it to become our center of gravity, we experience peace, joy, and tranquillity, as portrayed by images of the Happy Buddha, with his large belly of contentment.

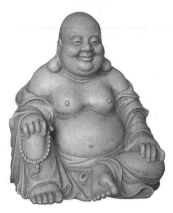

Happy Buddha

However, far too often our center of gravity is located at the level of our throat chakra, maintained by the belief that *as long as I think, I'm safe*. This leads to not only an overactive mind and resulting anxiety, but also stress and tension in the neck and shoulders. In addition, there are often difficulties with breathing and speaking, with the voice being forced from the throat and not expressed through the belly or uterus. Remember, in women, the uterus is "the utterer," which gives power to the voice, especially when we speak from the heart.

When a woman is disconnected from the dragon power in her belly, her words and actions are empty. She attempts to be heard by using the screech owl, residing in her masculine throat chakra, which relies on willpower and easily loses its strength and focus in a woman. If you want to understand this overuse of the throat chakra, I suggest you listen to some of the female figures in the media, politics, education, and the corporate world. You will quickly recognize which women are speaking from their deep feminine dragon power and which are relying on their masculine throat energy, which creates a shrill screech.

Simply lowering our center of awareness from the throat to the womb, or hara, and learning to speak from this place changes the level of transformation our words deliver. It often helps to place your hands over your sacral chakra to draw your attention away from the throat chakra, and to allow yourself one deep, out breath before beginning to speak. Sitting on the ground is also effective when you want a deep, meaningful conversation with someone. This posture is commonly adopted by indigenous peoples when serious decisions need to be made collectively by the community rather than by a lone authoritarian figure. Since the sacral chakra represents interdependent relationships while the masculine throat chakra reflects authority, when we speak from the womb we immediately send out a signal of inclusiveness and compassion, qualities strongly aligned to the Great Mother.

9 Hara Breathing to Calm the Mind

This practice to quiet the mind can be performed sitting, standing, or lying down—although, as already mentioned, for women, the best pose when working with Dragon Queen energy is to make sure the vagina is pointing down toward the earth. You may therefore prefer to stand or to kneel, resting your buttocks on a small stool or cushion.

- If you are standing, imagine that the soles of your feet have magnets attached to them pulling your body gently into the earth, until it feels that it is almost impossible to lift your feet.
- Gently bend your knees, which will immediately lower your center of gravity, and shift your awareness to the hara, about three fingers' breadth below the umbilicus.
- Place your hands over this area, joined at the tips of the thumbs and tips of the forefingers to form a downward triangle.
- Now, touching the tip of your tongue just behind the upper teeth, inhale through your nose for a count of five and slowly allow your breath, infused with qi, to enter the hara, beneath your hands.
- Hold your breath for a count of five, and then, removing your

tongue from the spot inside your mouth, exhale from your mouth for a count of five.

- Repeat this whole process, using slow and calming breaths, for at least five minutes, or until the area feels warm and your mind is quieter.

THE REALM OF SCORPIO

In esoteric medicine, the fertility organs come under the astrological sign of the intense and deeply passionate water sign of Scorpio, which is ruled by the goddess of the underworld, Pluto. The sign is named after the scorpion, which is easily recognizable with its pair of grasping claws and a segmented tail that arches over its back, at the end of which is its stinger. Because of its shape and its power to strike, Scorpio has also been associated with the dragon. Both the dragon and the scorpion inhabit dark places and often hunt by night.

Some of the most noticeable characteristics of the sign of Scorpio include:

- Exhibits a powerful and determined transformative force that is not easily dissuaded from its course
- Secretive, mysterious, intense, dark, and even dangerous
- Provides a cauldron for spiritual transformation that involves both death and rebirth
- Passionate, dramatic, and fully engaged, whether associated with people, food, or sex
- Self-blaming and self-destructive, often using a stinger against itself when things don't work out as desired
- Unable to forgive and forget the wounds of past experiences, holding on to grudges and dredging up old memories
- Sensually and sexually confident, revealed by the way it walks, the pleasure it has in its body, its playful flirting, and its wicked sense of humor

- Intimate relationship with death, often from an early age, and not fearful of its own death
- Often takes on the traumas of others, with an essential need to create healthy boundaries

The menstrual cycle bears the imprint of Scorpio, involving cycles of transformation through death and birth. The scorpion or dragon may also show itself during the premenstrual days, expressed as intense mood swings and a stinging tongue. Any woman whose astrological chart shows difficult aspects to her planets in Scorpio is more likely to experience issues with her sexuality or disease of her fertility organs. Since my Saturn, the planet of limitation and teaching, is in Scorpio, it is no wonder I am writing this book, which is based in part on the wisdom of my own hard-learned experiences.

ENTERING THE VESTIBULE: THE VAGINA

Moving through the vesica piscis–shaped doorway of the vulva, we enter the vagina, a hallway between the outer world of bustle, achievement, and desire for reward and the sacred and sanctified inner world of the womb. It's as if we've stepped into the vestibule of a church, where we naturally pause as our senses become accustomed to the dim lighting and hushed voices, and our mind shifts from an outer focus to an inner awareness. Many of these sacred protocols have been forgotten over time, and like the people who hang around at the back of the church in the hope of receiving a blessing without having to stay too long, we often find ourselves impatiently entering the vaginal opening. Whether inserting a tampon, stimulating the G-spot, or during penile penetration, we prod and thrust, with less than adequate sensitivity, eager to be in and out as quickly as possible.

Yet if we take the time to linger and listen, we will hear our womb calling us through her sweet song. If we stay awhile, we will inevitably be drawn inward, for our heart yearns to take time to rest and, once again, feel a deep sense of connection and communion. Just as there seems to be an energy that pulls you forward until you stand in the womb of a church or other sacred building, the vagina itself seems to assist in your passage. Such an active participation in the process can be understood through an appreciation of the structure of the vagina itself.

The Vaginal Environment

The vagina is a fibro-muscular tube that runs slightly backward from the vaginal opening in the vulvar vestibule and ends in a blind sac that surrounds the cervix, the neck of the uterus. The vagina is on average about three inches long and is angled about forty-five degrees to the uterus.

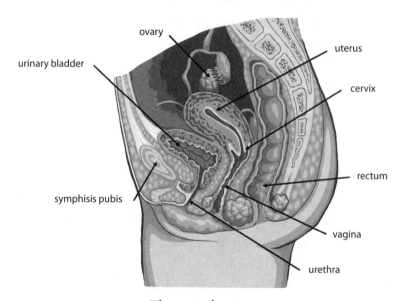

The vaginal environment

During sexual arousal, the muscles in the walls of the vagina cause it to expand in width and length, making it easier for sperm to enter the cervix, while the elasticity of the walls allows it to stretch during intercourse or labor. The vagina has a natural source of lubrication that keeps it moist and healthy, and therefore it does not need cleaning or sanitizing. At ovulation, under the influence of estrogen, there is an increase in the quantity of the mucus, which appears sticky and opaque, like egg whites. There is also an increase in the moisture during sexual arousal due to circulating testosterone levels.

Unfortunately, this pure environment can become distressed by a number of factors, including lowered estrogen levels at menopause, contraceptive chemicals, antibiotics, stress, and the candida fungus. Any of these factors can exacerbate a vulvar-vaginal area already made vulnerable from forceful entry during childhood sexual abuse. Even as an adult our body-mind can react to disrespectful entry into the sacred space of the vagina, leading to the potential for disease in this area. This problem can be likened to the ease with which you allow people to enter your home. If you are a private person and allow visitors to access only certain rooms, you may become disturbed if they ignore or disrespect your rules. In the same way, if someone fails to respect your body and attempts to enter without hearing your needs, this intrusion may immediately cause the vaginal mucus to dry up and the muscles to become tight, leading to vulvar-vaginal distress.

For many centuries women have been told that it is their duty to allow their husband to enter their vagina; otherwise he will become frustrated and take it out on the family or take a mistress. This has given some men the idea that it is their right to have sex without necessarily considering the needs of their partner. Whereas there are many sensitive and caring men, women today still take on the guilt and blame when they have vaginal soreness and have to say no to sex. If the condition is not easily resolved, chronic anxiety can develop, further contributing to dryness and tension. Only through honesty, sensitivity, understanding, and perhaps the help of a couples therapist can the relationship—and the vagina—heal.

This shift in energy from the open-armed and excited welcome of the base chakra to the often unspoken and mysterious needs of the sacral chakra may be confusing to visitors. Yet if your partner loves and respects you, he or she will pause and wait in the vestibule, allowing trust to develop, until you feel ready to let him or her proceed deeper.

During intercourse, this invitation is perceived through experiencing the tightening of the vaginal muscles, which grasp anything within the vault, pulling it toward the cervix. But wait, I hear you say; does this mean that the vaginal muscles have some power and are not merely flaccid bystanders? According to ancient Tantric tradition, young girls in India were taught, first by their mother and later by a Tantric guru, the art of sahajoli mudra (*sahajoli* means "strong" or "mighty" in Sanskrit). In this practice, which is highly valued by men, a woman is able to hold the man's lingam (penis) in her yoni, opening and closing the muscles at her pleasure.

The Tantric Vagina

In Tantric practices it is the woman, as Shakti, who controls the sexual process, creating the sacred space for the man's energy to rise within her. Once the man enters the vagina, he must decrease his thrusting and allow his partner's energy to pull him toward the cervix, using the strength of the dragon energy stored within her womb and in her vaginal muscles. The effect is achieved by centering her attention on her cervix, at the top of her vagina. This aims to prevent the release of her energy merely through an orgasm of the nervous system and collects the energy into the area of the cervix. It is easy for women who have been Tantrically trained from an early age to concentrate their awareness into this area; but for those of us who have little awareness of our body, we need to start by becoming aware of physical sensations, beginning with the perineal muscles, and then moving to the muscles of the vagina.

I am indebted to Andre van Lysebeth, a Tantric devotee, whose book *Tantra: Cult of the Feminine* brought sacred sexual practices alive for me.[3] Although the focus of the following practices is commonly associated with those in relationship, they are in fact essential for all women to ensure a continuous source of creative power and so can be carried out without a partner. By working in this way, we can reconnect with the dragon energy within Earth; heal and invigorate the base chakra where kundalini awaits; and move the energy into the powerhouse, the womb.

The exercises that follow are designed to be carried out in a sequential manner, as they move from the more physical outer muscles to more subtle inner muscles. The practices should not be rushed; they are not a competition but a loving reconnection to body-centered memories.

☾ *Mula Bandha: Strengthening Our Foundations*

Since the tightening of the muscles in this exercise is relatively invisible to people close by, it can be carried out standing, sitting, or lying down, whenever you have a few minutes available to practice.

- Begin by constricting the muscles around the anus, as if you are trying to refrain from passing a stool.
- Hold the contraction for five to ten seconds and then relax. Repeat five times.
- As you practice this, you will find that other muscles of the perineum and vulva are engaged, causing constriction to the vaginal and urethral openings as well as some clitoral stimulation, as the blood starts to collect in the erectile tissues. This is because the muscles are wrapped like a figure eight around the anus and the vulva, so that tightening one tightens the other. I suggest you enjoy the sexual arousal but allow it to dissipate after ten seconds rather than proceeding to an orgasm, as that is not the goal of these rituals.
- Keep up the practice until there is a smooth flow of muscle contraction from anus to clitoris and then a relaxation in the opposite direction.

This exercise is very similar to those created by Dr. Arnold Kegel, who showed that weakness of the hammocklike muscle of the pelvic floor was linked to both urinary incontinence and poor sexual response. By practicing Kegel exercises, or mula bandha, the muscles become stronger, reducing the risk of developing incontinence or prolapse—and your sex life improves!

↻ *Vaginal Strengthener No. 1*

Use a clean, smooth, plastic or metal cylindrical object that is long enough to protrude from the vaginal opening, such as a vaginal dilator, a vibrator, or any of the other products presently on the market used to strengthen the vaginal muscles. If none of these are available to you, you can use your own fingers.

- While lying comfortably on your back with your legs apart, insert the cylindrical object on a deep inhalation, holding onto its end.
- Hold the breath for three seconds, and then slowly exhale as you remove the object. Repeat this exercise five times.

Marvel as the sensations within your vagina increase as you repeat the exercise. With practice, you may wish to see if you can manipulate the cylinder so that it starts to circle, an art that will certainly enliven your sex life!

Since "energy flows where attention goes," the increased attention given to your intimate feminine area, with regular practice, will vitalize the organs and tissues, which is especially important after menopause.

↻ *Vaginal Strengthener No. 2*

This next exercise requires practice and patience, but it is well worth mastering. It not only heightens a partner's sexual experience but more importantly encourages us to move the sensations of sexual arousal from the area of the vulva and clitoris up to the cervix and into the dragon's lair, the womb, stimulating a deep orgasmic experience.

- First, see if you can separate the constriction of the anus from that of the vagina; this requires practice and focus, but eventually you'll be able to notice the ability to relax one set of muscles while engaging the other.
- Now, try practicing isolating the muscles at the opening of the vagina that constrict an object from those farther up the vagina that

move an object upward along the vaginal passageway. To begin, place a finger in the vaginal opening and hold it by using your vaginal muscles. Then attempt to constrict the "lifter" muscles of the vagina, so that you feel your finger being drawn farther into the vagina.

- When you feel you have mastered this part of the exercise, you can replace the finger with a similar object to that used in the previous exercise. The goal of this practice is to be able to move an object along the vagina, from the vulva to the cervix, using sequential groups of muscles.

One of the aims of this type of Tantric practice is to forestall a man's ejaculation so that he can hold his energy and experience a spiritual orgasm. If he is able to become still once he is within the vagina, as a result of your being able to "hold" him and "lift" him, he will find that these maneuvers of the vaginal muscle will not only help him maintain his erection but ease his need to ejaculate.

MEETING THE DOORKEEPER: THE CERVIX

Now we are facing another doorway, one that leads to the inner sanctum of the womb. If the uterus is a sacred temple or church, only those who fully respect and honor the Goddess are permitted to pass the doorkeeper, the cervix, and allowed into the sacred chamber beyond, the uterus. The cervix, or neck of the uterus, is about one inch in length and extends from the upper reaches of the vagina into the body of the uterus. Cylindrical in shape, the center of the cervix is transected by a canal that runs from the vagina into the cavity of the uterus. It is through this passageway that products of menstruation pass and sperm swim. This is also the passageway through which a baby squeezes on its journey into this world. During a woman's labor, because of uterine contractions, the shape of the cervix changes: just prior to delivery the whole cervix flattens out (complete effacement), with the canal dilating to its maximum of ten centimeters. It is at this point that the woman is encouraged to push the baby into the world.

The cervix naturally produces mucus, the appearance of which changes during the menstrual cycle. Just after menstruation, the external opening of the cervix into the vagina is plugged by mucus, preventing any sperm from entering the womb. However, around the time of ovulation, the mucus becomes much thinner, allowing sperm to pass. Women who advocate natural contraception use the presence of this peri-ovulation mucus as a sign to avoid intercourse. During pregnancy, the opening is plugged by a special antibacterial mucus that is dislodged at the onset of labor.

Despite the symbolic importance of the doorkeeper to prevent anything harmful or disrespectful to the Goddess from entering our inner sanctum, the cervix is one of the most underrated organs in the female body. It commonly takes on the pain we experience in the presence of emotional and sexual abuse, but because of its location—deep within the pelvis—the hurt often remains hidden and unspoken, until brought to light during a routine cervical examination. I was forty when my biannual cervical (Pap) smear revealed the early signs of cervical cancer. The diagnosis certainly made me look at my relationship with my cervix, which until then had been sorely lacking. It quickly became apparent that the cellular changes reflected some emotional battering I'd experienced in a few of my relationships—with both males and females—when I'd failed to stand up for myself because of my tendency to think I must be in the wrong. As I explored the origins of these beliefs and perceptions, I became aware of a profound sense of shame I was carrying in my sacral chakra, and yet the sum of the activities of my present-day life didn't warrant such intense emotions. Where did this come from?

Digging deep, I came upon a family story that spoke of a great aunt who had given birth to an illegitimate child. Even though this was a long time ago, the shame of her being branded a "wanton girl" who was "used goods" obviously had continued to influence the psyches of generations of women in my family. I remembered times when my mother would comment, "You must be grateful that someone wants to be your friend"—suggesting that I didn't really deserve such favors; this memory revealed the degree of ancestral shame that had been unconsciously passed down. On the one hand, it was a relief to realize it wasn't all *my* shame. However, I knew that emotional healing would occur for me only if I took time to sit with the pain and shame of my ancestor, imagining what it would have been like to have been her. Enveloping her in compassion, I immediately felt waves of love passing through my sacral chakra, bringing healing to both myself and my family. Strengthened with a renewed sense of self-worth and self-respect, I went about closing the doors on unhealthy relationships, focusing instead on those that nurtured my body and soul. Within a few months, the cells of my cervix returned to normal and have remained so ever since.

Since most changes to cells of the cervix do not produce symptoms, I'm a strong advocate for regular Pap or cervical smears. The availability of screening programs varies greatly between developed and developing countries, but all usually target younger women in an attempt to diagnose and treat the early stages of cancer. In most circumstances, the smear detects mild, abnormal changes to the cells of the cervix—cervical dysplasia, which is self-limiting and will go away of its own accord.[4]

More importantly, however, every woman should create an intimate relationship with her cervix, the doorkeeper. It is not only during sex that people enter your vagina. As the womb is a place of transformation and power, it is not uncommon for people to try to access the dragon's lair energetically, often called "energy vampiring." Through seduction—by both men and women—threats, or entreaties, a person may seek to steal your power of transformation, entering via the base chakra and moving along the vagina. Depending on the fortitude of the doorkeeper, they may or may not gain entry to the womb. If access is gained without your permission, they can take up residence, refusing to leave and often becoming more and more emotionally demanding. A ritual I carry out on a regular basis is to move my awareness into my vagina and check on who may have sneaked inside. I then grab hold of their feet and pull them out, saying firmly, "Get out and don't come back!" I often advise women to imagine a strong representative of a doorkeeper, such as a lioness or mother bear, and to ask that figure to symbolically guard their inner sanctum, the womb, allowing in only those who come with love and respect. I myself have a large female hippopotamus with beautiful long eyelashes who looks adorable but is immovable when challenged.

THE UTERUS: CAVE OF POWER

The uterus is made up of three layers: the outer coverings, the muscle layer or *myometrium,* and the inner lining or *endometrium.* Under the influence of hormones the endometrium undergoes various changes during the monthly cycle, with the eventual shedding of its surface during a woman's moon time, in the absence of a pregnancy. The myometrium is responsible not only for the power that propels the newborn into the world but also

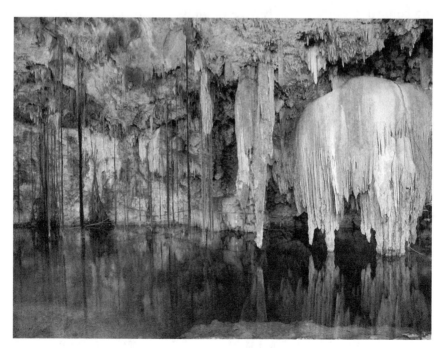

Cave of power within Mother Earth

for the transport of the sperm into the womb and the expelling of the products of menstruation. Abnormal contractility of the myometrium is responsible for pain during one's period (dysmenorrhea) as well as possibly certain spontaneous miscarriages and preterm births.[5]

When a woman reconnects to her womb and fills it with the wisdom and strength of dragon energy, she reclaims her power. Here she feels centered, grounded, and linked to all life. The womb holds the power of incredible transformation, not only in the creation of a human being but in the manifestation of our dreams and the evolution of consciousness for humanity, through cycles of death and birth. The womb's wisdom is deep, ancient, and grounded in what will sustain and nurture our families and communities now and in the future. Grandmothers from the indigenous tribes teach what our ancestral sisters always knew: *When the womb is healed and reconnected to the heart, sacred woman will stand in her power. Now she can become the vessel by which her man can start to heal his wounds, so that eventually they can stand side by side in equality. Then we will see peace and harmony on this earth.*

THE FALLOPIAN TUBES: CORRIDORS OF ENCOUNTER

Extending laterally from the body of the uterus are the fallopian tubes. Within these two very fine tubes are tiny hairs that waft the eggs toward the uterine cavity. The ends of the fallopian tubes are frayed or fimbriated. Since the ovaries are not attached to the fimbriae, it takes a leap of faith on the part of the egg to jump the gap and hope the sweeping motion of the fimbriae will catch it and draw it into the open tube. It is here that the egg typically meets the sperm and fertilization takes place, leading to the formation of a zygote. After about five days, the zygote reaches the uterine cavity and implants into the wall of the uterus about one day later, to develop into a fetus.

Occasionally, due to scarring in the fallopian tube from a previous infection, the zygote is unable to reach the uterine cavity and the pregnancy begins to develop in the fallopian tube instead. This is known as an ectopic pregnancy. Understandably, the tiny tube is ill-equipped to provide the nourishment or the space for a baby to develop, and so around the sixth week of pregnancy the tube ruptures, often causing acute pain. This is an emergency situation, for although there is little bleeding on the outside, there can be heavy internal bleeding. Depending on the damage, it is sometimes possible to save the fallopian tube; otherwise it requires removal, leaving the woman with just one tube.

The fallopian tubes are especially vulnerable to infections such as chlamydia. This bacterium enters the system through vaginal, anal, or oral sex and in 75 percent of women is without symptoms; hence it is known as "the silent epidemic." Chlamydia can also lead to a painful condition known as pelvic inflammatory disease, as well as scarring of the tubes, which can cause infertility or an ectopic pregnancy. Many countries now have screening programs in place for young people to detect and treat asymptomatic infections before a pregnancy occurs.

THE OVARIES: SACRED EGGS OF LIFE

The two oval-shaped ovaries are located next to, but not attached to, the fimbriated ends of the fallopian tubes. They are held in place between the pelvic wall and the uterus by ligaments. Physiologically, the ovaries have two main functions: to store and ripen the eggs, or ova, ready for release at ovulation, and to produce hormones.

A female, at birth, has all the eggs she will need for a lifetime—around two million—although due to natural decay, by the time a girl reaches puberty there are about 200,000 eggs in each ovary, and this figure declines as she ages. It is usual for only one egg to be released each month from one of the ovaries, in a random pattern, although if one of the ovaries is removed then the remaining ovary will produce an ovum on a monthly basis. Occasionally, in natural circumstances, each ovary releases an egg at ovulation, which can result in the birth of nonidentical twins.

Hormones

The ovaries produce three hormones: estrogen, progesterone, and testosterone.

Estrogen

Both men and women produce estrogen. There are three naturally occurring estrogens secreted by women:

- Estradiol, the main estrogen found in a woman during her reproductive years
- Estrone, weaker than estradiol, found primarily in postmenopausal women
- Estriol, produced by the placenta in pregnant women and found in small amounts in nonpregnant women and in men

Toward the end of the menses, the pituitary gland, under the influence of the hypothalamus, produces increasing amounts of follicular stimulating hormone (FSH), which stimulates a number of eggs within the ovaries to begin to mature within their sac or follicle. The developing follicle starts to produce estrogen, which acts on the endometrium, causing it to proliferate and thicken, while cervical mucus starts to thin. This follicular phase of the menstrual cycle lasts on average about eight days, with several eggs fighting for dominance, until only one is left.

Other than ripening the body for ovulation, the main function of estrogen is to promote secondary sexual characteristics at puberty, such as development of the breasts, growth of body hair, and increasing fat distribution. Estrogen maintains our features of femininity while also strengthening the bones and protecting the heart from disease. Estrogen also encourages creativity and outward expression.

In the past, doctors believed that the ovaries became inactive at menopause. This resulted in a fallacious tendency to remove the ovaries during surgery to remove the uterus (hysterectomy) in women over the age of forty, in the belief that this would reduce their risk of ovarian cancer. However, recent research questions this practice, as it has been shown that even though the ovaries stop producing estrogen, they continue to produce hormones from their inner core, or stroma, for several decades after menopause.[6] In particular, the stroma produces androgens, which are converted into estrone in the liver, adrenal glands, skin, muscles, and adipose tissue or fat stores—offering continual, if somewhat weakened, feminizing effects as our body ages.[7]

Returning to our discussion of the follicular phase of the menstrual cycle, the rising levels of blood estrogen eventually trigger the hypothalamus to stop producing FSH levels, leading to a surge in the secretion of luteinizing hormone (LH) from the pituitary gland, which causes the egg to burst from its follicle—ovulation. This announces the next phase of the cycle, the nurturing or luteal phase.

Progesterone

Progesterone is secreted from three sources: the now empty follicle, known as the *corpus luteum;* the placenta; and the adrenal cortex. Its role is to prepare the endometrium to receive and maintain the growth of the embryo. In the absence of pregnancy, progesterone levels fall and the upper layer of the endometrium is lost in the menstrual flow.

In the adrenal cortex progesterone is produced from cholesterol and is converted into both testosterone and the stress hormone cortisol. When a woman is experiencing stress in her life, the adrenal glands will "steal" progesterone from the body to generate more cortisol to deal with the stress, leading to increased potential for infertility and miscarriage. It is clearly imperative to find ways to lower stress levels in such a woman, rebalancing levels of progesterone within her body. Low levels of progesterone are also responsible for many of the symptoms of both PMS and perimenopause, made worse by concurrent levels of stress, where the body cannot keep up with the demand for cortisol, leading to chronic anxiety and fatigue.

Testosterone

Increased levels of androgens such as testosterone are secreted by the ovaries and adrenal glands prior to ovulation, causing an increase in a woman's libido so she can naturally seek fertilization of her egg. Though the production of androgens decreases over time, it is not enough of a decrease, even at menopause, to prevent a woman from having a healthy libido well into her later years.

THE NATURAL CYCLES OF THE MOON

Whatever her age and whether she has uterus or not, a woman's body and mind are programmed to respond to the phases of the moon and, in turn, to cycles of birth and death. Indeed, words such as *menses, menarche, menstrual,* and *menopause* all come from the Latin word for

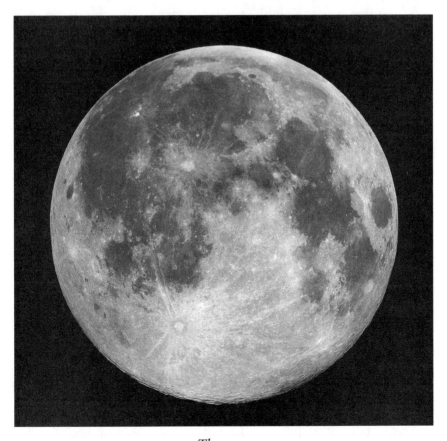

The moon

"month," which originally referred to the moon's phases as measures of time. The word *period,* commonly used to describe the monthly menstrual bleeding, originates from the Greek *periodos,* which means "going around," or a cycle, while also implying an ending. The Latin word for moon is *luna,* which gives us the word *lunacy,* a state of mind many men believe women enter just before a period and at menopause.

Like the moon, which starts out dark, waxes until it becomes full, then wanes back into complete darkness again, the menstrual cycle consists of three phases:

1. The menses, or moon time, is associated with the dark moon, a period of three days when no moon is visible in the sky. In the middle of these days, the sun and moon align, giving birth to a new moon, although the silvery sliver of the crescent moon is not visible for another thirty-six hours.
2. The follicular phase corresponds to the waxing moon, associated with the growth and maturation of the egg.
3. The luteal phase aligns with the waning moon, linked to the preparation of the uterus to receive and nurture the fertilized egg—and is followed by the next dark moon.

Moon Time

It was during a dark moon that our ancestral sisters would gather together to cleanse, share stories, and open themselves to divine wisdom, their periods often synchronizing to begin at the start of a dark moon. Representing a time of self-reflection, letting go, and surrendering to the mystery of death before opening oneself to the Great Mother's inspiration, this is the most important phase of the menstrual cycle and yet often receives the least attention, considered an unpleasant inconvenience for both women and men.

A girl begins to menstruate anywhere between the ages of eight and sixteen, on average, about two years after the onset of puberty. Factors such as heredity, diet, and overall health can accelerate or delay the first menstrual bleeding, or menarche. It is now known that girls who sit in front of the bright lights of television for long periods of time are more likely to have an early menarche. This is due to the fact that light inhibits the hormone melatonin, which otherwise would suppress menses and ovulation. In the same vein, girls who live where winters are longer, or in rural areas where there are fewer artificial lights, tend to start their menstrual cycles later than girls who live around the equator or in cities.[8]

I can still remember the day of my first period, when I was twelve. I was playing with my brother and his friends in a pool in the garden and noticed the blood. It wasn't that I was unprepared, but in that moment my life changed. My mother told me that there would be no more swimming until the bleeding stopped and that this event was something not to be shared with the men—it was our "secret," as though this major event in the life of a woman had to be hidden. Perhaps things would have been different if there had been a day of celebration, with all my aunts and grandmothers coming to our home to welcome me into the womb of womanhood. But I doubt that would have ever happened, especially as my mother referred to a woman's monthly period as "the curse" until her dying day.

Every woman's period is different. Although doctors often speak of a twenty-eight-day cycle, there are marked variations around this timing, all of which are perfectly normal. The amount of blood lost and the number of days involved also vary greatly. I was always a seven-day person, and from my mid-thirties onward I would bleed heavily for the first three days, often requiring both tampons and pads. My closest friend, on the other hand, bled for only three days and used the smallest-size tampon. Despite the fact that most women of reproductive age are programmed to bleed on a monthly basis, I find it strange how little the moon time is discussed among women. I've even noticed a degree of insensitivity on the part of other women when problems arise, such as pain or heavy bleeding, as if the patriarchal shaming around menses has suffocated the hearts of women toward their sisters. What a difference it would make if women would celebrate their cycles, coming together to share this unique gift with pride, as described in Anita Diamant's groundbreaking novel *The Red Tent,* whose title refers to the place where women gathered in biblical times during their cycles of birthing, menses, and even illness.

While we're on the subject, there is one profession that I think most women would agree seems totally oblivious to the needs of a menstruating woman: those who design women's restrooms. When are architects going to realize that since one in four women is likely to be on her moon, women need at least 25 percent more toilet facilities than those required by men? More importantly, who on earth designed those receptacles for used sanitary products? In my teens, women were provided with bags that were placed in a little incinerator in the restroom. Now you have to somehow dangle a blood-laden tampon through an almost horizontal hole into a bin that is already overflowing and often offensive. Come on, guys (if it is men who design the facilities): this is not rocket science!

But perhaps some young women have discovered the answer that modern "civilization" offers: using chemicals to suppress the natural cycles. In the past, a combination of hormones was used to treat endometriosis and painful and heavy periods; now it is being used for convenience, such as when the moon time coincides with an upcoming social event. For extended use, the commonest regime for these pills is eighty-four days on, followed by a seven-day break, although some regimes advocate just four moon times a year to correspond with the seasons. Breakthrough bleeding is not an uncommon side effect when taking these artificial menses suppressors, although it will be some time before we are able to assess the long-term side effects, especially to a woman's psychological and spiritual well-being.

The Creative Phase

Corresponding with the waxing moon, this phase of a woman's cycle is associated with the growth and maturation of the egg. During this time, because of increasing levels of estrogen, as well as dopamine, endorphins, and serotonin, we usually feel sociable, optimistic, confident, enthusiastic, and generally extroverted. Our creativity blossoms, especially when it comes to new ideas and plans. At the same time, our testosterone levels increase, giving us more energy, not only for projects but also, as we near ovulation, for sex. Now, as the egg is ready to burst from its follicle, the sense of well-being peaks as we share with the world our dreams so they may be fertilized by the rich experiences and encounters that follow.[9]

Disorders of this phase of the cycle involve the ovaries and endometrium and will be discussed later.

The Harvesting Phase

Following ovulation comes an immediate lowering of the excitatory hormones, including serotonin and dopamine, as well as increased levels of the nurturing hormone progesterone. Now the mood changes, as a woman begins to turn her attention inward. She becomes more self-absorbed as she nurtures herself with the fruits of her endeavors from the past few weeks and is able to reflect on what she will take from her experience and what she will release during her moon time. This symbolizes the inwardly focused energy of nesting, nurturing, harvesting, and introspection.

PMS: From Superwoman to Sacred Woman

Premenstrual syndrome, or PMS, is a collection of over a hundred physical and emotional symptoms; these include breast tenderness, weight gain, headache, bloating, constipation, neck pain, fatigue, irrational anger, tears, irritability, mood swings, low libido, depression, and sugar cravings. It is estimated that about 60 percent of women experience varying degrees of PMS anywhere from ten to three days before the start of their period. Preexisting conditions, particularly those linked to the health of the immune system such as candida, often flare up during this time, since progesterone lowers the immune response.

Those who live or work with a woman suffering from PMS commonly observe the immediacy of the transformation. One moment she is hypersensitive and irritable, picking fights with everyone, and the next she is curled up, crying into her favorite ice cream over what appears to be a trifle to everyone else. At other times, she shape-shifts from a happy and confident person to a highly temperamental monster. All these signs may be accompanied by low self-esteem, self-loathing, self-destructiveness, forgetfulness, disorientation, and exhaustion. Linda Crockett, a medical herbalist who has worked with many women with PMS, comments, "What is intriguing is that women adamantly refuse to accept that this darkness and negativity is coming from within them, preferring to blame their hormones or diet."[10] The Dragon Queen is clearly trying to get our attention.

In the past, as a homeopath, I would commonly prescribe the remedies sepia and lachesis for PMS. Sepia is the ink of the cuttlefish, produced when the fish wants to hide away and have some privacy; lachesis is snake venom, released when the serpent feels cornered and lashes out to get free. Both of these remedies describe perfectly the feelings of a woman during the luteal phase. We don't want to start new projects or take on more responsibilities; instead we want time alone to relax, to be nurtured, and to nest—the same way we would feel if we were in the final stages of pregnancy. Yet, despite the fact that over half of women in their reproductive years complain of symptoms from PMS, modern medicine has no clear idea as to its cause. Recent research has shown that the previously held view—that PMS is merely due to high levels of estrogen and low levels of progesterone—is far too simplistic. It is much more likely that several factors are involved, including low levels of serotonin, vitamin B_6, magnesium, and melatonin. However, unless scientific research is taken to a much deeper level, one that involves reconnecting women to the female mysteries of their ancestors and the teachings of the Great Mother, I don't ever see us "curing" PMS.

The luteal phase, like the waning moon, is not a time to plant crops. It is a time to gather the fruits and grains, store the seeds, and feed ourselves to withstand the passage through the underworld and celebrate a successful harvest. This phase of the moon is basically a time to return to our hearts for nurturing—something we, in our modern, busy world, are poorly equipped to address. This truth was brought to my doorstep many years ago after I had spent several days in the spring planting my garden with a variety of beans. When autumn came, I found myself far too busy to pick the vegetables, which slowly died on their stalks from neglect. I realized only then how quickly I can become fired up by a new project without ever giving time to harvesting and celebrating my successes. This is borne out socially, where the most common questions we are asked are, "So what have you been *doing* recently? Are you busy?" If you mention that you have been resting and enjoying the fruits of your endeavors, a puzzled look comes over the face of the inquirer, who eventually offers some sympathy: "That's okay, I'm sure things will pick up soon."

No wonder women are so wounded around this phase of their cycle. PMS levels have increased dramatically as women have entered the workforce full-time. Add to this the responsibility for caring for children, employees, parents, and even spouses in some cases, and it is no wonder that so many women reach screaming point at this time when what they really need is solitude and reflection. PMS is undoubtedly worse in a woman whose mother was a poor role model in terms of exhibiting good self-esteem and the ability to self-nurture, or if she was a martyr type, all too willing to sacrifice her personal needs. It may feel as if there is no way out of all the pressures being placed on you at this time. But small steps make a big difference, especially if you have family or friends who want to support you during this time, allowing you to transition from superwoman to sacred woman. The luteal phase is all about preparing you to descend into the cauldron at moon time, but first you need to feed your heart and soul for the journey.

Here are a few suggestions for aligning yourself with the luteal phase of your cycle, which on average begins around day seventeen from the start of your last period. These ideas are based on the agricultural cycle:

- *Collect the fruits and grains.* Spend some time each day in self-reflection, looking back over the month and making notes in a journal of some of the major themes both at work and at home. What seeds, dreams, or ideas did you plant this month? The most important events are those where you feel emotionally involved.

- *Separate the seeds from the weeds.* From your list, decide what pearls of wisdom or sense of accomplishment you want to take away from these experiences, and what dreams or projects you are ready to release as weeds, choosing not to give them any more energy.

- *Plow the fields and mend the fences.* This is a time for honesty. Which relationships or activities nourish you, and which leave you drained, dissatisfied, or unfulfilled? What needs to be said, and where do you need to build stronger fences to protect your precious time and space, starting now?

- *Nurture yourself and celebrate the harvest.* Make a point of making time, even a whole day, to celebrate and pamper yourself. Many of us don't know how to celebrate ourselves; it's time to learn.

Strengthened by this preparation, inwardly nurtured and ready to release those things that are complete and to receive new waves of creative inspiration, we are now ready to enter the dark moon phase and begin the cycle anew.

PREGNANCY

Giving birth is often described as one of the most profound experiences in a woman's life. Despite the pain and discomfort, the final push is orgasmic, resulting in the most precious moment in the world. As you hold your beautiful child against your breasts and look into its eyes, an instant bond of love flows between you. After nine months of being nurtured and nourished in the most sacred of waters, its soul is ready to be seen by the world.

Despite the long-held and widespread cultural belief that a woman's role is to give birth and hence to protect the ancestral line, getting pregnant is not a foregone conclusion for women these days. In 2008, 20 percent of American women between the ages of forty and forty-four were childless, some by choice and some because of infertility issues. Some women are desperate to get pregnant, while others become pregnant despite every precaution. Today many women enjoy expressing their creativity through their work and opt not to bring children into the world. Many women choose single parenthood, adopt, or use a sperm donor rather than live with a male partner. Perhaps we should remember the Inca belief that it is the soul that chooses the parents, not the other way around.

The Sacred Nine Months

Just as the menstrual cycle is divided into three phases, so are the nine months of pregnancy.

First Trimester

Many women who miss their period by around a week or so already know they are pregnant even before they get the results of their pregnancy test. The early signs include fatigue, tender breasts and nipples, morning sickness, bloating, and frequent urination. A pregnancy test measures the presence of the hormone human chorionic gonadotropin (HCG) in the urine, which is produced by the newly developing placenta as the fetus implants in the uterus. HCG stimulates the corpus luteum to continue to secrete progesterone and estrogen, encouraging the endometrium to thicken and prepare to support the pregnancy.

This is a very busy time for both mother and fetus, as the mother starts to adapt to the presence of a new life within her womb, and the few-celled zygote changes into a tiny being. By eight weeks, the baby's heart is beating and its features starting to form—tiny ears, a nose, and a mouth.

Fifteen to 20 percent of pregnancies between five and twenty weeks end in miscarriage, with 80 percent occurring in the first trimester; in such cases, pathological findings often show abnormalities in the baby or in the placenta that would have prevented the development of the fetus. In an otherwise healthy woman, there is no reason why she shouldn't try again if she so desires.

Second Trimester
The next three months are generally calmer, with the woman feeling more energetic and confident in sharing her news with friends and family, especially as the pregnant uterus is now usually visible just above the pubic bone. At four months, the placenta takes over the production of progesterone and estrogen. These hormones, along with prolactin, prepare the breasts for milk production. Progesterone and another hormone, relaxin, encourage relaxation of pelvic ligaments and muscles to make space for the growing fetus and eventually for childbirth. By twenty weeks, most mothers have felt the first movements of their baby within their womb—the quickening—increasing the sense of bonding and connection.

Third Trimester
After a pleasant few months, feelings of tiredness and discomfort commonly return because of the rapidly increasing size of the developing child. A woman will continue to gain weight and her breasts will swell; other symptoms may include backache, heartburn, frequent urination, shortness of breath, and varicose veins—what joy! Emotions also become more unsettled, often experienced as anxiety, weeping, sleeplessness, and food cravings. Only one thing is for sure at this point: there is no going back!

Labor and Delivery
Now comes the moment of truth. Most women will have attended birthing classes and have a birth plan in mind, although it is important to plan for the unexpected. In a normal, natural delivery, the water usually breaks first, followed by the onset of contractions, which cause the cervix to start to soften and thin, enhanced by the pressure of the baby's

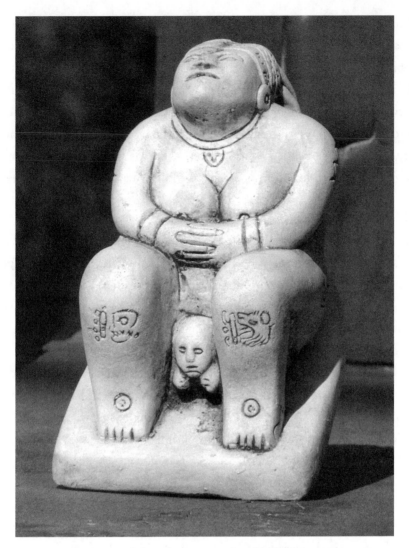

Mayan woman giving birth

head. Eventually it is time to push, as the baby is propelled along the vagina and out into the world.

For the mother, this will probably be one of the most magical moments of her life, especially if she is able to go through labor without an epidural and deliver vaginally. If the woman is able to concentrate on breathing with the waves of contractions rather than fighting them, she can be carried up along her own serpentine path toward her crown chakra. There the woman's soul will meet and embrace the baby's soul in a final moment of unconditional love before the child's birth, and the separation of the two souls begins. As the contractions increase and the desire to push increases, the mother's focus once again descends to the sacral chakra, bringing with her the soul of the baby, which she anchors into the baby's physical body. Then, with the woman's ecstatic, orgasmic cry, one that has echoed the joy of creation for women from the very beginning, the child is born, ready to begin its own unique life's journey.

C-Section

An increasing number of babies are being brought into the world by Cesarean, or C-section. When I worked in obstetrics thirty years ago, we did everything in our power to help the mother deliver naturally, via the vagina. I was fortunate to work with some wonderful midwives whose cultural backgrounds gave them the experience to know when to observe and support and when to intervene. We never took risks, and we carefully monitored the well-being of both mother and baby. I can still remember sitting at the bedside of a dozing mother listening to the pulse of the baby on the fetal monitor, feeling that I was hearing the voice of the baby's soul, directing my actions on its behalf.

Yet today, many women choose a C-section, not because of birth complications, as was true of this procedure in the past, but because of the opportunity it provides to have a pain-free delivery at the convenience of both the mother and the doctor. In 2008, 32 percent of newborns were delivered by C-section in the United States—up 50 percent from 1996. This means that one in three first-time mothers are being delivered by C-section.[11] Although clearly there are advantages to performing a C-section when the life of either the mother or the baby is at risk, any operation brings its own complications, including infection, hemorrhage, and decreased bonding time because of the mother's extended recovery time.

Vaginal delivery, in which the baby experiences the pressure on his body as he passes through the vagina and into the open air, prepares the child for life. In a fascinating book, *Birth and Relationships,* authors and rebirth experts Sondra Ray and Bob Mandell find that a child born by C-section can suffer from a variety of challenges depending on the reason for the procedure.[12] Those who were born at the convenience of the doctor or mother may have difficulty making their own decisions, resentful of being manipulated because of the needs of others. On the other hand, those who were delivered by an emergency C-section due to fetal or maternal distress may suffer from "interruption syndrome," where, however hard they try to push forward on their own course, they find they are constantly facing unseen interruptions. Most children delivered by C-section crave touch and hugs, as they never received this during the passage through the vagina.

Today, many women are choosing more natural ways to give birth. And increasing numbers of hospitals are working to accommodate their choices, recognizing that the most important factor is the well-being of the mother and baby. When I worked as a junior obstetrician in the early 1980s, we tended to confine the mother to bed once labor started in earnest, with just her husband or partner present. Now women are encouraged to move around; they have many choices, such as practicing relaxation and breathing techniques, receiving assistance from a doula or labor coach, or soaking in a warm tub to ease the pain of the contractions. Most births do not need medical intervention. With this understanding, everybody involved with the birthing can make it a positive experience for all concerned with the safe, calm, and loving delivery of the incoming soul—recognizing that this birth will influence this person for the rest of his or her life.

MENOPAUSE

If there is any confusion about the underlying purpose of the average woman's thirty-five years of menstrual cycles, there is probably even more confusion around what follows after her monthly periods end. Menopause generally occurs between the ages of forty-five and fifty-five, with perimenopause, or climacteric, beginning approximately five to eight years before the last period. Although some women experience no side effects of this part of the natural life cycle, more commonly a woman's symptoms include hot flashes or flushes, fatigue, weight gain, bloating, mood changes, and tender breasts. These symptoms can sometimes be followed by more long-term problems, such as thinning and drying of the vagina and osteoporosis.

Fueled by advertisements aimed at a woman's self-esteem—suggesting that she doesn't want to become a dried-up old hag with brittle bones as she ages—many women have been persuaded to undergo hormone replacement therapy (HRT) to reduce or even eliminate the inconvenient symptoms of "the change." These women are usually unaware that if and when they stop this treatment they will have to go through menopause anyway, often in a more acute manner. In addition, concerns have been raised about an increase in breast cancer seen in women who take HRT, which has caused many women to seek alternative approaches to reduce their symptoms of menopause, with herbal and biochemical remedies coming onto the market as viable alternatives.

According to Linda Crockett, author of *Healing Our Hormones, Healing Our Lives,* the infamous hot flashes are far more pronounced when the adrenal glands, the source of the postmenopausal hormone estrone and progesterone, are exhausted from chronic levels of stress. Crockett makes a strong correlation between menopause and the luteal phase of the menstrual cycle, both of which represent a time to focus within, relax, and receive intuition. If external circumstances prevent such inward reflection, or if we were not taught to honor our need for relaxation, then when we reach menopause and progesterone levels fall, it becomes far more difficult to adapt to the change.[13] There are many ways to reduce stress and revitalize the adrenal glands, including such practices as yoga, tai chi, and meditation. In the end, getting to the root of what stresses you and addressing it in a proactive way is the start of your own healing.

In traditional Chinese medicine, hot flashes are associated with an excess of yang, or fire energy, and an inadequacy of watery yin energy.

According to Master Nan Lu, it is the amount of energy, or qi, stored within the kidneys that determines the quality of menopause. If there is an imbalance between the amount of energy used and that generated through rest and restoration, we are more likely to develop symptoms.[14]

There are those within the medical profession who view menopause as a pathological condition attributed to a lack of estrogen and progesterone—despite the fact that menopause has been occurring in women at around the same age as far back as records exist, with many of our ancestors living well beyond their centennial birthdays. I cannot accept that the Great Mother, who built us in her image, just ran out of hormones and said, "I'll give each woman enough for fifty years and then she can just fend for herself." No, this change of life was designed perfectly, not as a pathological event, but as a sign of maturity. I suggest that by this time in our lives we have stored enough power and wisdom in our wombs that we do not need to continue the menstrual cycle's monthly flow, for now we are imprinted with the memory of the eternal nature of our existence.

This frees the sacred postmenopausal woman from living within the confines of familial and tribal messages that had defined her when she was younger. Now she can make choices based on her own desires, her inner wisdom, and the inspiration that comes from her heart, and not on the rules and expectations of others. As a younger woman, she entered the valley of death over four hundred times, where she was embraced by the love of the Great Mother in the void, before being reborn. Now her connection to the deep wisdom and strength of the Mother is natural, pure, and direct, enabling her to teach, heal, and lead from a position of feminine power. No longer producing eggs, she can now devote all her creative energy to other projects, especially those that are artistic, restorative, and expansive, feeding her heart with pleasure and great satisfaction. This is a great time to clear out the closets, passing on to others those things that will never again fit, never be read, never be learned— those things that were never comfortable and, frankly, you never liked.

It is to the grandmothers that indigenous peoples have always looked for guidance, wisdom, and discernment, knowing that their judgment would be just and unbiased, for they no longer have a need to please others merely to enhance their own self-esteem. Embodying the archetype of the Crone, these elders have clear insight, a no-nonsense approach, eternal wisdom, and the interests of the greater good always in their sights.

However, such qualities are not a foregone conclusion. Perimenopause represents another death, when the Mother within transforms into the Crone, and so the transition must be honored. This is one of the greatest opportunities for transformation in our lifetime; it leads up to the second time the planet Saturn returns to the place it was in our astrology chart at the time of our birth. Carrying our spiritual blueprint, Saturn demands that between the ages of fifty-six and fifty-nine we look inside and ask ourselves, *Am I fulfilling my soul's destiny?* Even a woman who goes through menopause in her forties will still experience this nudge from Saturn in her late fifties.

If we fail to make the most of the change, then we will probably carry forward unhealthy patterns of behavior or beliefs that can certainly influence our health and well-being as well as our relationships. During menopause we are given a chance to look back at events that occurred around another transition period in our lives, puberty, when we began our transition from Virgin to Mother. Any wounds that we are still carrying from this time will become exaggerated during the Saturn return period, in our soul's search for healing. Menopause gives us the opportunity to delve deep within our psyche, open the pages of old and painful stories, retrieve the bones of wisdom, and move on. An easy menopause does not always mean that there is no unfinished business, merely that the past is well hidden. This is a great time to face the past, clear the clutter from our womb, fully connect to the Great Mother's wisdom within the earth, and become the role model that younger women so desperately need now.

So whether you are still passing through the climacteric or are post-menopausal, here are some simple suggestions:

- Remember that you are now free to follow your own heart and dreams.
- Create sacred time and space in your day, just for you.
- Do things that you would never have done when you were young.
- Whenever possible, stand barefoot, sit, or lie on Mother Earth and relax into her warm embrace, filling your sacral chakra with her energy.
- At the time of the waning moon, make a list of the thoughts, emotions, activities, and even relationships you are ready to release. Read the list as you hold a glass of water, and then pour the water onto the earth or into flowing water such as a creek or stream, asking the Dragon Queen to receive and transform the energy.
- With each new moon, become aware of your heightened intuition. Open yourself to new insights, drawing them into your heart and then into your womb so they can be nurtured and eventually birthed. Have fun—you have achieved what everybody seeks: the freedom to be yourself!

CONDITIONS OF FEMALE IMBALANCE

When patriarchal conditioning and programming of the female psyche continue over many generations, it is inevitable that the distortion of the truth will eventually present itself as physical illness. In this section we will explore some of the most common conditions that affect the fertility organs of women.

Cervical Cancer

Cancer of the cervix is the second most common cancer in women worldwide, with about 500,000 new cases and 250,000 deaths each year. In the United States, about 12,000 women are diagnosed annually with cervical cancer, with 4,000 women dying from the disease. Globally, almost 80 percent of cases occur in low-income countries, with virtually all cervical cancer linked to a genital infection of HPV, or human papilloma virus.[15] Apart from HPV, other known factors in the development of cervical cancer include sex from an early age, multiple partners, and smoking or using drugs; the disease rate is also higher in those from a lower socioeconomic background. The relatively lower incidence and mortality from cervical cancer in developed countries is largely credited to effective screening programs as well as to the recent addition of a vaccine against HPV, offered primarily to teenage girls.

However, I doubt the virus alone is the root of the problem; it is more likely that a weakened immune system allows the virus to proliferate. As we have discovered, cancer in any organ is usually associated with an inadequate sense of love and acceptance of the self and a dependence on others for one's identity, which can negatively impact the immune system. Studies have shown that women diagnosed with cervical cancer often have low levels of sexual arousal, are less likely to experience a vaginal orgasm, and may even have an aversion to sex. It is not uncommon to find a history of sexual or emotional abuse.[16]

Some researchers have also found that they can predict whether a woman with several abnormal smears will progress to cervical cancer by the way she responds to stressful life events. Women with cervical cancer have a tendency to be more passive, codependent, and self-blaming when things go wrong. This is in contrast with women whose smears never show any signs of cancer, who are more likely to take control of a situation and set healthy boundaries in their relationships, especially when it comes to knowing what is their responsibility and what to expect from others.[17] As mentioned earlier in the chapter, to facilitate the healing process, it is helpful to install a strong symbolic doorkeeper who knows how to recognize abusive behavior in others, when to draw the line, and when to close the door on relationships that fail to honor and respect the Goddess.

Fibroids

A fibroid, or myoma, is a benign tumor of the uterus affecting one in five women in their childbearing years. Commonly thought to be dependent on estrogen for their growth and survival, fibroids usually completely disappear at menopause unless a woman decides to take an estrogen-based hormone replacement therapy. They are often asymptomatic, although they can cause heavy bleeding, bleeding between periods, and menstrual cramps. As fibroids grow, they can eventually start to press on the bladder and rectum, causing incontinence, constipation, and even a prolapse. In the United States, fibroids have been found to be three times more common in African American women than in Caucasian women, although the reason for this difference is unclear.

One of the first questions I ask when I meet a woman with fibroids is: "Who takes care of you?" I am often met with tears in response. This is because the uterus, which usually gives power to the voice of one's heart, is most likely devoid of Dragon Queen energy, which means the woman's voice has gone unheard. It is saying, in effect, *What about me?!* Disempowered, such a woman's heart and womb start to cry, and this is expressed as heavy menstrual bleeding.

Healing begins when we start to build healthy structures around our time and space and invite the Dragon Queen to visit. The first thing we need to do is create sacred space, which usually involves letting certain members of our family and circle of friends know that they cannot take up permanent residence in our womb! As we draw dragon strength into the hara, our voice will become stronger, encouraging us to share our needs while also opening us to receive love from others.

Endometriosis

In this condition, the cells that line the uterus are found away from their normal location, such as in the muscles of the uterus, on the ovaries, and even outside the pelvis itself. Since these cells are affected by monthly hormonal changes they also bleed during menses, leading to inflammation and scarring within the pelvic cavity. Endometriosis can lead to infertility and can be asymptomatic or painful, especially around ovulation and during menstruation.

The disease's etiology is still under debate. Some researchers suggest that the problem is present from birth, while others believe that the disease represents a conflict between a woman's drive to be in the masculine world and her desire to express her feminine self. In my experience with women with endometriosis, I have found it very important to look at ancestral beliefs surrounding femininity, especially motherhood, as I see these factors deeply impacting a woman's willingness to embrace her fully feminine self.

Endometrial or Uterine Cancer

This is a commonly diagnosed gynecological cancer, although fortunately the prognosis is good with appropriate treatment. It is rare before the age of forty and usually presents with abnormal or heavy bleeding in women who are peri- or postmenopausal and between the ages of fifty-five and sixty-five. Its appearance has been linked to the intake of therapeutic estrogen without compensatory doses of progesterone, and it is more common in women who never had children or whose menopause occurred after the age of fifty-five. A total hysterectomy is often recommended, although it is important for a woman with endometrial cancer to look at any issues she may have that are connected to an imbalance between her masculine and feminine energies, reflected by her emphasis on work and the time she allows herself for rest and self-care.

Polycystic Ovaries

All disorders of the ovaries are associated with the expression of creativity, fertility, and femininity. Benign ovarian cysts are relatively common during the reproductive years; most are asymptomatic or cause pain that resolves with time. Occasionally these cysts require treatment.

In the past, polycystic disease of the ovaries was regarded as relatively uncommon; however, with enhanced imagery techniques it is now clear that increasing numbers of girls and women are affected by this disease. It is a complex disorder, with multiple causative factors, including underlying emotional distress and hormonal malfunction. Physiologically, the symptoms are seen to be the result of abnormally high levels of the male hormone testosterone, which leads to masculine features such as excess facial hair, as well as acne, weight gain, and recurrent infections, especially candida. Due to inadequate levels of female hormones, the ovaries fail to mature and release their eggs, leading to amenorrhea, infertility, and the appearance of multiple unripe cysts on the surface of the ovaries.

Psychologically, many women with this condition express a deep wound to their femininity, often associated with feminine degradation, sexual abuse, abandonment, and betrayal, causing the masculine aspect of the woman to rise up to protect itself. This leads to heightened levels of circulating stress hormones, which in turn can lead to insulin resistance and the potential for diabetes. As medical herbalist Linda Crockett describes, it is not uncommon for a woman with polycystic ovaries to appear as if she is protected by a hard shell of defensiveness and aggression, yet inside there is a wounded female child and an exhausted male protector.[18] They both need the care and attention of the woman's own inner Dragon Queen, who can offer them nurturing and protection, while the girl within begins to blossom into the woman her body wants to be.

Ovarian Cancer

Ovarian cancer is the fifth most common cancer in women and yet causes the most deaths among the cancers of the fertility organs. This disease most commonly affects women over the age of fifty-five, and its symptoms are unfortunately vague, with the cancer often not being diagnosed until it is well advanced. Symptoms include distension of the abdomen, abdominal pain, constipation, easily becoming full when eating, nausea, sudden weight gain or loss, and persistent lower back pain. Conventional medicine believes there are few, if any, known causative factors. There is little evidence that hormone replacement therapy, the pill, or fertility treatments increase the risk of ovarian cancer. It is more common among Caucasian women and has a much higher incidence in countries like Scandinavia and Switzerland, where the galactose in dairy products such as cottage cheese and yogurt appears to increase the incidence of the disease. Depending on the staging of the cancer, the conventional treatment usually includes removal of the womb and ovaries plus chemotherapy.

I suggest we look at cultural patterns before we decide to isolate a particular food item as the cause of the condition. Since diseases of the ovaries are associated with suppression of our creativity or our dreams, cancer in this area suggests a belief that someone or something is preventing us from planting our seeds, or that our seeds are somehow damaged. This suppression of our natural creativity leaves us feeling frustrated, and yet, as is so often the case with cancer, we feel powerless to change the situation. I have met several women with ovarian cancer whose confidence in their creative abilities had been constantly undermined by critical comments such as "Who do you think you are?" or "You'll never amount to much." Eventually, convinced of their worthlessness, they suppressed their gifts and talents, accepted jobs beneath their skills and passions, married unsupportive men, or stayed in situations far beyond the "sell-by" date.

Heather was fifty-six when she developed ovarian cancer. As a young woman, she was vibrant, clever, and adventurous, but she was never allowed to forget the circumstances of her conception. During her childhood, her mother repeatedly told her that she had been conceived as a result of a loveless one-night stand, which had caused her mother much shame and embarrassment, which she projected onto her daughter as criticism. Heather married a man who continued her mother's disapproval, but she kept any feelings buried under a cheerful and determined demeanor until around the time of her menopause. Then, as she passed through her dark night of the soul, all the emotions of unworthiness, shame, and rejection that had infiltrated her eggs as she lay in her mother's womb erupted in a highly aggressive form of cancer.

She immediately underwent surgery and started chemotherapy, although her doctors weren't optimistic about the outcome. But she was surrounded by a group of amazing women friends who truly loved her in ways she had never allowed herself to feel before the cancer. Through their gentle probing, she began to share all the deeply buried emotions, especially the anger she felt toward her mother, who, now dead, had never seen Heather as anything but a loveless mistake. She wrote letters she never sent to her mother and to her unknown father, both of whom had abandoned her, making her feel worthless. She also started to accept that her own marriage was loveless and certainly void of respect and honor for the beautiful and desirable woman she was. She stayed with her friends during the treatment, strengthened by their love and understanding to the point that she started divorce proceedings.

One of her friends had an art studio, and Heather found herself spending more and more time there, rekindling a love of painting and drawing that had been lost due to a lack of encouragement in her family home. She found that she could express her feelings far more easily on canvas than in words, painting with wild moves and bold colors in great contrast to her previously demure character. In time she found a perfect apartment where she could continue her art, entertain friends, and decorate exactly as she chose. She lived another ten years after the diagnosis—many years beyond her doctors' expectations—happy, content, surrounded by the jewels of her own creation and friends who loved her unconditionally.

This story reminds us how important it is for parents to set aside their own expectations for a child and instead provide the incoming soul with love, encouragement, and nurturing, so that the creative flower within that young person's soul can flourish and find full and joyous expression in the world.

THE TRANSFORMATIVE POWER OF CYCLES

We are spiritual beings born of a unified field living in a world of dual-ity, and our purpose is to move energy or consciousness between the two different planes of existence. The two basic processes that assist us in this transfer of energy are known colloquially as sex and birth: Sex moves our awareness from self-identification and individuality to union within the collective consciousness of the Great Mother, remembering that every relationship is a sacred sexual experience. Birth, both physical and inspirational, moves our awareness from the unified consciousness of the no-thingness to self-identity. Women are natural vessels for both of these currents, which are expressed in cycles of three, just as there are three trimesters of pregnancy, three main phases of sexual arousal, three stages of menstruation, and three aspects of archetypal womanhood, the Virgin, the Mother, and the Crone.

> **The Virgin** represents new beginnings, inspiration, focus, excite-ment, desire, and creativity, as seen during the first trimester, the follicular phase of menstruation, and the excitement or desire phase of sexual arousal. This takes place in the sacral chakra dur-ing sex and the crown chakra during birth.
>
> **The Mother** reflects acceptance, trust, openness, comfort, and nur-turing, as seen in the second trimester, the luteal phase of men-struation, and the plateau phase of lovemaking. This stage always occurs in the heart chakra.
>
> **The Crone** symbolizes powerful release, ecstasy, purification, and ful-fillment, as seen during the third trimester, the moon time, and the orgasmic phase of sexual union. This stage takes place in the crown chakra during sex and in the sacral chakra during birth.

Cycles of Life

So why does it matter that we cycle? Alignment with our natural cycles ensures our creativity, connectivity, and transformation. Everything in nature follows a cyclical pattern. From our perspective, the sun appears to rise in the morning, reach its maximum height by noon, and then set in the evening. It is then hidden from view at nighttime before reemerging at dawn. The moon follows a similar pattern over twenty-eight days. Its light grows in size until it appears in all its glory at full moon, then it wanes until there is only darkness for a period of three days. The four seasons of the year are similarly divided into a time of nurturing, growth, and creativity in the spring; full blooming in the summer; harvesting and storing in the fall; and silence and darkness—metaphorical death—in the winter. What is consistent in each of these examples is that full expression is later followed by death, and death is always followed by birth. Even our breath shows the same pattern: inhalation (birth) follows exhalation (death) and so on. You cannot have one without the other. Birth and death are inextricably linked, and they are intrinsic to the purpose of the uterus. Indeed, the womb of great goddesses like Isis, Artemis, and Kali was seen to be both a womb *and* a tomb, a place of birth and death.

The ancients clearly understood that this is our covenant with the Great Mother. She promises to continually fill us with pure inspiration from her primordial waters, so that through creative manifestation we are fed and nourished. But this agreement is made on one condition: although we can enjoy and be expanded by our creations, we should never try to possess or become possessed by them. As with the dying sun and moon, there will come a time when we will be required to offer back to the Great Mother the seeds of our experiences, better known as wisdom, so she can grow in consciousness. Once the seeds are implanted in the womb of the Mother, then the experience itself dies, for it has fulfilled its purpose. Nothing is permanent; this is a Universal Law.

Our ancestors agreed to this covenant by reenacting the death-to-life scenario through sacred ritual. In this case, a man would be chosen to sleep with the priestess who represented the Great Mother so that he could plant his seed in her womb. Once this was done, he symbolically died, for he had completed his mission. Her eggs were fertilized with his seed, and new life emerged out of the void. If, like our ancestors, we accept these conditions, we will experience a life without fear, with all our soul's needs met as we pass through cycles of death and birth. If, however, we forget our promise and choose to hang on to our creations rather than relinquish them to the Goddess, then we will face continuous anxiety, greed, poverty, and hunger, and eventually the flow of inspiration will cease because it cannot find space for birth.

Many great civilizations have imploded because they didn't follow the basic rules of life. Enjoy, celebrate, and be nourished by the fruit of your endeavors, but remember that anything or anyone you try to possess—your children, material goods, your stories, even your beliefs—will eventually prevent your inner growth and expansion. Once we start to live in fear of loss, hoard our achievements, attempt to control the future, or try to acquire what is not ours through force, then we are on the slippery slope to our own destruction. This is not divine retribution, it is causation; if we try to hold on beyond the expiration date, then death will come to find us and we will be made to let go.

The irony is that on a spiritual level, our greatest desire is in fact to die to the experience so we can once again surrender to the wisdom and love of the Great Mother, until it is time to be reborn. Here we experience everything and no-thing; we are boundless and totally at home. It is here that we can sense the inner strength of deep connectivity, where any decisions we make impact not only our own lives but all of humanity, the planet, and the universe. We can experience this magical place now, by breathing in, exhaling, and floating in the pause at the end of a full exhalation. For these few seconds, before the next inhalation, we are held in the timeless mystery of nothingness, and all is well. Death and birth are merely two sides of the same coin, similar to night and day. It is our ability to live between the two because we have no fear that creates the magic.

This understanding of the covenant sheds new light on the story of Adam and Eve. It was Eve who, it is said, ate of the fruit offered to her and whose eyes were first opened to the knowledge of death and birth. Because of her courage in following her intuition despite punitive threats, she, and all the women who have followed, was chosen to carry the wisdom of eternal life through the acceptance of these cycles of death and birth, as manifest in the menstrual cycle and as stored within the womb. This is a divine gift. With such wisdom comes tremendous power and strength, for when you consciously enter the darkness every month and are reborn, there is no fear of death.

The Creatrix decided that when a woman has passed through three cycles of her moon's passage between the sun and Earth, or approximately three cycles of eighteen years, she no longer needs the physical reminder of the covenant—the menstrual cycle—for now she has embodied the wisdom of immortality. This is the reason why the average woman completes menopause around the age of fifty-four, for astronomically it takes this amount of time for the moon to return to the exact place it was at the time of one's birth; in astronomy this is known as a triple saros cycle.* It has nothing to do with failing hormones—rather, it is the readiness of the postmenopausal crone to step forward as an inspirational and transformational leader, strengthened by the knowledge that death holds no sting, for without it there is no growth.

The Great Mother knows that a woman's innate desire for connection with her ensures that she never forgets the covenant; and yet we have seemingly forgotten. We women of the modern world have abandoned our eternal nature, and like men we live in fear of death, holding on tightly to our creations, whether they be objects, thoughts, emotions, stories, relationships, or fantasies. This disharmony manifests in both mental and physical illnesses that will not be healed until women, individually and collectively, remember their covenant with the Great Mother and start to share this knowledge with their families.

---

*The saros is a period of approximately eighteen years and eleven days when Earth, the sun, and the moon are aligned and therefore can be used to predict eclipses. In astrology, it relates to the north and south nodes of the moon in our natal chart and is commonly used to predict our soul's destiny in this lifetime.

Cleansing and Purification

The cycle naturally starts at what is often thought to be the end, the menses or moon time. I believe this is why the timing of a pregnancy begins on the first day of the last period; all birth starts with a process of cleansing and purification. As a young obstetrician, we would always perform a D and C (dilation and curettage) after a miscarriage, clearing away all the products of the last pregnancy before a woman tried for a new baby. We need to be willing to scrape away from our wombs remnants of unfulfilled dreams, hurts, disappointments, and regrets; otherwise there is no space for new life.

Although the description below focuses on the menstruating woman, every woman needs to go through the same procedure on a regular basis whatever her age, or whether she has a uterus or not, to fulfill her destiny as a sacred woman. The best time for this is during the three days of a dark moon.

According to Native American healer and seer Jean Reddemann, every month during her reproductive years, a traditional native woman gathers from her family and tribe all that is dead and finished into her womb, saving the seeds of wisdom and releasing the feelings of sadness and grief in her menstrual blood. This includes the energy from unfulfilled dreams, finished relationships, and disappointments. This is the reason why many native women, when possible, stay away from other people during their moon time, as this is the time a woman cleanses herself and her family of unwanted energy; she doesn't want to return it to them through the food she's prepared or the people she touches, so she sequesters herself. Unfortunately, this has led to the mistaken (patriarchal) belief that a menstruating woman is "unclean" and therefore to be shunned or shamed. In truth, she is at the peak of her power during this time, as her womb is acting as a fiery cauldron, breaking down everything into its essential form so it can be either given up to the Great Mother as wisdom or released back to Mother Earth.

Indigenous women have different viewpoints on whether a woman on her moon should have intercourse with a man. Most agree that at

the very least, at the beginning of the period, when the flow i
a woman should stay away from men and refrain from sexual
She is, in effect, processing dead energy; she is also in her greatest
power, which can drain a man's energy. However, in the later stages of
the moon time, as a woman focuses her receiving inspiration, it is then
possible—only if the woman desires sexual contact—for a man's awareness to be carried up along his partner's serpentine energy pathways
during intercourse so that he too can enter the Great Mother's abundant source of inspiration.

Once a woman stops menstruating it is even more important for
her to find time every month to release unwanted energy into the earth,
so that she can be cleansed and make space for new inspiration. If she
does not make time for cleansing, she may find her body discharging
unwanted energy in other ways, such as through a cold, vomiting, or
diarrhea. The uterus has even been known to start to bleed again, several years after menopause, due to the body's need to discharge accumulated grief.

Although inherently men are dependent on their women to cleanse
the emotions and stories of the past, there are times when a man may wish
to retreat from the outer world and spend time alone, to remind himself
of the impermanence of life. Traditionally, this takes place in caves or on
hillsides, both of which resemble the features of the Great Mother. For
the Lakota, the *inipi,* or sweat lodge, is representative of the womb of
the Great Mother, with all members of the tribe entering its womblike
confines for the process of purification and renewal.

☽

RITUAL NO. I
Cleansing and Purification:
Separating the Gems from the Compost

Whether during menstruation or during the dark moon for postmenopausal
women, the first step to the cleansing process is to share the stories. An ideal
scenario is for women to gather together in sacred circle, perhaps creating a

"Red Tent" menstruation hut, or simply a place of nurturing where food and creature comforts are in abundance, although this process can also be carried out alone. Since we know that women are the embodiment of the Great Mother, the creator of all life, the first condition of telling a story of our life is to take ownership of its creation. This is one of the most challenging parts of the process, programmed as we have been by the patriarchy to see ourselves as victims of our lives against which we must struggle, suffer, or battle. Unless we understand that our soul has created the experience or story for a purpose—even if that purpose is not yet understood—then we can never be in the position to make choices to change the circumstances of our life.

It sometimes helps to ask the following questions to stimulate our thoughts before sharing—concentrating, in particular, on events of the past month:

- What dreams or fantasies am I holding onto that will never be fulfilled?
- What friendship or relationship cannot be revived?
- Where am I giving love in the delusional belief that it will reciprocated?
- What expectations do I carry that can never be fulfilled?
- Where am I procrastinating? What am I afraid will happen if I make a decision?
- What activities no longer stimulate me or enable me to grow?
- Where am I still attached to my own stories from the past because they evoke emotions such as anger, pain, disappointment, and shame?
- What seeds of wisdom do I need to glean from the situation that will allow me to move on?
- What beliefs am I holding onto that are limiting the freedom to be me?
- What situation am I clinging to that offers security and little else?

If we are in circle, once we start to share our story our sisters act as witnesses, remaining silent, listening with open and compassionate hearts. It is important to share how we feel—whatever the sensations—as emotions allow for full expression of our creation. If we are alone, we may wish to write our story in a journal. However, after a set period of time, the telling of our story must end. A period of silence ensues, and in the case of a circle, then the next sister starts to share. This helps us remember that we are not our story and that at the end of this process we need to ask ourselves, "Why did my soul create this experience?" and "What pearls of wisdom am I going to take from the situation?" Remember that the only reason to manifest our dreams or ideas is to collect the gems of wisdom or consciousness and give them lovingly to the Great Mother so her consciousness can expand.

At the end of the sharing, we are left with a collection of gems or pearls, which we place in our hearts to be offered to the spiritual Great Mother when we ascend to the crown chakra. We are also left with a pile of emotions, beliefs, and unfilled dreams, which we are ready to discard to the Dragon Queen. You may wish to mirror the actions of the traditional native women and gather the unwanted energy from your family—even from those who are deceased— collecting into your womb their pain and regrets. Now it is time to ask the great Mother Earth to receive these emotions and this completed energy from the dying stories, knowing that she is able to transform anything, just as she transforms fallen leaves into compost.

The next step of the ritual is best carried out by a woman wearing a skirt (preferably without underwear) or even naked. However, it is important to feel comfortable and not self-conscious during any female ritual, or else deep emotions such as shame can be evoked, which dilute the purpose of the practice. If you are menstruating, you may decide to find a sacred place in nature and, squatting down, bleed some of your blood into the ground as an offering to Mother Earth. Otherwise you can join the postmenopausal women or those who do not bleed on a regular basis and, taking a glass of pure water, infuse it with all the energy you wish to release. Then, whether squatting or standing with your feet firmly on the earth, say a prayer as you pour the water or the blood onto the earth, saying: "Mother Earth, as I cleanse and purify my womb so I may receive new inspiration, I ask with gratitude that you should accept this blood/water filled with old emotions (tears, anger, anxiety, etc.) and redundant beliefs on behalf of myself, my family, and the generations still to come."

As we die to our old stories and empty our wombs or vessels into the earth, we find our energy naturally connecting with the womb of the Great Mother, deep within the earth. Here, in the moments after the cleansing prayer, we find ourselves bobbing on slowly moving waves of molten energy—the pure transformative energy of the Dragon Queen or the primordial waters. We may wish to lie or sit on the earth or, more appropriately, enter water, where we can gently let the water support our weight, or even lie on an airbed.

Bobbing on the Mother's Ocean

In this place of death, we are embraced by ancient grandmothers who instill in us a reassuring peace that there is nothing that we have experienced in our life that hasn't been experienced by generations of women throughout the ages. There is no emotion that we have felt that hasn't been felt before. This collective knowing, endowed with compassion, is the ancient wisdom of all women. It is as if the Great Mother is saying, "You and I are one; your tears are my tears, your story is my story. Like waves in an ocean, there will be times of highs and lows; these are all part of the cycles of life that flow through your body. In the sharing and release come healing; rest awhile in my warm embrace."

My most precious memory of meeting such ancient wisdom and love is from about ten years ago when I was privileged to swim among mother and baby humpback whales in the Caribbean. There was one magical moment when I found myself floating on the surface of the ocean as two large mothers rose up beneath. Awed by the gentle strength these mighty creatures possessed, I didn't move but felt their combined energy explode into my base chakra and then move swiftly along my spine, causing an amazing orgasmic release. I knew this was my initiation in ancient woman wisdom.

Sometimes, when our heart is full of sadness or we feel overwhelmed with anxiety, we cannot wait for a dark moon or our menses to cleanse and purify. Then the whole process described above can be carried out at the end of the day, asking the setting sun to carry our tears or anxiety into Mother Earth, giving an offering, as before, of water infused with gratitude and unwanted emotions.

Cleansing the Tears of the World

There are times when our womb becomes the cauldron for the tears of the world. On a gorgeous sunny day in 1996, I was on a ferryboat crossing the deep and sacred waters of Lake Atitlan in Guatemala. This stretch of water is among the most beautiful in the world, formed from the eruptions of several sacred mountains, all seats of the Dragon Queen. As the boat moved through the choppy blue waters, I felt a wave of anguish and despair rise up and settle in my sacral chakra. Immediately, a tremendous sadness mixed with despair and confusion passed through my body, and my womb began to weep with blood, uncontrollably. Totally unprepared for this impromptu bleeding, I changed my plans, and instead of going sightseeing with the rest of the group I found myself entering the home of a sweet and caring Mayan woman, who found me sanitary pads and soothed my soul. Only later did I realize that my uterus was being used to cleanse, purify, and release

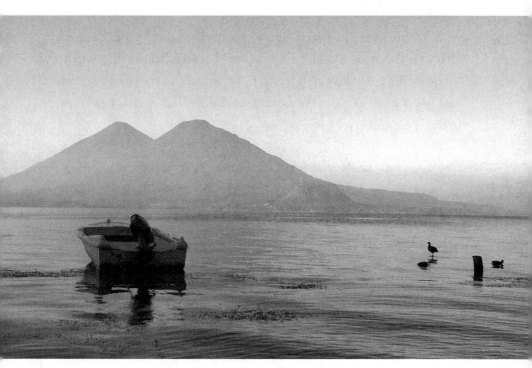

Lake Atitlan, Guatemala

the great sadness that had settled around the lake from 1960 to 1996, when an estimated 200,000 native people died in unspeakable atrocities during a civil war that ravished the country.

Another memorable occasion when my uterus wept, not only for myself but for millions of people, was on the day that Princess Diana died. This woman epitomized in her short life so many different faces of the Great Mother. I was listening to the sad news as I drove home from a seminar when I felt a surge of emotion enter my body, and all of a sudden blood was flowing down my legs, across the car seat, and onto the floor. Somehow I made it to the women's room, stripped as best as I could, and started to wash my bloody clothing; all this time I was surrounded by other women, all of whom were obviously numbed by the shock of Diana's death. As the bloodstained water drained away, it felt as if it was carrying all the sadness and pain back to the primordial waters from which all events arise, even death. In that moment, it was clear I did not have to cry alone, nor did I have to carry the world on my shoulders.

Over the years, I have come to accept that there is only one thing that everybody needs, and that is love. I remember the day when the Great Mother spoke very clearly to my heart: *Remember, your love is enough. Let go of the need to understand or fix the situation. Love is always enough.*

You can remain bobbing on the ocean of the Great Mother for as long as you choose, allowing all the stress and concerns of your life to dissipate into her eternal waters. I often hear her reassuring words, "This too will pass." When you are ready, it is time to revitalize and empower the womb and sacral chakra with dragon energy and reawaken the slumbering kundalini in the base chakra by reconnecting it to the source of its power. If your practice is taking place during the dark moon, the cleansing, purification, bobbing, and revitalization should all take place on the first day. If this ritual is occurring at sunset, this is the last process before the practice is complete for the night.

☉

RITUAL NO. 2
Revitalizing the Womb with Dragon Energy

Stand on the earth barefoot, if at all possible, with your feet slightly apart so that the vaginal opening is facing the ground. In this position your legs act as the piercing stone mentioned previously, attracting the serpent energy to start to climb up your legs, just as a serpent curves around a stick. Gently bend your knees and take your awareness to the root chakra, about twenty-four inches under the soles of your feet. This is where the dragon energy from the primordial waters gathers in our auric field.

Now, inhaling through the nose, slowly start to draw the dragon energy up your body, aware of how it naturally wants to wind around your legs. On exhalation, allow the dragon energy to retreat slightly back toward the root chakra, creating a wavelike motion with your breath. On the next inhalations draw the dragon energy farther and farther up your legs—not rushing the process, for the Dragon Queen is in control. You are just the snake charmer, using your breath as sweet music to entice the serpent to climb.

As the fiery, fluidic dragon energy reaches the top of your thighs, it starts to gather around the vulva and you may find yourself becoming sexually aroused. Try not to allow these sensations to evoke an orgasm, for at this point it will only affect your nervous system. But as the energy increases in the vulva, you will feel your whole magnetic field start to light up as the dragon energy ignites your erogenous zones. This is your signal that mastery of this energy is now in your hands; the Dragon Queen has relinquished her control to you.

Place your hands together with thumbs and fingertips touching to create a downward-pointing triangle over your sacral chakra to bring attention to the fact that this is the new lair or home of this energy. As the now serpentine energy passes through the vulvar opening, use the techniques of contracting and relaxing the vaginal muscles learned in the previous exercises to gently draw the energy, in a circular or spiraling manner, if possible, toward the top of the vagina and the doorway of the womb, the cervix. If you are still becoming familiar with these muscles, using visual imagery to imagine the movement can be just as effective. Once again use your breath to assist the speed of the process, remembering that a slow, wavelike motion of contraction and relaxation is preferable.

As the energy builds around the top of the vagina, kundalini joyfully awakens after thousands of years of disconnection from her mother, the Dragon Queen. For so long she has been under the control of the patriarchy; now she stretches and enjoys the freedom of her own power. As she playfully encircles the cervix, your doorkeeper becomes stronger and more confident. Then, with the doorkeeper's permission, slowly allow the serpent energy to pass through the short passageway and begin to curl around the inside of the womb, just as it does inside a mighty mountain. Continue the process, using your breath to modify the speed, until the energy of the sacral chakra underneath your hands feels warm and full.

Finally, with your hands still over the hara, imagine an umbilical cord that stretches between the root chakra deep within the earth and the sacral chakra, ensuring a pure and steady connection between your womb and Mother Earth, from which you draw your feminine energy. Beginning at the hara, inhale and then exhale slowly and deeply down along this umbilical cord and into the root chakra. Repeat the breath three times. At the end of the third exhalation, pause and experience a vast peace as you are washed in the waves of mystery, nothingness, and thousands of years of women's wisdom.

Now, inhale and draw the energy back up along the umbilical cord and into your sacral chakra under your hands, repeating the process until your womb is full. Feel the strength and joy as the energy vitalizes and nurtures your energy field. Feel the inner power, knowing you are eternally connected to the full creative force and wisdom of what it is to be a sacred woman.

Even though throughout this process we have been focusing on a dark moon (or perhaps sunset) ritual, I find that after so many thousands of years of disconnection, it is invaluable to renew and strengthen this connection every morning when I first place my feet on the ground. Each time I am rewarded with a deep sense of love and wisdom from all the grandmothers who have gone before.

The serpent will rest in the womb until the next chapter, when we move into the heart chakra.

Today our world faces many of the same crisis points that other civilizations have reached in the distant past before their collapse, when they failed to reinstate the feminine to her rightful position. Now we are being given the same choice. Let us, as women, whatever age we may be, remember the covenant with the Great Mother and honor the cycles, freeing ourselves from the fear of death and teaching our children the mysteries of eternal life.

A woman's body is an alchemical vessel that possesses the power, wisdom, and knowledge to bring about transformation and enlightenment. For far too long we have submitted to patriarchal thinking and rejected our body's seeming imperfections, illogical rhythms, and chaotic expressions. Yet when we stop fighting our body and allow it to do its work, we find ourselves embodying its mysteries and becoming a formidable force that refuses to be hidden or suppressed any longer.

PART THREE

The Mother Cow

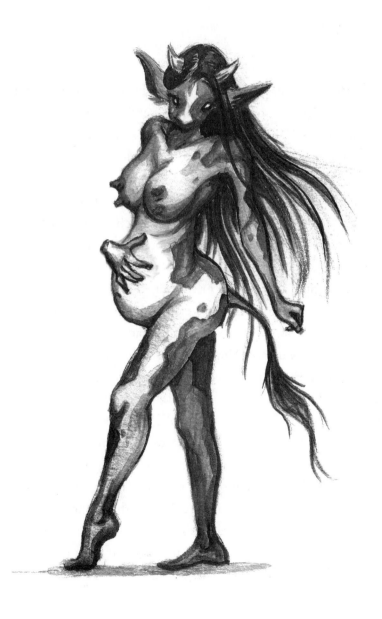

7

BREASTS, BEAUTIFUL BREASTS

O f all the organs in the body, it is the breast that most commonly differentiates women from men, serving as the primary symbol of femininity in most cultures. If you ask the majority of women to describe the role of their breasts, they would probably say that it is the feeding and nurturing of children first, followed, to a lesser extent, by sensual pleasure. Yet how many of us are taught to appreciate our breasts as sacred temples of love through which the nectar of immortality flows? How often do we show appreciation of our breasts with a compassionate look at them or the soft touch of our hands? Do we give ourselves time after a bath or shower to massage our breasts, perhaps with aromatic moisturizing creams, to enjoy their perfect shape and size? Or is it only during a self-examination that we squeeze and prod them in the fear of finding that sinister lump?

And if a lump is discovered, how much do we know about the complex relationship a woman has with her breasts, especially when faced with cancer and the possibility of a mastectomy? It wasn't until my diagnosis of breast cancer that I became passionately attached to my breasts, savoring their every little curve and wrinkle. I learned, in retrospect, that there was a moment just prior to my surgery when the radiologist shared his doubts with the surgeon that a lumpectomy alone would be sufficient. I am so grateful for the confidence and skill of my surgeon, especially when I woke up and saw the swell of two breasts beneath the bandages.

As we will discover, our breasts are part of a deep collective mythology linked to love, nurturing, trust, and transformation, which stretches far beyond the individual and into the bosom of the Great Mother herself. In the presence of breast disease, these are the issues that require our attention. Over thousands of years, as the memory of the sacredness of the female body has faded, many women have come to see their breasts as vulnerable organs, linked to feelings of powerlessness and inadequacy. This perception emerges not only from a perceived flaw in terms of their shape and size, but because of the very aspect that makes them beautiful: their soft and sensual nature.

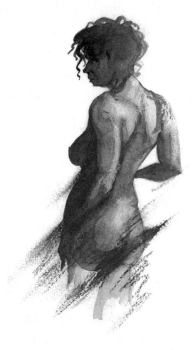

The soft and sensual nature of the breast

Unlike our four-legged mammalian sisters, whose teats are safely hidden on their underbelly and protrude only when the mammary glands are full of milk, the human breasts are exposed all the time. If we compare the physical strength of the breast with that of other organs, mammary tissue is practically defenseless, containing minimal muscle and no bone or cartilage. The breast is supported entirely by the overlying skin and fibrous ligaments that anchor it to the muscles of the chest wall. Because of this lack of protection, the breasts have been subject to more physical abuse than any other organ in the body. However, even though we cannot change their physical vulnerability—except perhaps by wearing a steel bra, which I highly discourage—we can increase the inner strength of our breasts by honoring them as uniquely perfect and sacred in every way.

When I first began to research these precious feminine attributes, I was surprised by the scarcity of information available except as it applies to three specific areas: eroticism, augmentation, and cancer. This focus on extremes is, I believe, because of centuries of misinformation about the divine nature of the breast, which continues to the present, despite the liberation years of feminism. Such a distortion of the truth is highly relevant when it comes to looking at the causative factors associated with breast disease. The lack of ownership of these feminine icons is explored in an inspiring and detailed book by Marilyn Yalom called *A History of the Breast*. In the introduction, she asks, "Who owns the breast?" Then she questions:

> Does it belong to the suckling child whose life is dependent on a mother's milk or an effective substitute? Does it belong to the man or woman who fondles it? Does it belong to the artist who represents the female form or the fashion arbiter who chooses small or large breasts according to the market's continual demand for a new style? Does it belong to the clothing industry who promotes "training bras" for pubescent girls, the "support bra" for older women and the Wonderbra for women wanting more noticeable cleavage? Does it belong to religious and moral judges who insist that the breast be chastely covered? Does it belong to the law, which can order the arrest of "topless" women? Does it belong to the doctor who decides how often breasts should be mammogrammed and then when they should be biopsied or removed? Does it belong to the plastic surgeon who restructures it for purely cosmetic reasons? Does it belong to the pornographer who buys the rights to expose women? Or does it belong to the woman for whom breasts are parts of her own body?[1]

I have to admit that my breasts and I haven't always had a close relationship—that is, until relatively recently. This was partly influenced by the messages I received from my mother, whose breasts were large and voluptuous, probably a size 40DD, and who stated until her dying day that if she ever won the lottery she would pay for a breast reduction. As a child I never saw any problem with her bosom; I was proud of how she dressed in showing great respect for her symbol of femininity. Yet as I matured into womanhood, I came to understand her challenges: the difficulty of finding bras that fit properly, the weight of the breasts causing the straps of the bra to dig into her skin, and the strain on her back.

Mum was delighted that my sister and I inherited our smaller breast size from the other side of the family, although it was evident that clothing requiring a cleavage was not for me. But with my mother's focus on the problems that went with having large breasts, I learned little from her about the reverence they deserved and the pleasure they could give. As is the case even for many teenagers today, the discussion surrounding breasts in the 1960s was whether they were too small or too large, and of course the big question was: would they attract the opposite sex? I can still remember doing exercises to increase the pectoral muscles of my chest, in the mistaken belief that my breast size would grow as a result. I also remember being embarrassed that my perky nipples were clearly visible through my clothing, especially when it was cold, causing me to pad my bras so I wouldn't appear too "forward."

Despite the easy recall of these memories, I cannot remember any conversation about the positive experiences of possessing breasts, apart from the opportunity to feed future babies. So, when researching this book, I asked my close "bosom" friends, "How do you feel about your breasts? Do you like them, and has this always been the case?" I was surprised by their answers, not because their opinions were particularly uncommon among women, but because I'd known these women for over twenty years and I had never heard their breast stories.

One friend told me that her husband approved of the size of her breasts only when she was pregnant, which was the only time she felt confident enough to wear a bikini. At all other times he ignored her completely as a sensual and desirable woman. Another vivacious friend told me that when she was in her twenties, her breasts were so voluptuous that when she walked along the beach she was followed by comments and whistles from men. This made her so self-conscious that she constantly wore baggy shirts to hide her natural curves.

Both of these tales revolve around the opinions of men, and yet I perceive that this isn't merely because their views are dominant, but because we women are confused about the appropriate relationship we should be having with our own gorgeous breasts. So here are some questions I want to ask all women:

- Who taught you that your breasts are sacred?
- Who taught you that when you focus positive attention on your breasts, your heart opens to receive love?
- Who taught you that your breasts' signature curves and softness ensure that care, compassion, and trust are the basis of all true human relationships?
- Who taught you to celebrate their unique shape and size, just as they are?
- Who taught you that these wonderful icons of femininity maintain a loving connection between our spiritual and earthly life?
- Who taught you that the breasts nourish not only a newborn baby but also your dreams and visions, enabling the consciousness of the human race to grow?
- Who taught you that the exquisite sensitivity found especially around the nipple is the elixir that creates a loving bond between mother and baby?
- Who taught you that stimulation of the breasts' sensuality usually leads to the activation of other erogenous zones, causing your whole body to be revitalized?
- Who taught you that since the breasts are sacred temples, nobody

should touch or surgically alter them without first receiving permission from the Goddess within?

THE HEART CHAKRA

It is no coincidence that the breasts are situated on either side of the heart chakra, which sits in the center of the chest. It is through this sacred center that we maintain our connection to the Great Mother's love and are reminded that through a healthy balance of loving ourselves while loving and nurturing others, the eternal fire of creativity is kept burning. It is also through the heart chakra that we connect to the pulse of our soul and our intuition, which keeps us true to the destiny we have chosen in this lifetime.

As we will learn, the heart chakra is the site of transformation within our chakra system, the place where energy shifts take place between spirit and matter, dreams and reality. All of this is dependent on the pure love that radiates from the heart chakra and is amplified by the breasts, encouraging us to surrender, trust, and bond to all that we can be in this life.

THE DESIGN OF THE BREAST

Before we proceed into this subject, we need to understand how these representatives of soft benevolence and love were transformed into objects of lust, dissatisfaction, and disease. To answer these questions, let's go back to the basics and review the perfect design created by the Great Mother.

The Developing Breast

During the fourth week of gestation, the human fetus, like all mammals, develops two mammary ridges, or milk lines, that run from the inner groin to the armpit. Since the number of nipples in the animal kingdom relates to the number of expected offspring, by the fifth week of gestation all the unnecessary breast tissue disappears, leaving in most humans only two primary mammary buds, located at the level of the heart chakra. In approximately 3 percent of men and women, however, the milk line does not dissolve completely, leading to the presence of extra breast tissue, including nipples, along the milk line's length.

Over the next few months, these mammary buds continue to develop in both sexes until, at birth, each breast consists of fifteen to twenty lobes of glandular tissue, each with its own lactiferous (milk) duct, opening into the nipple. On the surface, the nipple is surrounded by a pigmented areola, the whole area being highly sensitized through a rich nerve supply. It is not uncommon to grow hairs around the nipple that have their own glands that produce sweat and pheromones, similar to the hairs in the armpits and in the pubic area. It has been shown that a baby around six weeks of age can differentiate between the aroma of its own mother's breast and that of a stranger, a natural survival instinct.[2]

The Blooming Breast

After a child is born, its breast tissue remains relatively quiescent until the influx of hormones that herald puberty. In a girl, this can occur anywhere between the ages of seven and thirteen, depending on ethnicity and environment. During this time, under the influence of estrogen from the ovaries, the breasts begin to fill out with fat and fibrous tissue, and the simple duct system starts to develop multiple branches. With the onset of menstruation some one to two years later, maturation of the breasts continues, with each lobe forming multiple lobules and secretory alveoli, the eventual source of milk. This feature of acquiring fully formed mammary organs long before the need to suckle a child is unique in humans.

I was eight years old when the puberty switch was activated within my psyche. I desperately wanted to go swimming in the sea, and yet, despite my parents' encouragement, I felt suddenly embarrassed, as I had nothing to cover my breasts. Until that day, being topless hadn't been an issue, but suddenly I felt self-conscious, even though there was very little to see of my developing breasts.

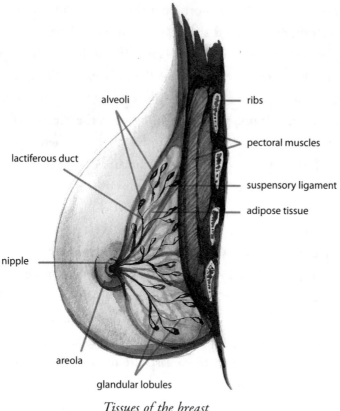

alveoli

lactiferous duct

nipple

areola

glandular lobules

ribs

pectoral muscles

suspensory ligament

adipose tissue

Tissues of the breast

Development of the breasts continues under the influence of hormones such as estrogen, growth hormones, and prolactin, until about five years after the onset of puberty, when fat tissue accounts for between 80 and 85 percent of the total structure. In many cases, breast development is asymmetrical. This usually corrects itself, although up to 25 percent of women have a persistent, visible breast asymmetry and may seek surgical reconstruction. It is noteworthy that symmetrical breasts are an indicator of fertility and may in fact influence a man when choosing a suitable mate.[3]

The Cyclic Breast

Except for during pregnancy and immediately afterward, when breast-feeding, the breasts maintain their basic shape and size, with minor changes occurring due to hormonal shifts, especially before a period. Each month, during the first half of the menstrual cycle, estrogen stimulates growth of the milk ducts. Then in the luteal phase, progesterone stimulates the development of the milk glands in preparation for pregnancy and the production of milk, causing the breasts to marginally increase in size. If pregnancy does not occur, the breasts will return to their normal size. Up to 80 percent of women experience premenstrual swelling, pain, or tenderness in their breasts during their reproductive life, often associated with other symptoms of PMS.

The Sensual Breast

Despite the fact that a woman's breasts are commonly considered icons of sexuality, especially by the opposite sex, the woman herself may not experience them as erogenous zones, with sensitivity to touch varying greatly among different women. For some women, breast stimulation alone, especially of the nipple, can lead to an orgasm, especially at certain times of the month when the breasts are more sensitive; other women are numb to such contact. These variations from woman to woman are not anatomical. Whether your breasts are large or small, they contain the

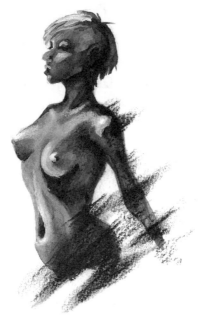

Breasts are commonly considered icons of sexuality.

same number of highly sensitized nerve endings, with the greatest concentration being found in the nipple, areola, and upper quadrants of the breast. Any desensitization, therefore, is rooted in a woman's psyche, and it is usually the result of dissatisfaction concerning one's own breasts as well as a past history of insensitive or abusive touch.

As the sensitivity of a woman's breasts naturally changes from day to day, month to month, and year to year in response to her hormones, it is essential that she communicates the quality of caress she requires to satisfy her needs. The more relaxed and safe a woman feels, the more she will experience sexual pleasure and arousal through stimulation and massage of her breasts.

The Breast during Pregnancy

A few weeks after a woman conceives, a variety of changes occur, beginning with a growing tenderness of the breasts and nipples, a darkening of the pigmented areolae, and an increased erection of the nipples. Under the influence of estrogen and progesterone, the milk ducts and glandular tissues expand, leading to a marked increase in the size of the breasts, often by one or two cup sizes.

Despite these changes and the fact that most women are designed to breast-feed, it is not a foregone conclusion. Problems with the baby latching on to the breast, sore nipples, and engorged breasts can leave mother and baby feeling frustrated and despondent. During pregnancy, the secretion of prolactin, mainly from the anterior pituitary gland, stimulates the mammary glands, or alveoli, to prepare to produce milk—although, because of the high levels of circulating progesterone in the mother, actual milk production is inhibited until just after the baby is born. Often called "the mothering hormone," prolactin produces a calming and protective effect, causing the woman to act like a mother lion who serenely shields her offspring from intruders. It has been noted that there is also a rise in the expectant father's prolactin levels, by 25 percent, encouraging him, perhaps, to be a more protective and loving partner.[4]

As soon as the placenta is delivered, prolactin levels fall unless the nipple is stimulated by the suckling of the baby at the breast. When this occurs, prolactin secretion leads to the full production of milk as quickly as twenty-four to forty-eight hours after childbirth. As long as lactation continues, prolactin levels remain high, inhibiting the production of estrogen and hence ovulation. This form of natural birth control is estimated to be 98 percent effective—much more successful than a diaphragm or condom—and has been used by women for thousands of years. It is probably the reason why women of nobility were discouraged from breast-feeding during the Middle Ages, as the high level of infant mortality required a woman to produce many children in order to maintain the family lineage. Instead, the baby was passed along to a wet nurse, whose breasts provided milk and comfort for the child. Of course, in those days, people did not understand that an infant has a greater chance of survival if it receives its own

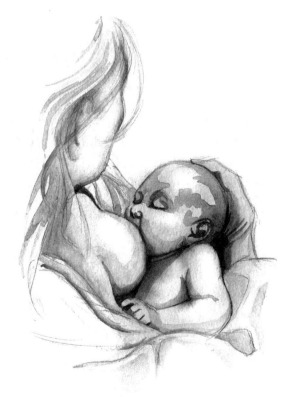

Breast-feeding

mother's milk, especially the richly immune-protective colostrum that is produced in the first few days after birth. However, even though this knowledge is available today, many women still choose not to breast-feed. In 2006, the rates for American mothers who breast-fed, even once, varied from 43 percent in those under the age of twenty to 77 percent in those over thirty.[5]

The other significant hormone in breast-feeding is oxytocin, which is released mainly from the posterior pituitary gland in response to the baby sucking on the nipple. Oxytocin leads to the "let-down reflex" in lactation, which describes the contraction of the muscular tissue within the alveoli, causing milk to gush along the ducts and out of the nipple and into the mouth of the newborn. Oxytocin is also responsible for the contraction of the uterus and cervical dilatation in the final stages of labor. As the *love hormone,* oxytocin enhances human bonding by decreasing fear and increasing trust, especially during lovemaking and in the early months of a child's life. This action is believed to occur because of the hormone's inhibition of the emotional centers in the brain that relate to fear and anxiety. It is not uncommon for a woman to feel sexually aroused while she is breast-feeding. This is thought to be due in part to oxytocin's role in both events, as well as a convergence of sensory nerve fibers in the brain that arise from the vagina, cervix, and breasts. It has even been found that giving new fathers a whiff of oxytocin causes them to be less hostile and more willing to engage with their infant.[6]

Low levels of oxytocin are associated with an increased risk of post-partum depression, reinforcing the importance to both mother and child of cuddling and feeding at the breast as soon after the birth as possible. Since oxytocin is secreted during sexual arousal, returning to sexual activity or receiving intimate massage as soon after delivery of the baby as possible decreases the tendency toward depression. All stud-ies show that a child benefits both physically and psychologically from breast-feeding, especially if it is continued for at least six months. One recent study from Australia showed that children who were breast-fed, especially boys, exhibited higher academic scores by the age of ten than those who were not. The variation between the sexes is believed to be because boys are more reliant on positive maternal bonding than girls.[7] Many studies have also revealed that during breast-feeding, the mother experiences calmness, confidence, and connectivity, which coincide with the effects of raised levels of prolactin and oxytocin.

The Cuddling Breast

There is clearly great value in receiving maternal milk in the early months of life; however, what is even more important for any child is to be held close to his or her mother's or father's heart in a protective and tender cuddle. Indeed, as an infant grows, breast-feeding is less about the milk and more about being embraced and cushioned within the softness of a parent's breasts. As we will see, it is through such a maternal heart that we reconnect to the loving heart of the Great Mother, the source of our existence. Through this eternal link we receive and are nurtured by the milk of immortality, synonymous with the continual flow of love and inspirational consciousness available to all of us.

As adults, we experience these same feelings of trust, safety, and compassion when we are held in a loving embrace and during the intimacy of lovemaking. It is during these moments of tenderness that we release our hold on our individual identity and seek union with the compassionate heart of another. Today, many people of all ages go months without being touched or receiving a hug. Fortunately, our mind can come to the rescue in such cases, for even the memory of such an embrace causes our body to physiologically react as if the hug were real.

In simple terms, there are two main purposes of breast-feeding and cuddling. The first is to provide the newborn with love, connection, and sustenance; the second is to deliver a sense of security and confidence so that eventually the child can let go of his or her dependency on the breast and step out into the world as a self-assured person. Even though the two functions usually work in harmony, there are fictional tales that speak of the breast that gives nurturing as the loving breast, while the other breast is seen as poisonous because it pushes the child away. It is most probable that the writers of these tales believed that they were ejected too early from their mother's breast—an issue that is certainly relevant when we begin to review the psychological factors linked to breast disease.

The Wise Breast

At the completion of breast-feeding, the breasts return to their normal, nonpregnant size, if not slightly smaller, as they are once again under the control of the hormones of the menstrual cycle. After menopause, without the benefit of estrogen and progesterone, the glandular tissue starts to shrink and is replaced by fatty tissue. The fibrous connective tissue loses its strength, which leads to sagging of the breasts, and at this point it appears as if the function of the breasts is complete. Yet how many of us can remember the comfort and safety we sensed when wrapped in the bosom of a precious grandmother or elder aunt? Her

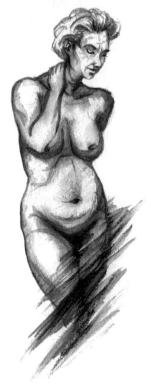

The wise and giving body of the crone

love felt unconditional and all-inclusive, as if we were the only person who mattered in that moment. I believe that such a level of bonding can occur with a crone because of the reduction in glandular tissue, which causes the breast to be less dense and more giving and forgiving. At the same time, the womb of the older woman has been released from its hormonal changes, allowing the breasts and the womb to work together to radiate powerful waves of love, common sense, wisdom, and inspiration.

The Cosmetically Enhanced Breast

In 2009, over one and a half million women around the world received breast augmentation, with the United States, Brazil, Thailand, and Holland among those at the top of the list. Meanwhile, with more disposable income available to women in China and India, plastic surgeons there are getting busier all the time. The worldwide market for breast implants is roughly $820 million a year and is growing annually by 8 percent, according to industry figures.

Implants have been used to enhance the size or shape of breasts as far back as the late 1800s. In those days, various substances were employed, including some that were extremely dangerous, such as paraffin and even glass. Nowadays saline or silicone is used to provide a natural-looking shape and soft flexibility. Many advances have taken place in recent years to avoid leakage of these substances outside the implant, and recent studies have shown minimal links with systemic disease.

While most women seek plastic surgery for the purpose of enlarging their breasts, there are many women who wish to reduce their breast size; the most common reasons given include the elimination of neck and back pain associated with overly large breasts, skin irritation, discomfort when exercising, and embarrassment at the overly large size of their breasts. Other reasons why a woman may seek breast surgery are to enhance self-esteem; for reconstructive purposes, to restore body image after a mastectomy; and to correct asymmetry or other deformities of the breast.

Most breast surgeries are successful, with women feeling happier and more confident with their new body image. Most plastic surgeons offer careful counseling before the surgery to ensure that expectations are realistic. In particular, they advise against the procedure if a woman is going through a stressful event such as a divorce, if there are deep-seated emotional issues, or if there is a desire for the perfect body. Many surgeons along with other health professionals are concerned about the increasing number of young, healthy women who have been encouraged by magazine articles that overemphasize the positive effects of breast augmentation, such as sexual attractiveness to men, and underplay the risks of undergoing invasive surgery.

The Breast of Male Obsession

We cannot omit from this discussion of the breast the subject of men and their fascination with the female mammary glands. Whether they are called "boobs," "jugs," "orbs," "a rack," "hooters," "tits," "puppies," "knockers," or any number of other appellations, large, voluptuous breasts are an obsession for many men, as any adult television sit-com or movie targeted to adolescent boys confirms. However, such an obsession does not exist in all cultures. In a study carried out in the 1950s by anthropologists Clellan Ford and Frank Beach, it was found that of the different cultures they studied many favored a "plump body build" rather than perfect breasts. When the breasts were considered, the preference ranged from "long and pendulous" to "upright," with only a quarter preferring them "big."[8] Margaret Mead, the cultural anthropologist, revealed that young women in New Guinea would try to stretch their breasts so that they were long and pendulous like those of their mothers; then they were considered "long enough to be thrown over the shoulder and feed the baby who was riding behind."[9]

When anthropologist Katherine Dettwyler told women in Mali that American men think breasts are sexually arousing, they were horrified. "You mean men act like babies?" the African women asked, collapsing in laughter at the thought.[10] Indeed, in many African tribes, women walk around bare-breasted, which is taboo in Western cultures.

To African women, however, their breasts are a symbol of fertility and have a strong connection to Ra, the life force, which is why they consider breast-feeding essential, enhancing the well-being of the growing child.

While there is no definite explanation for the emphasis placed on the breast as a sexual object in Western countries, one possible hypothesis is the fact that they are concealed under clothing, essentially making them forbidden fruit. In the United States, where freedom is supposedly worshipped, topless sunbathing is prohibited in most public places, unlike European countries, which have a much more relaxed attitude toward the naked breast. Similar issues of freedom occur around breast-feeding in public in the United States, even when there are laws in place to protect women who are breast-feeding.

If we are to assume that the concealment of a part of the body makes it more sexually desirable, then there are plenty of other areas of the body that should, by this definition, be considered sexual—for example, the abdomen. No, it is something specific to the breasts themselves that causes men to stare and women to seek augmentation in increasing numbers.

As was noted earlier, symmetry of the breasts has been linked to higher levels of fertility, which certainly may explain why a certain amount of gawking may be necessary when a man is searching for a mate. If size is the attracting feature, then, as the only difference between large and small breasts is the amount of fat present, a male may be inherently driven to choose a woman with large breasts because her fat supplies increase her chances of survival. Larger breasts are also associated with pregnancy, which sends out a signal that this woman is fertile. Yet, paradoxically, it also confirms her lack of availability, which would cause a man to select the smaller-breasted woman, as she is still awaiting a mate.

Freud was convinced that a person's sexual life begins with infant breast-feeding, and that men perpetually seek to return to that one great encounter of bliss. Yet this theory doesn't account for the obsession by men who were not breast-fed, nor does it explain why other cultures turn their sexual attention to parts of the body other than the breasts, even though they have high levels of breast-feeding. No, it is my belief that men do have a desire to return to the breast, but not merely the bosom of their physical mother; they want to suckle at the breast of the Great Mother to receive her milk of immortality. To do this, to manifest their unconscious desire, men must learn to respect and honor the Goddess, to whom the breasts of all women belong. And that conversation needs to take place face to face with a woman, and not face to bust!

HISTORY AND MYTHOLOGY OF THE SACRED BREAST

Many of the feminine figurines from 4,000 to 30,000 years ago show that there was no need for breast augmentation in those days, as there was an emphasis on an abundant flow of fertility and nourishment. Indeed, several of the archetypal images of the Great Goddess show her supporting her ample breasts with her hands, as if sending out an invitation to come and enjoy her exquisite milk. This is certainly true of figurines found in the Mesopotamian region, which portray such goddesses as Inanna, Ishtar, and Astarte in this way. When depicted in their breast-offering pose, these goddesses were called Mother of the Fruitful Breast, Creator of People, Mother of Deities, and River of Life—names that highlight their role as the provider of endless fertility. Could this be the hidden interpretation behind the seductively "forward" pose of female models who adorn the pages of modern magazines?

Egypt was ruled by the great goddesses Hathor and Isis. Both were known as the Great Mother Cow and were usually portrayed wearing a headdress shaped as a throne, clearly indicating that it was through their grace that the pharaoh received his power and strength. To the Egyptians, the milk of the Goddess provided more than mere physical sustenance; it promised a continuous connection to immortal or eternal life. Such was the value placed on the Great Mother's gift that images

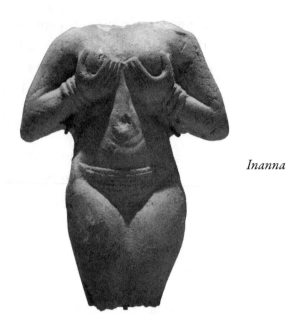

Inanna

of Isis often show a proportionally smaller pharaoh sitting in her lap, receiving milk from her breasts. The size of the pharaoh doesn't change, even though the statues symbolize him in different stages of his life—birth, coronation, and death; this indicates his continual reverence for the Great Goddess, despite his powerful position as head of the society.

Breasted Gods

Despite the subjugation of women from around 1500 BCE onward, the power of the breast to confer immortality was not lost on the rising religion at the time, whose figurehead was Yahweh. He was awarded another title, El Shaddai, meaning "god of the breast," suggesting that it was this deity who, through his own male breasts, provided spiritual nourishment.[11] The ancient Egyptians also wanted to convey the fact that nourishment could be provided just as easily by a male deity as a female, and therefore they strapped breasts onto their god of fertility, Hapi. However, this representation conveyed a deeper significance when it is understood that Hapi (or Hep) was the pre-dynastic name of the River Nile, which was seen to flow through the underworld of the dead before arising between two mountain peaks to provide water, food, and the yearly inundation of the agricultural fields. It is clear that the two mountain peaks are symbols of the breasts, while the flow of fertility from death to life shows a healthy acceptance of the feminine dominion over resurrection and rebirth.

The Breasts of the Milky Way

As we move forward in time to ancient Greece, we discover that the word *galaxy* comes from the Greek word for milk, *gala,* and that there are many legends that relate to the naming of our galaxy the Milky Way. The oldest of these describes the stars that comprise our galaxy as a herd of dairy cows whose milk produces the creamy appearance. This story probably emerged during an age when fertility, nurturing, and creative abundance were seen as a blessing from the multinippled Mother Goddess.

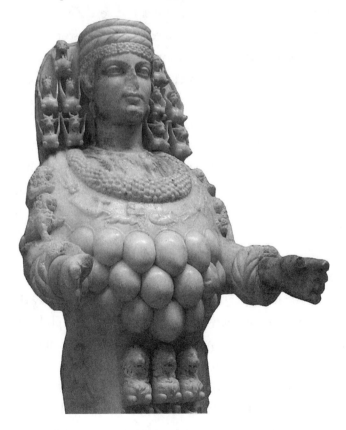

The goddess Artemis (Selçuk Museum, Turkey)

It amuses me that some male archaeologists still find it difficult to accept that the pendulous appendices attached to the chest wall of the goddess Artemis are indeed breasts; somehow, they prefer to see them as dates, eggs, and even scrotal sacs! Gentlemen, trust me: they are gorgeous, ample, sensuous breasts.

Another story connected with the Milky Way tells of the conflict between Rhea, the primordial Mother, and her brother/husband Cronus, the god of time (later known as the Roman god Saturn). Cronus was seen as all-devouring and destructive, keeping mortals trapped through the illusion of time and thus unable to experience the grace of eternal life. Warned that he would be overthrown by his son in the same way that he had deposed and castrated his own father, Ouranos (Uranus), Cronus swallowed all the children born to his wife, Rhea. However, wishing to save her last son, Zeus, from this fate, she hid him from his father and offered Cronus a stone wrapped in swaddling linens instead. Before Cronus swallowed the child, he asked Rhea to feed the child one last time; the milk, failing to penetrate the stone, spurted across the sky to become the Milky Way. I believe this story reveals Rhea's determination, as the Great Mother, to save her children from the bondage of time, reminding them of the continuous nurturing available to them all when they step beyond three-dimensional limitations and remember their universal origins. Interestingly, the stone became the omphalos stone of Delphi, a symbol of the fruitfulness of Mother Earth.

Hera, the Disenfranchised Goddess

There is one last tale about the formation of Milky Way that also relates to Zeus, who has by now become a powerful and philandering god. To set the scene, we must meet his much-maligned wife and older sister, Hera, for her archetypal wounds play a significant role in the disharmony experienced by many women today.

The goddess Hera is much older than the deities who occupied the pantheon of classical Greek mythology. As a loving and powerful pre-Hellenic deity, she was known as the Queen of Heavens, representing right and sacred relationship, whether this was with a partner, the nature kingdoms, other people, the universe, or aspects of the self. She is mentioned as having an orchard in the far west corner of the world, in which she grows golden apples of immortality that are protected by the great serpent-dragon Ladon, who winds around the tree. Sound familiar? Whether we are talking about golden apples or pearls, we are referring to dragon energy, and it is through its mastery that we will access eternal life.

Following the invasion of lands previously inhabited by people who worshipped Mother Earth by people who placed male gods at the top of their pantheon, Hera was demoted, married off to the supreme god Zeus. With this union, all equality was lost, destroying the concept of sacred marriage over which Hera had previously presided. At this point, as a subjugated wife, Hera is often portrayed as a woman degraded and humiliated by the adulterous activities of her husband. Greek mythology has little sympathy for her, preferring to side with Zeus, who is, after all, "just being a man." Hera is therefore described in Greek mythology as a vengeful woman who took every opportunity to strike back at her husband and his illegitimate offspring.

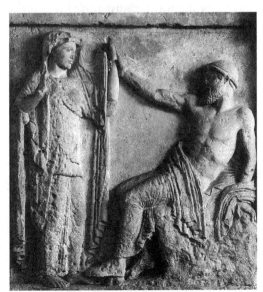

Hera and Zeus

Hera's downfall and her archetypal wound live on in the collective unconscious of women today. Hera was disrespected, disempowered, abused, and disenfranchised—a situation replicated in the workplaces and homes of many women around the world today. Mythology tells us that she did retaliate by having her own affair, although this merely resulted in further scorn and humiliation, with Zeus receiving sympathy for being burdened with such an "ungrateful" wife.

Yet Hera also sowed the seeds of a way of regaining power, one that is still used by modern women. She decided that if she supported her husband's rise to fame and success, she would, by inference, also benefit. She thus became "the power behind the throne," a situation I certainly saw in my mother's generation, when women were more likely to stay at home and depend on their husband's efforts to achieve fulfillment, even if this was at the expense of their heart's desires. This was the message I received as a child—boys are more important than girls—and this was the reason given as to why my parents focused so much attention on my brother's education, while the achievements of my sister and I were minimized.

One has only to look at television programs and films from the 1950s to see that a woman was expected to be a dutiful wife, creating the perfect meal in the perfect home for her husband's boss in the hope that this would lead to his promotion. A woman would, perhaps, convince herself that even though her man appeared to be master of their home, she was the one who was in control, using manipulation or withdrawal of support to remind him who really held the keys to his success. And if her husband failed to meet her dreams and expectations, then she would divert all her attention to her firstborn son, and he would eventually become her pride and joy.

Despite the fact that twenty-first-century women have accomplished much within the workforce, the archetype of the wounded Hera still lives on in many women today. The disenfranchised feminine is particularly visible when a successful woman places unrealistic expectations on a male partner or colleague. Unfamiliar with the role of being honored in her own right, she can become scornful and critical of the man's failure to meet her expectations. Eventually he shuts down, recognizing that he can never please her. At some level, he may become aware that the real imbalance is not with him, but between her inner masculine and her inner feminine, where her well-developed masculine is replaying Zeus's role of being scornful of the feminine. One solution to this problem is that if a woman wears the pants in a relationship, then she must allow her partner to provide a nest for her energy rather than chiding him for not "being a man."

But the greater issue is the disrespect many women feel toward their own inner feminine, often citing the flaws of their mother, whom they saw as weak, inadequate, and helpless. This is an echo of Hera's fall from power, for in the past the strength of women came from their inherent sense of cooperation and desire for community. Whatever their differences, sisters would stand together and support one another for the sake of their families. They didn't need to compete to win the favors of men, for as with cows, there was only need for one bull, and only at certain times of the year, for the females to be fruitful. It was the bulls who jostled with one another to be the chosen one.

As women have sought to distance themselves from the wounded Hera, they have often done so by detaching from any woman who reminds them of their own scars and shame. Yet the healing we seek can never be fully achieved through separation. As we open our hearts to the vulnerability and sensitivity of our inner feminine, there will hopefully be a day when, without judgment, we can embrace our wounded sisters with compassion, whether physically or energetically.

With the emergence of more single-parent families, we are witnessing another of Hera's subtle attempts to regain her power through the transference of a woman's expectations from a husband to her child, especially if that child is a son; if a mother is not careful, it is easy for her to burden her son with the responsibility of succeeding not only for himself, but also for her. In this codependent model, the son relies on his mother for nurturing and support, while she is dependent on him for her own fulfillment. She may see him as needy and immature, while he sees her as overbearing and suffocating.

I am always concerned when a woman describes the love of an intimate partnership as the same as the love that flows between her and her child: "I don't have a partner at present, but my children love me." It can sometimes be difficult to differentiate between the two, but a mother is not in an intimate relationship with her child, nor should her child be forced to act as her partner. This is the disempowered and wounded Hera speaking. There is clearly a need to be able to recognize the difference between the two types of affection, freeing children to open their hearts, form their own relationships, and fall in love. Children are not here to fulfill our unrealized dreams or to repair the damage of past unsuccessful relationships. It is time for all of us to heal the wounds of our inner Hera, which will begin only when our own inner masculine shows respect and adoration for the indwelling feminine.

Hera and Heracles

Now, let us return to the story of Hera and her link to the naming of the Milky Way:

> Heracles, or Hercules (meaning "Hera famous"), was the child of Zeus and a mortal woman named Alcmene. Even though Zeus impregnated many mortals outside his marriage to Hera, he was particularly fond of the half-human Heracles and wanted to confer on him immediate immortality and other godlike qualities. He therefore decided to allow the infant to suckle on the breast of the sleeping Hera so he would receive the milk of immortality from the goddess. However, the fierceness of Heracles's sucking awakened Hera, who, annoyed that she was breast-feeding another of Zeus's illegitimate offspring, pushed him away, causing her spurting milk to flow across the heavens, leading to the creation of the Milky Way.
>
> Yets Heracles received enough of the goddess's milk to become strong, although not immortal. Hera was furious and vowed that she would make his life difficult from that moment on. In time, Heracles married Megara,

and together they had children and were extremely happy. However, through Hera's vengeance, Heracles became crazy and killed his family. In his despair, he called on Apollo to send him twelve labors, which he would perform to cleanse his soul, each task subsequently made more challenging because of Hera's continuing retaliation.

Finally, with his labors complete, Heracles was free to marry again. In this moment of happiness, he was given a cloak that was covered not in a love balm, but in a caustic poison, and he became wracked with pain. Longing to die, he lay down on a funeral pyre and prepared to do just that; however, Zeus saw him and called on Hera to finally relent. At last she forgave him and lifted him from the pyre to Mount Olympus, where he was immortalized in the summer sky as the constellation known as the Strong Man.

What is the meaning of this story? The twelve labors of Heracles are the twelve stages or doorways of life through which we must pass to know ourselves as immortal beings. At each doorway we collect a pearl or seed of wisdom, which makes us stronger. These are the seeds of consciousness we eventually offer to the Great Mother so we can gain access to her ocean of abundance and possibility at the crown chakra.

Zeus, wishing to spare his son from the trials and challenges of earthly life, thought that a few sucks at Hera's nipples would confer him with immortality and he could avoid the discomforts of human life. The underlying message of this story suggests that unless a person is adequately prepared to receive such high-frequency energy, the end result is destructive madness. Heracles's labors required him to become strong, both physically and mentally; he had to use intellect and guile to complete his tasks. Yet his immortality was not granted merely because of his deeds, but as a result of his eventual willingness to surrender his will and strength to the Dragon Queen. As he lay on the fire, Heracles was lifted up by the love of the Great Mother and finally could lay on her breast.

Could this tale explain some of the attraction men have for women's breasts, where, like Heracles, they just want to suckle at the breast of the goddess and receive instant immortality without doing any of the hard work? The story of Heracles offers a warning: should a man subconsciously believe he has the "right" to take whatever he wants, without permission or respect for the Goddess—including the milk of immortality—then, as Heracles discovered, such beliefs or desires will inevitably drive him crazy!

The Olympian Breast

Over time, as the power of the patriarchy increased, there was a corresponding decrease in the depictions of the size and appearance of the Goddess's breasts. For instance, Athena, the goddess of wisdom, was wrapped in heavy drapery by the Greeks, with a helmet on her head and her chest covered by a breastplate adorned with snakes.[12] This change in emphasis does not include all goddesses; Athena's sister, Aphrodite, goddess of love (the Roman goddess Venus), is commonly portrayed in a state of near-complete undress, leaning forward to offer her breasts while coyly covering her genitals.

In ancient Greece, Aphrodite was the only goddess depicted life-size and with her breasts exposed, highlighting a theme that continues to this day: when it comes to the amount of breast that can be revealed, there is one standard for a wife and quite another for a mistress!

Aphrodite's archetypal energy, which represents the pure love of life, became distorted by the Greeks and then by the Romans into lust and sexual desire. In just a few centuries of patriarchal rule, she was demoted from a highly revered goddess to a whore. This shift in attitude echoed in the attitude toward women in general. By the fifth century BCE, Athenian women were expected to stay indoors and segregate themselves from men other than their husband and the men in their immediate family. In the house, they were expected to wear a long shirtlike tunic; when outdoors, they wore a cloak for warmth with a veil or shawl to cover their heads. Ancient drawings show little evidence of breasts or breast-feeding, with wet nurses being commonly employed to

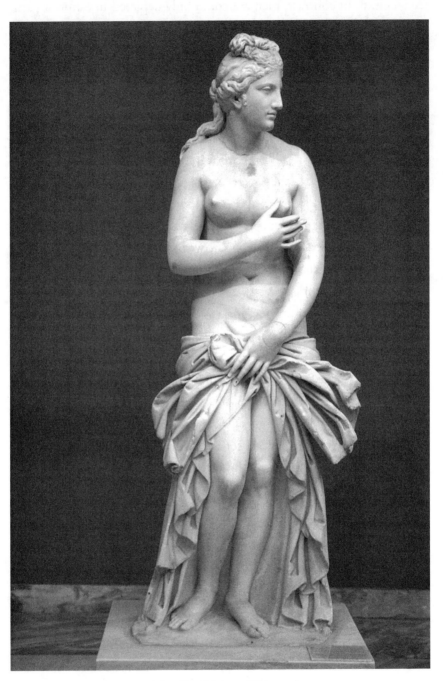

Aphrodite (Athens Museum)

feed a child. In contrast, men are commonly depicted in outdoor gatherings, exercising naked in gymnasiums, or satisfying their sexual needs in brothels, where they had the choice of either young men or women. It was here, in the brothels, that Aphrodite's human representatives would be found. Known as *hetairai,* or courtesans, these women were often well-educated, accomplished musicians and sociable companions, who, more often than not, would have sexual relationships with the patrons—although providing entertainment was their main purpose. In classical Greek art, they were often represented as fully naked or clothed in a sensual manner, and always with breasts exposed.

I am certain that Hera must have wept to see the disempowerment of the classical Greek woman, with a complete loss of equality within her relationships, whether as a wife or a mistress. Of course, our ancestors found subtle ways to regain the illusion of power, through seduction, manipulation, denying a partner's needs, infidelity, physical attacks, and, the most common, emotional abuse. Many of these same techniques are used today to gain power over men, mirroring the example set by the patriarchy in a quest for domination. But this was never Hera's way; she seeks equality, wherein each person is respected and honored for the contributions she or he brings to a relationship. It is only when we place this respect at the center of any liaison that we will find real peace, not only at home, but throughout the world.

The Amazons

There are many stories and much mystery surrounding the legendary female warriors known as the Amazons, who are believed to have emerged from countries surrounding the Black Sea, including present-day Libya and Turkey. They are said to have worshipped the Greek god of war, Ares, and the goddess Artemis, portrayed in her virginal aspect as the successful huntress. Greek mythology embraced the presence of such powerful combatants in battle, where women rode horses like men and were described as bloodthirsty and fierce.

Beyond this, there has been much speculation about the Amazons' way of life. Some ancient texts propose that they lived in an all-female society and that once a year they slept with foreign men to perpetuate their race. It is also written that any male offspring were either sent away or kept in slavery, while girls were trained as warriors. One other focus of discussion of the Amazons concerns their breasts. Some writings suggest that the right breast was cauterized at birth to prevent its growth to allow an arrow to fly unimpeded as it left the bow. Other stories say that such depictions are mere fantasy, and that the name Amazon comes from two Greek words, *a* (without) and *mazos* (breast)—simply implying that their breasts were covered.

Perhaps the Amazons represented the projected nightmare of Greek men, who, having castrated women of their power, feared the outpouring of feminine rage and vengeance. Of course, the men could only envision such dreadful figures by delving into their own subconscious fears. Therefore, they portrayed them as demons without breasts, with a lust for blood and total disrespect for the opposite sex—in other words, the dominant male archetype.

Even today, a woman who acts like a man—i.e., without breasts— can be threatening to both genders. In such a woman, the natural feminine desire to find a way to work and live together has been shattered by competitiveness and a focus on individual needs. Women will always fight to protect their home and loved ones, encouraged by the release of the hormone prolactin. However, unlike the recent flurry of well-publicized "cat fights" that show women behaving like men, the feminine lion never fights to possess and win, but only to reestablish a cooperative community for the survival of the generations to come.

The Breast in the Last 2,000 Years

As we move forward in time through the era of Roman domination and the rise of Christianity, we witness an ever-increasing disrespect toward a woman and her body. From the writings of this era, we hear of breast mutilation as a punishment for any woman found engaged in lewd acts or displaying her breasts in an erotic manner. Such accusations were often grossly inaccurate and almost never mentioned the man who was enjoying her company. There is little evidence of breast-feeding, with the employment of wet nurses being standard.

It wasn't until the sixteenth century onward, particularly in Europe, that there was a shift in attitude toward breast-feeding and how much female flesh should be exposed. At this time, many women reinstated themselves as the nurturer of their child, probably appreciating the intimate bond that develops between mother and child. There were also increasing concerns as to whether the milk of the wet nurse could infect the child with dangerous toxins and even pass on negative personality traits.[13] Since then, interest in breast-feeding has waxed and waned, as has the attitude about the amount of breast that should be shown.

In the early 1900s in the United States more than two-thirds of mothers breast-fed their babies. By 1950, this figure had dropped to only 25 percent. The lowest figure was reached in 1971 when 22 percent of women were recorded as having initiated breast-feeding. Research suggests that the fall was probably due to a number of factors, the main one being the introduction of formula milk and a worldwide campaign that sold it as being more hygienic and convenient for the working mother. Formula's selling power was enhanced during the twentieth century by a few headline cases of breast-feeding failures such as infant starvation and the transmission of a mother's illness through her breast milk.[14]

But the tides turned again in the 1980s, with increasing numbers of women returning to breast-feeding. They were encouraged by a widespread promotion drive by doctors and midwives claiming that breast-feeding not only was safe and hygienic but provided important nutrition to the newborn baby as well as invaluable psychological benefits to both mother and child. In 2007, 75 percent of babies were breast-fed at least one time, with 43 percent continuing for six months, and 22 percent for one year. However, exclusive breast-feeding levels are only 33 percent at three months, which suggests that women are probably having to adapt to busy lives and the convenience of supplementing with bottle feeds.[15]

The Mountainous Breast

Many cultures considered mountain peaks as places where the Great Mother poured her milk of immortality into the breasts of Mother Earth, to nurture and feed her people. Such mammary peaks are described as holy mountains; they include Mashu, in the Epic of Gilgamesh; Ninhursag, in Sumerian legends; the Breasts of Anu, in Irish tradition; and Gaea Olympia, in Greece.[16] This awareness of the powerful feminine nature of Mount Olympus, as being an expression of Mother Earth herself, was lost when the Greek pantheon took control of mythology and denigrated the mountain to the status of residence of their masculine gods.

One of the reasons why ancient people honored many of the mightiest mountains as the milk-giving Goddess is because the glacial water that flows from them commonly appears milky in color. This explains the sacred name of the tallest mountain in the world, which was renamed for the climber Sir George Everest. The actual name of this mountain is Chomo-Lung-Ma, which means "Goddess Mother of the Universe," referring to one of the oldest Tibetan deities. Another beautiful Himalayan peak is Annapurna, whose name means "Great Breast Full of Nourishment."

I will never forget the sublime peace and contentment I felt when trekking in Annapurna's foothills, as if there was nothing I needed but to be in her presence. The goddess Annapurna is the Hindu deity of food and cooking, capable of supplying unlimited sustenance. She is one of the incarnations of the Hindu goddess Parvati (aka Shakti), the wife of Shiva. Temple art in India often depicts Lord Shiva with his begging bowl, respectfully asking the goddess to nourish him so that he may achieve knowledge and enlightenment.

THE ASTROLOGICAL BREAST

The breasts are linked to the water sign of Cancer, the crab, which is ruled by the moon. Since everybody has a placement of the moon in their natal astrological chart, each of us has specific needs when it

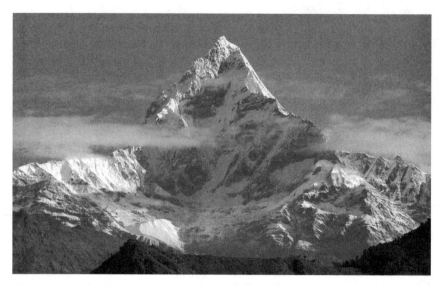

Annapurna, Great Breast Full of Nourishment

comes to caring and nurturing. However, the presence of a planet in the sign of Cancer reveals specific characteristics, which include:

- A great love for the family, children, and home, as in "home sweet home"
- Creativity (especially around the home), intuitiveness, and a strong imagination
- Sympathetic caring and compassion and enjoyment of hugs and "homey" comforts
- Emotionally sensitive, romantic, and sentimental, leading to an easy flow of tears
- Desiring for everybody to be happy, with a strong psychic sensitivity to the unhappiness of others
- A tendency to withdrawal to within the proverbial crab's shell in the presence of conflict
- Moodiness—one minute warm and clingy, the next silent and defensive
- Denial that any problem exists: "Everything is beautiful; have a nice day"

When the sign of Cancer is emphasized in a woman's astrological chart, she will have had to learn how to care for others while also being sensitive to her own needs, hence achieving a healthy balance of give and take. There are also indicators within such a natal chart that suggest the potential for problems in the area of nurturing, which could manifest as breast distress. Such signposts include:

- Saturn in Cancer, where care and nurturing may be limited, both in the giving and in receiving
- Mars in Cancer, where there is a passion for and maybe even obsession with caring for others, which can be claustrophobic for the recipient
- Moon in Cancer with a difficult aspect to the planet Saturn, in which the instinctive need to be nurtured is limited, in particular by conditions laid down by the mother

Even though these astrological placements hold the potential for breast disease, nothing is set in stone when it comes to whether a disease will actually manifest in our lives. I have been for some time aware that in my natal chart, Saturn is square to my moon, and therefore I should perhaps have done more to reduce the control my mother's opinions have held over me. Yet it was only when I felt brave enough, because of the discovery of the breast lump, to face some well-hidden emotions that I saw how much I had abandoned my own inner urgings. They say forewarned is forearmed, and I hope this brief astrological overview may encourage other women to explore their true feelings and not just attempt to keep everybody happy, in true Cancerian manner.

The other astrological factor strongly associated with the breasts concerns placement of the moon in one's natal chart. This celestial body has a powerful cyclic influence on the watery emotions and represents our instinctual nature. The position of the moon in our natal chart shows us how to best care for ourselves, especially during times of stress, so that we can steer ourselves back to calmer and happier waters. Like the breasts, the moon reflects the sensitivity of a loving mother who knows instinctively our emotional needs.

My advice would be to commit to following the instinctual desires of your astrological moon-sign placement, at least once a day, so that you will always be able to find the way home to your heart. These instinctual needs include:

Moon in Aries: new ventures, adventure, movement, and competiveness

Moon in Taurus: comfort through good food, music, touch, and financial security

Moon in Gemini: someone to talk to, good books, information, and change

Moon in Cancer: hugs, a place to cry, being with family, at home, and away from conflict

Moon in Leo: approval, praise, being noticed, humor, and risk taking

Moon in Virgo: beauty, cleanliness, analysis, and making things just right

Moon in Libra: harmony, relationship, fairness, and consideration of all the options

Moon in Scorpio: intensity, expression of deep emotions, and sensual pleasures

Moon in Sagittarius: expansion, movement, travel, and searching for the truth

Moon in Capricorn: order, planning, challenges, integrity, and feeling in control

Moon in Aquarius: time alone, understanding, unusual interests, and objectivity

Moon in Pisces: creativity, daydreaming, star-gazing, and honoring psychic awareness

And always remember: when the moon is happy, you are happy!

BREASTS THAT FLOW WITH LOVE

In our search for the sacred identity of womanhood, what can we learn from goddesses such as Inanna, Isis, Hera, Annapurna, and Aphrodite? Why were pharaohs and gods like Shiva so willing to bow down in their presence for the gift of being suckled at the breast or of receiving divine nourishment? We have learned that Lord Shiva wanted to experience enlightenment, but what was the nourishment that he needed for his journey? How can the anatomy and physiology of the breast help us understand our divine inheritance?

Here are some key points:

- The breasts are prominently positioned around the heart chakra, which radiates unconditional love.
- They are not hidden away like other female organs, but clearly visible.
- The breasts are soft and round, with no noticeable defenses, suggesting qualities of trust and openness.
- Prolactin, the mothering hormone, promotes relaxation, loving protection, and nesting instincts.
- Oxytocin, the love hormone, encourages bonding, trust, and a decrease in fear and anxiety.

The purest energy flowing through the breasts is love, wherein love means a deep connection to every part of our existence, our eternal self. Surrounding the heart chakra as they do, the breasts provide a safe and comforting resting place where we can move our awareness between the realms of spirit and matter. Here we drink the abundant love that radiates from the heart chakra; thus cocooned, we surrender our hold on old paradigms of living, and with trust we allow new awareness to develop. It is impossible to imagine a more perfect place in which to surrender than in the soft embrace of the breasts of the Great Mother. Since love is the sustenance that allows us to move with ease between spirit and matter, it is the elixir of immortality.

This transition between different dimensions is similar to the shift between the states of sleeping and wakefulness. As we fall asleep, we surrender our attachment to the physical world and open ourselves to multidimensional experiences while our body rests. When we awaken, we leave behind the dream state and become fully functional and engaged here on Earth. The more secure and safe we feel, the easier it is to sleep.

If we were to see the three faces of the Great Mother, our own birth mother represents her transformational aspect, supplying a vitally important link between the Queen of Heaven and Mother Earth. Without maternal love as expressed by the breasts, it would be impossible for a soul to incarnate here on Earth and for a person to receive spiritual sustenance at various times during his or her life. The newborn, whose soul has lived within the watery spiritual realms for nine months, must adapt to living in the physical world. Through the nourishment provided by breast-feeding and cuddling, the infant starts to adjust to its earthly surroundings.

When the child is deemed ready, the mother weans him or her from the breast and anchors the child to the material world by offering food harvested from Mother Earth. In time, the child learns to stand on his or her own two feet, to make new friends outside the family, to develop a healthy sense of self, and to metaphorically leave the breast and create his or her own life.

For the Hawaiians, this emotional weaning traditionally occurs around the age of five, when, in many cultures, a child begins school. Until then, the upbringing of the child is often shared among the women in a family or tribe, so that they can all instill him or her with the love, confidence, and security the child needs to walk his or her own path, knowing that the nurturing of these collective breasts is always available should the need arise. For there are times in our life, when, like the pharaoh, our soul seeks inspiration and restoration within the ethereal and primordial waters of the Great Mother.

On these occasions, the shift in energy travels in the opposite direction, to that of the newborn baby, moving from the physical world to that of spirit. Instinctively, we move our awareness inward and away from our busy lives, creating an environment that represents the loving bosom of the Great Mother. We probably find ourselves spending more time in nature or surrounded by loving friends and family, intuitively drinking in the warmth of heartfelt connections, trust, and loving protection. Though we do not attach to a physical breast as an infant does, we still enjoy the closeness of hugs and loving embraces, which bring us in contact with the heart chakra and breasts of a beloved person. As our outer energy becomes quiet, we become more aware of our own heart calling us home, wrapping us in tender love for ourselves.

This surrender into love, the elixir of immortality, allows our consciousness to move from the denser material world toward the lighter and finer frequency of the spirit realms, where our awareness is eternal and unrestricted. With the spirit now free, we become immersed in the pure waters of divine inspiration, receiving nurturance for the soul as it reconnects to its divine purpose. Refreshed and restored, the soul then begins its descent back to Mother Earth. It passes through the heart again, where insights are transformed into dreams, to eventually manifest as reality. Without this ability to set our spirit free, it is easy to become depressed, dis-spirited, dis-heartened, and uninspired. Without our willingness to plant our dreams firmly on this earth, we may become delusional, shallow, fanciful, schizophrenic, and unfulfilled.

A very similar path is taken during the sacred act of sex when we release our hold on the physical world and, through an orgasmic release, surrender into a pure state of bliss. However, if sexual arousal is not associated with intimacy and the opening of the heart—whether with another person or alone in an act of self-pleasuring—then the orgasm will remain on the physical level, with little or no restoration for the soul. Fortunately, we don't need to have an orgasm to feel ourselves being transported to the pure waters of the Great Mother; all we need is love.

During a healing session, I received one of the clearest messages about the importance of returning to the heart to receive nurturing.

I saw my breast lump as a module that was floating out in space, having been sent out on a mission from the mother ship many years ago. I intuitively knew the ship represented my heart. Initially, the module had been successful in achieving its goals, but in recent years its effectiveness had begun to wane, and it was time for the spacecraft to return to the mother ship for restoration and an upgrade. However, during its time in outer space, the module had become encased in dense emotions, much as a boat becomes coated with barnacles. I heard myself giving all manner of excuses to my heart as to why I couldn't return to the ship: "I haven't finished what I'm doing." "There are more people I can help." "I think I can make them understand if I make some changes." And "Don't you realize there are so many people living in pain?" Yet, despite my protests, I had to reluctantly acknowledge that over the past few years, my inner martyr and prostitute had been working overtime, causing me to give more effort for less reward, in the mistaken belief that this would ease the pain of humanity. I knew this perception was inaccurate, but I've always been stubborn and arrogant enough to believe I could make a difference.

In the first few days following my diagnosis, I had toyed with the idea that perhaps I was meant to sacrifice myself for the sake of the message. Always with a tendency for the dramatic and aware of the origins of my first name, I saw myself as Jesus hanging from the cross. But just as quickly as the idea had popped up in my mind, I heard the message, If they didn't understand his message then, your sacrifice isn't going to make a bit of difference. *Swiftly yet gently put in my place, I knew that I didn't fear death; I feared living a life disconnected from the love of my soul, which could be accessed only through the expansiveness of my heart.*

From the moment the lump appeared it had ached, and now the pain increased, as if it were being pulled in two directions. I longed to return to the mother ship so I could reconnect with my spiritual origins and be refreshed. Yet because of my natural tendency to feel the emotions of others, I empathized with the despair of humanity. I had clearly become too psychically attached, which was not helpful or healthy to anybody involved, especially me.

I'd experienced similar pivotal points in my life previously, when I had visualized myself standing on a window ledge, being encouraged by my heart to jump and fly free. Yet all I could do was look back at the people in the room behind me and ask, "But what about all these people who need help?" With great clarity and patience, my inner guidance replied, "Look ahead and see the people who are waiting for you to jump; they need you more." At least four times I had trusted these voices and jumped, successfully changing jobs, partnerships, and even countries, to fulfill my soul's destiny, and now here I was again, on a ledge.

The commander of the mother ship, my heart, gave me wise advice: This spaceship cannot move forward until we bring every part of the soul back on board, including the module. If you want to help, your consciousness must be expanded, and yet this cannot happen while we are immobile here in space. *I knew it was time to move and immediately saw my ego-self, the module, being brought back on board the mother ship, relinquishing its hold on a perception of reality that could no longer sustain my soul. With the maximum thrust of its engines, the mother ship took off into space at hyperspeed, to explore new horizons, while I took full advantage of the ship's facilities to rest, play, and heal.*

In that moment, a wave of relief passed through me as I saw how I'd been clinging to control, desperately attempting to make things work, when all I had to do was return to my heart and accept the support of my soul. Once I surrendered to this far more expansive power, the aching eased, and I relaxed into a deep and healing peace that I hadn't experienced for a long, long time.

It's time for women to acknowledge that without the love that emanates from their breasts, the evolution of humanity is doomed. Creative ideas and dreams will fail to be downloaded onto Earth, and the soul will be unable to return to the spiritual realms for restoration and renewal. For such love to flow, we as women need to develop a pride in our breasts that goes far beyond their appearance. As this happens, vulnerability and softness become strengths, facets of one of the most powerful forces in the world: love. As a woman's self-love expands, her enjoyment of the pleasures of Mother Earth will increase, while at the same time she will experience a heightened sensitivity to the nonphysical, spiritual realms. Then and only then will she be ready to assist in another person's sacred transformation, and then only if that person genuinely wishes to reconnect to his or her soul's dreams.

Hera offers this advice: "Anybody who seeks to nestle into your metaphorical breasts and drink the milk of immortality must, like the pharaoh, surrender his ego and approach with honor and respect, for without this there is no bond of trust, and true spiritual transformation will be impossible." Those who choose not to let go of the pride and ego but still want to receive the milk of human kindness may attempt to do this through energy vampiring, similar to those who steal energy from the womb. This time their approach is via the solar plexus chakra, which is where we store self-esteem and self-assurance. "Vampires" who wish to latch on to the breasts to receive transformation to the spiritual realms will look for a weakness in your confidence and use it to their advantage—what we may call emotional blackmail. They often start by lauding you with praise or compliments to encourage you to open your solar plexus and let them in. Then, in an instant, they turn off the sweet talk and make a comment that leaves you feeling inadequate, worthless, guilty, or criticized—and, quickly, while you're still reeling in confusion, they latch on to the breast. When you have the courage to ask them to leave, you are met with further demeaning comments such as, "If you were really a loving person, you wouldn't ask me to leave. I thought you cared. You're really not a nice person after all. You of all people should understand. I thought you were my friend."

Energy vampiring at the level of the breast is insidious in many relationships and is particularly problematic when your sense of self-confidence is weakened by an upbringing where you were immersed in guilt, anger, and criticism. Rather than attempting to wear a steel bra to protect the breasts from vampires, the first step is to strengthen feelings of self-worth, which come from knowing it is absolutely perfect to be you—without any justification or apology. Then, it is important to connect to your own spiritual or inner self, which is accessed through the heart chakra in the center of the chest. You can feel this energy by placing your hands over the center of your chest, on top of each other in the shape of an X. Now there is no room for any form of emotional blackmail or energy vampiring, and you can choose who will be allowed to suckle at your breast and for how long.

As I always say, "You can suckle from my breasts while there is a need, but once you begin to bite, you're off!"

8

THE DISTRESSED BREAST

Having gained a deeper understanding of the breast, let us now consider what happens when the breast becomes distressed.

BREAST CANCER

Up to 80 percent of women experience premenstrual breast tenderness and generalized lumpiness in the breasts sometime during their life; this temporary condition usually disappears during or after the menstrual flow. Thought to be due to a hormonal imbalance, the symptoms are exacerbated by stress, chocolate, and coffee, all of which stimulate the effects of estrogen. This benign condition is commonly diagnosed as fibrocystic disease of the breast, and it usually disappears after menopause.

In the United States in 2010, a woman was eleven times more likely to die from heart disease than she was from breast cancer. Yet from the media attention surrounding breast cancer, it would appear that the ratio was reversed.[1] Breast cancer is a very emotive disease, probably because of the deep and complex relationship we have with our breasts around such issues as love, trust, and nurturing. Although both genders can develop this disease, women are a hundred times more likely to be diagnosed with breast cancer than men. In 2008, it was estimated that worldwide, 1.38 million women were diagnosed with breast cancer, accounting for around a tenth of all new cancers, and nearly a quarter of cancers in women.[2] The incidences of female breast cancer vary considerably, with the highest rates found in Europe and the lowest in Africa and Asia.[3] Indeed, the lowest rates are found in East Africa, which includes some of the poorest countries in the world, including Kenya, Tanzania, Rwanda, and Uganda.[4] In fact, it is the relatively small country of Belgium that currently has the highest incidence of the disease in the world, with 109 cases per 100,000 women, followed by France, Denmark, the Netherlands, Italy, and the United Kingdom. The prevalence of breast cancer in the United States is now at 76 per 100,000 women, double that of Brazil and triple the rate in China. These statistics have been age-standardized but obviously need to be seen in the light of reduced life expectancy in many of the poorer countries, as well lower detection rates because of limited health and testing facilities. However, that said, these statistics clearly show that breast cancer is far more prevalent in the wealthier and developed countries of the world than in the poorer nations, suggesting that poverty is not a determining factor in the disease.

Looking at the United States alone, one 2006 study showed that 12.15 percent of women—one in eight—will be diagnosed with breast cancer during their lifetime. The risk increases significantly with age until around the age of sixty-five, when the incidence starts to drop off and becomes less of a factor in the actual cause of death. In 2010, breast cancer was the leading killer among all other cancers, with approximately 200,000 women being diagnosed with the disease in that year alone, and some 40,000 deaths.[5] The incidence of breast cancer has increased in most countries worldwide in the last decades, with the most rapid increase occurring in the developing countries. There was, however, a fall in prevalence after a study released in 2002 showed there was double the risk of a woman's developing breast cancer if she took hormone replacement therapy (HRT) for five years, causing many women to stop taking the drugs.[6] Many medical studies—which, needless to say, exclude a psycho-spiritual component—conclude that the factors in breast cancer include reproductive behavior, the use of hormones, obesity, lack of exercise, and excessive alcohol consumption. Scientists suggest that in developed countries, the incidence of breast cancer could be halved if women had more children earlier and breast-fed for longer. Clearly, this suggestion is a limited "solution" to what we know is a much, much bigger issue.

Still, despite the increase in the prevalence of this disease, the survival rates from breast cancer are much improved, with two out of three women diagnosed still alive after twenty years. However, there is much work still to do, as no breast cancer is the only acceptable statistic.[7]

Breast Love

The obvious place to start when attempting to unearth factors that may be associated with breast cancer is within the psyche, for as we know, our perceptions and emotions deeply influence the health of our cells.

Natural childbirth is often described as one of the most blissful and extraordinary experiences of a woman's life, when opioids and other hormones flow through her body, transforming her into the embodiment of the sacred woman. By designing this heightened experience at the time of birth, the Great Mother wanted to create an instant bond between the newborn child and the mother, so that the child can be marinated in love as soon as he or she arrives on the planet. After childbirth, the breasts play a vitally important role in the next stage of the infant's journey. They provide closeness and protection, keeping the child safe and connected to his or her spiritual roots while nourishing and encouraging the child's confidence so that one day he or she can be weaned from the breast as a self-assured individual. This is where things become more complicated.

For a woman to be able to give her child both spiritual and physical sustenance, she needs to feel loved by the people around her, by her spiritual family, and, most importantly, by herself. If, for whatever reason, she feels unloved, then she will have greater difficulty sharing her love with others, or she will give in excess in the hope that she will receive love in return. Both of these emotional states commonly lead to disappointment, frustration, and hurt, all of which may contribute to the onset of breast cancer, as we will soon discover.

Unfortunately, many people do not receive the love and care they need from their mothers and are physically and emotionally ejected from the breast too soon and forced to fend for themselves from an early age. There are other people who do receive their mother's love but then are not weaned from the breast at the appropriate time— an unhealthy situation for both mother and child. The difficulties in achieving this delicate balance between holding and releasing, both of which involve love, is the basis of the mythological tales that speak of one breast offering love while the other is poisonous.

Understandably, mothering is not an exact science, and parents do the best they can under their particular circumstances. Over time, most children adapt to their situation by creating ways to find love as well as to develop self-confidence. But for certain people, the wounds of earliest childhood do not go away, mainly because of issues related to the heart chakra, leading to the potential for illnesses such as breast cancer. To understand this process, we need to look at two different scenarios.

Lack of Love

When an infant fails to receive comfort from being held close to her mother's breast, she experiences not only the immediate disconnection from her own mother, but disconnection from the archetypal spiritual bosom of the Great Mother (this of course applies to male children too, who suffer the same consequences). Cut off from the ethereal nourishment in which she marinated during her time in the womb, the infant is quickly set on the course of finding nourishment from the physical world. Such a child must learn to fend for herself from an early age and is forced to learn that she cannot rely on others for nurturing. Because of her early experiences, she may have a tendency not to trust love, keeping other people at a distance and often harboring an unconscious belief that the reason her mother didn't love her was because she is unlovable. When such a person does reach out for love, she may still keep herself somewhat at a distance or develop relationships with people who are similarly unavailable. Sadly, she may also experience the loss of other loved ones during her lifetime, reinforcing the belief that she is unworthy of love. Because such a woman learned survival skills early on, she is often successful in the outer world, receiving accolades that boost her self-confidence, while the deeper wound of being unloved remains unhealed. Amy was just such a woman.

From the outside, no one doubted Amy's self-assurance. She was gregarious, fun to be around, and always there for others. But she made certain that few people entered her own inner sanctum, which still contained the scars of living with a mentally ill mother who was rarely present during her early years. Although Amy was married, she and her husband lived relatively separate lives, and she always maintained she was too busy to have children. When she developed breast cancer, she dealt with it as she would a project at work, focusing on how she could remove the intruder from her life as quickly as possible with minimal emotional involvement. Following her allopathic treatment, she was given a clean bill of health—until the cancer returned three years later. Amy was finally forced to stop working in the outer world and, with the help of a good therapist, courageously began to take down the wall around her heart so she could at last feel, and only then release, the pain she had held in her heart since earliest childhood.

Women who lose their mother early in life, for whatever reason, may find themselves playing out the Persephone archetype. This Greek goddess was the daughter of the Mother Goddess Demeter. One day, as Persephone was playing, she was captured and taken by Pluto into the underworld, where she remained for some time. Meanwhile, Demeter became distraught and began searching for her daughter, a journey that ultimately led to Persephone's return.

This myth outlines the archetypal wound, not only of a grieving mother, but of a daughter who has lost the love of her mother. In an attempt to rekindle that love, the woman who carries the Persephone archetype will often take up a role in a caring profession, where she can "mother" other wounded daughters in the hope that this will heal her own wound.

Such caring for others to procure a lost love for oneself is also seen in the woman who dedicates herself to her family, especially her children, in the hope that if she showers them with love, one day she will feel loved herself. Unfortunately, we can never give enough love to fill our hearts if the door to our heart is locked by painful experiences from the past. Even if we're showered with love, we will probably not be able to feel and accept it, because we carry the anguish and belief that we don't deserve love. This reminds me of Sylvia:

The oldest of eight children, Sylvia was quickly ejected from the maternal breast by the birth of her sister. With her mother's attention now focused elsewhere as more and more children came, Sylvia grew up quickly, becoming responsible for the welfare of her younger siblings. As soon as she could, she left home to become a nurse and, in time, married and began her own family. All went well as she found happiness in the upbringing of her children and caring for other people. But things started to deteriorate when her children began to leave the nest. She had become so dependent on their love and their presence that she found herself attempting from a distance to get involved in every aspect of their lives, just to be close to them. She would expect them to call every day and increasingly became disappointed and hurt by what she felt was their lack of consideration. The more she demanded, the more they pulled away. Eventually, she developed breast cancer, which gave Sylvia the opportunity to take a good, hard look at herself and especially her relationship with her children. As she lay in a hospital bed receiving treatment, she could see how needy she had become, because, somewhere along the line, she had lost interest in herself. She remembered all the things she wanted to do for herself but that she had put aside for the sake of the family. These dreams came from deep within her heart, and as she started to give them an opportunity

*to be voiced, she found a new type of love entering her body—not from
outside but from her own soul connection.*

*As a teenager, one of the ways she would escape the demands and
chaos of her home was to take herself to town and wander around antiques
shops, imagining how the treasures she found could be brought together
to create a beautiful home. As her body healed, now with plenty of time
on her hands, Sylvia returned her attention to this hobby, which in time
became an occupation as more and more friends, valuing her opinion,
asked her to find treasures for their homes. Her children, delighted at the
transformation in their mother, increasingly found time to visit, enjoying
listening to their mother's enthusiasm as she described her new life.*

Another issue that can emerge from a lack of a mother's breast love
is the potential for not trusting the connection to the spiritual realms,
and especially to the love of the Great Mother, or God. A woman may
even believe she's been abandoned here on Earth, harboring feelings
of hurt and resentment and perhaps a sense that she must have done
something wrong. Such a woman may try to reconnect through prayer
and meditation, and yet healing begins only when we realize that it is
impossible *not* to be loved by the Great Mother, for we were made in
her exact image. At times like these, Mother Nature can play a vital role
by showing us the gentle and beautiful ways that plants and animals
seem to accept life here on Earth, and in time we can find ourselves
drinking the same sweet nectar of love.

Suffocated by Love

Now let's look at the child who did receive love and nurturing in early
childhood, but who stayed on the breast far longer than is deemed
healthy. Here, I am not necessarily talking about the physical sustenance
involved in breast-feeding, the duration of which, as already mentioned,
can vary from no breast-feeding for some children to staying on the
breast until four or five years of age for others. The issue is really about
emotional nutrition and whether there can be too much of a good thing,

especially if codependency develops between the mother and child, both believing that the weaning process will cause pain to the other. This is particularly common in single-parent families and where a child feels responsible for the mother's welfare, especially when he or she perceives the mother to be vulnerable and unable to cope on her own. The child may also unconsciously remain emotionally immature so as to provide the mother with permission to continue to "feed" him or her.

Unlike the child who was removed abruptly from the breast and hence from the safety and security of her spiritual home, the child in this situation often remains firmly connected to her spiritual roots and fails to make the full transition to Earth. Later, this person may develop a keen interest in spirituality, especially the New Age movement, for this is where she feels inherently at home.

From the standpoint of traditional Chinese medicine, the area most involved in these kinds of situations is the stomach meridian, which helps us create secure bonds with Mother Earth through the food we eat and the relationships we develop outside our family. Under normal circumstances, this ensures a healthy self-confidence and a willingness to stand on our own two feet. However, if a mother wants to keep her children close, perhaps to fulfill her own needs, then she is less likely to hand a child's care over to Mother Earth, thereby discouraging independence, self-assurance, and the forming of new relationships. As I discovered during my time of healing and introspection following my diagnosis, this is my own story. I certainly don't blame my mother for what happened; the situation suited us both.

As a child, I was super-shy, hypersensitive to the energies of other people, and my mother was strong and protective. The youngest child, I hid in her shadow, and although she encouraged all three of her children to get "out there," she also enjoyed the mutual dependency that she and I had, which allowed her to step forward and shine. I'm not sure there was anything she could have done differently to boost my confidence when I was young except as she did, to encourage me in areas where I excelled, which was academia and sports. My intuitive skills quickly taught me how to get on with people by being helpful, kind, and conscientious. But for most of my teenage years, I didn't have a clue as to who I was, and therefore I became reliant on strong characters—like my mother—to give me direction.

Our dependency became more complicated when I was seventeen and my father died. All of a sudden, the roles were reversed, and I was the one taking care of my mother. In that moment, I felt as if I had lost the two people whom I relied on the most to give me a feeling of security here on Earth. There were no other adults around to comfort me, so I focused all my healing energy on the person who was my rock, my mother, and she responded well to my attention.

It was during this period that the lump that eventually became a cancer thirty-five years later first appeared in my right breast. Some might say that it developed because of the trauma of my father's death, but I know it was linked to my emotional dependency on making my mother happy in order to survive. I underwent various tests at the time, all of which showed nothing sinister, and the lump slowly disappeared.

As the years passed, I moved in and out of relationships, and my mother was always there to comfort me when things fell apart. On one of those occasions, I was making lunch after returning from having a mammogram and biopsy of the same lump in my breast, the results eventually revealing a benign tumor. I posed what I believed was an innocent question (if there is such a thing) to my then husband: "What do I need to do to make you happy?" Simply and without emotion, he replied, "Let me go." It sounded like such an easy solution, and I wanted to say, "No, really, tell me something else to do." In that moment, my world was ripped apart—not because we had to worry about custody of children and division of animals or property, but because I couldn't believe you couldn't love someone enough to make them happy. Looking back, I can truly appreciate how resistant I was to admitting how unhappy I was in the marriage, as I had been subliminally driven by our familial adage you make your bed and lie on it. *My emotional identity was so intertwined with his that I truly believed that I couldn't be happy until he was happy—resulting in an impossible scenario for both of us.*

*Returning to my mother's love was safe and dependable. There were
times when her love felt suffocating, but I was also terrified to let go of
her metaphorical breast. As I became more and more successful in my
career, it became clear that my personal self, the "I" located in my heart,
between my breasts, had become lost between my spiritual desire to make
a difference in the world and the needs and wishes of other people. I was
a proficient pleaser, rescuer, and chameleon and had never fully grounded
in the full power of what it is to be Christine.*

*In December 1999, a few days before the new millennium, my
mother died suddenly. Despite the initial shock and grief, there was no
doubt that Mum had decided it was time for her to leave and for me to
stand on my own two feet. Whether she set me free or pushed me from
the bosom, I don't know, but love was definitely involved. Within a few
months, I made the decision to come to the United States, something I
would never have done if she was still alive. But it took until 2012 and
the diagnosis of breast cancer for me to finally stand in my power on my
own two feet, loving every part of myself. As the surgeon removed the
tumor, she also cut the emotional tie of dependency that had been so
strongly linked to other people through the solar plexus, freeing me to
make decisions that were best for Christine, the lovely woman whom I
see every day in the mirror.*

As I write, I am sure this story will resonate with other women,
especially those I've met who have become dependent on a relationship,
male or female, because, like me, they hadn't as yet fully embodied their
personal power and identity. In such situations it is so easy to cling to a
relationship, a metaphorical breast, even when the dysfunctional activities that take place within the relationship (often involving energy vampiring) merely enhance the intrinsic belief in one's own unworthiness.

*Margaret was one of the nicest people I had ever met. She was considerate
and charming and always had a smile on her face, which was surprising
as her husband of thirty years did nothing but treat her with disapproval*

and disrespect. He was constantly criticizing her for minor faults and rarely had a good word to say about her. The problem was that Margaret couldn't see anything wrong with his attitude, and like all codependent persons, she just kept making excuses for his bad behavior. This was mainly because she had experienced the same sort of criticism as a child, from her mother, who now lived around the corner from her marital home. When Margaret developed a lump in her breast, she kept it quiet, as she didn't want to bother anybody and knew she would probably receive little sympathy anyway. When she eventually went for help and was admitted on an urgent basis for immediate surgery, her husband merely looked up from his paper and said she was being inconsiderate to leave him at home to cope by himself. That comment was the tipping point for a rage that had never seen the light of day. As sick as she was, Margaret reached over, pulled down the newspaper, and announced, "Things are going to have to change or you're going to find yourself having to deal with more than just a few days of inconvenience." I'm not entirely sure what happened at home over the next few months, but suffice it to say that by the end of the year she filed for divorce and her empowerment was well under way.

As with other forms of cancer, those with a malignancy of the breast are often nice people who wish to please others in the subconscious hope that they will receive love in return. However, when their inner needs are not met, it is not uncommon for them to express anger and resentment, although being nice people their feelings are often veiled and may emerge in other ways, such as in passive aggressiveness, moodiness, or withdrawal of attention. Anger is linked to the liver meridian, which runs right through the breast tissue, and whose major role is to maintain the flow of qi or energy around the body. When anger is repressed, qi becomes stagnant, leading to a greater risk of developing breast disease.

This last story illustrates the complex feelings of anger, hurt, and rejection that can underlie a diagnosis of breast cancer.

Nancy was a fifty-six-year-old grandmother from the East End of London. She had been diagnosed with breast cancer three years earlier and had been successfully treated with allopathic medicine. But by the time she saw me, the cancer had returned, presenting as an unusually hard tumor in the same breast. When I asked, "What was happening in your life when you developed breast cancer?" she came straight to the point: "I know why I have cancer. Three years ago I visited my daughter. As a single parent, I've done everything for her, and now I'm helping with her children whenever I can." As she spoke, she touched her breasts as if to emphasize their flow of love. "We were sitting at the table and my grandson misbehaved. I naturally told him off. Immediately, my daughter attacked me, accusing me of trying to control her life and being critical of the way she's bringing up her children. Well, she might as well have stabbed me with a knife!" With that, she stabbed her hand into her left chest exactly at the site of her cancer. "I haven't spoken to my daughter since then," she concluded, clearly still deeply resentful of her daughter's reaction to her attempt to help. "Considering the seriousness of your condition, do you not feel it is time to talk and even make up?" I proffered. "No," she retorted. "I want her to come to my deathbed and see what she did to me!" Quietly I told her, "Your attitude is as hard as your cancer."

Fortunately, the next time I saw Nancy, her attitude had softened considerably. She had been to see her daughter, she told me, and they had shared many truths that had opened the door to a more honest and mature relationship between mother and daughter. Nancy's cancer did not instantly disappear, but she was no longer facing further treatment and recovery alone, for now she was supported by her family who loved her.

Factors Associated with Breast Cancer

Like any disease, there are many factors involved in the development of breast cancer. One question that arises is why the prevalence of the disease is so high in countries that possess some of the finest preventive-medicine information, screening techniques, and treatment regimens. Some researchers argue that it is because the intense level of screening shows cancers more frequently and earlier. However, as we will soon see, there may be other factors specific to these highly developed countries that should be brought into the equation.

Genetic Predisposition

For some years now, scientists have recognized that both genders have an increased risk of developing hereditary breast cancer if they are carrying certain mutations of genes known as BRCA1 and BRCA2 (breast cancer susceptibility genes 1 and 2). In normal cells, these genes help prevent uncontrolled cell growth. However, based on our understanding of the science of epigenetics, even when a mutated gene is present, it still requires certain environmental factors to switch it on. It is clear that further research is needed to understand the familial and psychological triggers that potentially contribute to the onset of this disease.

Family History

There is a definite higher risk of breast cancer where there is family history of the disease or a history of cancer in other female organs. Whether this is because of gene patterns as yet not discovered, or more likely because of patterns of behavior that have been running through the ancestral lineage for many generations, we have yet to clearly discern.

Age

Breast cancer is much more common in women whose first menses occurred before the age of twelve and whose menopause didn't take place before the age of fifty-five. It is also known that women who have never had children or who started their family after the age of thirty are at a greater risk of developing breast cancer. In fact, a woman who has her first child after the age of thirty-five has twice the risk of developing breast cancer as the woman who gives birth to her first child before the age of twenty.

Ethnicity

A study conducted in the United States found that the highest prevalence of breast cancer occurs among white women, with Hispanic and Native American women showing much lower levels of the disease.[8]

Breast-Feeding

Some organizations cite the reduced incidences of breast cancer among those who breast-feed as a means to persuade expectant mothers that they should breast-feed their babies. However, studies show that any such benefit occurs only after twelve to eighteen months of breast-feeding, the protective effect probably attributed to the bonding that naturally occurs between mother and child over such a length of time.[9]

Estrogen

Seventy-five percent of breast cancers occur in women over the age of fifty, and most of these tumors are estrogen dependent—in other words, highly susceptible to circulating estrogen in the body. Whereas HRT is obviously culpable, soy products and high doses of vitamin E are both known to be estrogenic and hence potential factors in the causation of cancer.

Obesity and Exercise

Being overweight or obese certainly appears to increase the risk of breast cancer, especially in postmenopausal women whose fat tissues becomes the source of estrogen supplies. However, the issue is not clear-cut, as those who gain weight during adulthood have been seen to have a greater potential for developing breast cancer than those who have been overweight since childhood.[10] Similarly, those who store their fat around the waist seem to be at greater risk than those with fat thighs. In the midst of this uncertainty, the experts recommend the maintenance of a healthy weight and body mass index (BMI) at all times. Regular exercise, in which the body reaches a peak level of aerobic activity for at least twenty minutes a day, has also been shown to help keep the body healthy and cancer-free by enhancing the efficiency of the immune system.

Foods and Vitamins

Many studies have attempted to isolate the foods that appear to contribute to the onset of breast cancer, but without success. Part of the problem is that we cannot isolate a food item from the value a culture places on eating and mealtimes. At the same time, there has been no conclusive evidence that shows that extra minerals or vitamins make a difference, although research continues in these areas.

Alcohol

Several studies have shown a link between an excessive alcohol intake (anything over one glass a day)* and breast cancer, thought to be because of the way a woman's body metabolizes alcohol. However, there has been little research that has looked at the incidence of breast cancer and a woman's drinking patterns. Does she drink to celebrate or commiserate? Is it a social event or shrouded in secrecy? It is known that women have a greater tendency to drink at home and alone, as well as to use alcohol to reduce the stress of troubled relationships.[11] Could excessive alcohol intake merely be a symptom of a much deeper issue of low self-esteem?

The Pill, HRT, and Fertility Treatment

The contraceptive pill is known to increase the risk of a woman developing breast cancer, although the risk disappears ten years after she has stopped the pill. As mentioned previously, women who take HRT also have a much higher risk of developing breast cancer, and the American Cancer Society suggests that these risks should be taken into account before HRT is recommended. There is ongoing research to decide whether fertility hormones, usually prescribed for much shorter periods than the pill or HRT, may increase the risk of ovarian and breast cancer, although at present the association has not been incontrovertibly established.[12]

---

*For clarity, a standard glass of wine is seen as a 5-ounce pour, which is equivalent to one shot of hard alcohol or 12 ounces of beer.

Melatonin

As we will learn in the next chapter, the hormone melatonin is essential to maintaining normal sleep cycles as well as affecting the timing of menarche because of its effect on ovarian function. It has been shown that women who develop breast cancer between the ages of sixty and sixty-five are more likely to have receptor sites to melatonin on the cell membranes of their breasts, although the deeper meaning of these findings is still unclear.[13]

Antiperspirants, Pesticides, Smoking, and Breast Implants

All these substances have been studied at one time or another as potential factors in the causation of breast disease, without any concrete link being established.

Brassieres

The wearing of a bra has been intertwined with functionality and social status as far back as the seventh century BCE, when women athletes of the Minoan culture wore a bralike piece of clothing to increase their chances of athletic success. From the sixteenth century onward, the bra was part of a woman's corset, pushing the breasts up from below to emphasize her beauty. In the early twentieth century, the bra and corset were separated, and today the selling of brassieres is a multibillion-dollar industry, with the bra as much a fashion item as something worn for its functionality.

Experts believe that over 70 percent of women wear poorly fitted bras. This is thought to be partly because of the fact that we make choices based on fashion rather than on comfort. There is also a tendency not to notice the fact that even if our cup size remains the same as we age, our chest circumference expands. Many women wear a bra because of a belief that if they don't their breasts will sag. Yet researchers in Japan and France have shown that rather than causing the breasts to sag, going braless actually causes the breasts to become more shapely.[14] In 2003, Dr. Laetitia Pierrot and Jean-Denis Rouillon asked

250 women who practiced sports to stop wearing a bra for one year. By the end of the study, 88 percent of the participants reported improved comfort, while the measurements showed firmer, more elevated, and perkier breasts overall.

From a health point of view, there is no doubt that a mismatch between our natural contours and the fit of our bra can lead to skin irritation, back pain, and headaches over a period of time. In 2000, two British breast surgeons asked a small group of premenopausal women with moderate breast pain to go braless for three months. Not only did the pain reduce significantly, but the women's moods became more positive. The surgeons also used thermography, which showed that wearing a bra increased the heat of the breast. Unfortunately, the research did not go far enough, and it failed to study whether the heat actually caused cellular changes in the breast.[15] An earlier study carried out by Harvard researchers, published in the *European Journal of Cancer* in 1991, revealed that women who went braless had a lower rate of breast cancer than women who wore bras, although the investigators would not go so far as to suggest that wearing a bra causes cancer.

Vocal exponents of the link between the wearing of a bra and breast cancer are medical anthropologists Sydney Ross Singer and Soma Grismaijer. In their book *Dressed to Kill,* published in 1995, they claimed that the restrictive nature of the bra—especially those that are underwired—constricts the lymphatic vessels, preventing adequate drainage of the breast tissue, leading to unhealthy fluid and toxin accumulation in the breasts.[16] Their claims have been disputed by most of the major cancer organizations, who cite inadequate standards of research and the lack of consideration of other known risk factors. Medical specialists also state that 75 percent of the lymph from the breast passes to the lymph nodes in the axilla, or armpit, rather than passing under the tight band of a bra into the abdomen, making the bra irrelevant to the issue. However, in my mind there is no smoke without fire, and there must be good reasons why so few studies have been carried out to answer these fundamental questions:

- Are bras healthy for me or not?
- Should I limit the wearing of a bra to less than twelve hours a day?
- Would an annual professional fitting for a new bra reduce my health risks?
- What are the risks from wearing underwired bras?

Intuitively, I have never felt inclined to buy or wear an underwired bra, despite the difficulty of finding bras without wires from many lingerie retailers. During my research for this book, I was surprised to learn how many of my friends had made similar personal decisions, either wearing nonwired bras or no bra at all.

Wiring began in the 1950s in the belief that greater support could be offered to the breast, although, as noted above, this is truly a myth. Today the metal used is mainly steel, and although as a teenager I couldn't pinpoint my concerns, I knew that any wires had the potential to stop the flow of energy around my body. This has been confirmed by acupuncturists, who express concern that the underwiring of bras may restrict the flow of energy partly because of the tightness of the material used and partly because of the actual wire, which interferes with the flow of qi. This is a particular issue for the stomach and liver meridians, which ascend from the abdomen into the breast. For this reason, energy medicine authority Donna Eden advises all women to wear bras that are free of wire (whether metal or plastic) so that their energy can flow unimpeded.[17]

Cultural and Religious Factors

One area that seems to receive little attention is the cultural and religious differences between various countries and the incidence of breast cancer. What do countries with the highest incidences of breast cancer, such as Belgium, Holland, Malta, Great Britain, and the United States, have in common? Or, looking at it from another perspective, what do cultures with low incidences of the disease, such as Japan and China, have in common? The answer to the second question is, I believe, the fact that these countries were less affected by the spread of patriarchal doctrines rampant during the days of the Greek and Roman civilizations, which in turn were supported by the birth of religions such as Christianity. Any religious teachings that maintain a basic lack of reverence for the feminine while suggesting that their followers should doubt the unconditional and eternal love of the Divine Mother must negatively impact the cellular activity of breast tissue. Such false beliefs include:

- It is better to give than to receive.
- A woman's role is to love and take care of her family.
- Your family's happiness is your reward.
- Service and sacrifice are good for the soul.
- Self-love is selfish and not spiritual.
- You must give in order to receive.
- Think of others before you think of yourself.
- Celebration of one's achievements is egotistical.
- Love of your body is the work of the devil.

These beliefs have accumulated within the personal and cultural collective unconscious of women over many centuries. They will never be transformed until women return to their sacred roles within society.

I also suggest that a common feature in countries where the incidence of breast cancer is low is the prevalence of a strong sense of tribal or family connection, where the needs of the family or group are still considered important. Have women in the West become so intent on self-sufficiency and self-identity that we have forgotten that our greatest source of nurturance is found within community and especially with our close, bosom friends? There is clear evidence to show that a woman who has close women friends and confidantes has far less of a chance of becoming ill and is able to maintain good physical health well into her later years.[18]

So what does the Mother Cow want us to know?

- Our breasts represent the loving bosom of the Great Mother.
- They are symbols of trust, openness, softness, and sustenance.
- Through their prominence and shape, our breasts focus the transformative energy of the heart chakra.
- This center is a transitional point between the spiritual energy of the Queen of Heavens and the physical essence of Mother.
- When energy flows between the Queen of Heavens and Mother Earth. Earth, assisted by the energy that flows through the breasts, we are guaranteed love, confidence, and a strong sense of self-identity.
- It is a woman's role to maintain the link between Heaven and Earth, which is achieved through her own sense of self-love and connection.
- The energy that radiates from the heart and breasts is love, also known as the milk of immortality.
- When a child is born, the breasts support its transition from the spiritual world until it is ready to nurture itself on the riches of Mother Earth.
- There are times in our lives when we will return to the breast of the Great Mother, and by drinking her milk of immortality, we will travel to the source of inspiration and restoration.
- At these times, we probably need to turn within, spend time in nature, be in the presence of someone who offers motherly love, or seek the warm embrace or reassuring hug of a loved one.
- Once our soul has been renewed, we need to release our hold on the metaphorical nipple and return to the outer world with confidence and a new sense of purpose.
- The breasts remind us that the love of the Great Mother is eternal, offering us abundant joy if we just open our hearts.

Our breasts are beautiful, they are precious, and they belong to us.

he great-grandmothers, including Hera, Isis, Annapurna, and Artemis, are standing before us now holding their breasts toward us. They urge us to release our tendency to feel separate, so that we may nestle into their breasts, linking our hearts together. As we bond, we are filled with the milk of immortality, which nurtures every cell in our body and then radiates out through our breasts. This creates an aura of confidence, contentment, and connectivity, which encourages others to know such love as well.

୨

RITUAL NO. 3

Surrendering into Love with Mother Cow

It is now time to return to the serpent curled up comfortably within the uterus and encourage it to ascend once again so that it may trigger the heart to pour out its joy, laughter, and playfulness, just as a child will laugh when he or she feels loved and secure. Such pleasure in innocence naturally encourages our adult ego to release its hold on separation, pride, and seriousness and snuggle into the breast of the Great Mother so we can be lifted into the place of mystery and inspiration at the crown chakra.

If this ritual is taking place during the dark moon, this practice is best achieved on the morning of the second day. It can also take place at sunset if you are following the sun's movement through the sky over a day. The first part of the exercise can be carried out sitting, lying, or standing—whatever is most comfortable, as we are going to work with love and nurturing.

Close your eyes and inhale. On the exhalation, breathe all the worries and concerns of the head and heart down into Mother Earth, asking her to receive and transform them. Repeat the inhalation and exhalation until you feel calmer.

Breathing normally, take your awareness to the heart chakra and breathe in and out of the heart, mixing the breath with compassion. Now, through your heart's mind, imagine that you are sitting in a wonderful, sensually comfortable chair where you can relax, perhaps curling up inside so that the chair totally supports you. Relax deeper and deeper into the chair. The chair represents the softness and strength of your own heart, a place to feel completely safe and nurtured. Relax. As you allow yourself to be cossetted in love from your own heart, watch as those who love you in your present life approach the chair and shower you with more love. Behind them follow those who love you from the spirit world: family, friends, guides, angels, and spiritual teachers. Allow yourself to absorb their love and compassion unconditionally, filling all the cells of your body, especially those that are distressed or diseased, until you feel satisfied. Bathe in this gorgeous state until you are ready to come back to full consciousness. Sending love and gratitude to those who have visited you as you relaxed in your chair/heart, allow the visions to dim and open your eyes. Take some time to enjoy this feeling of love throughout your body, but especially in your heart.

With the heart now open to receive, you are ready to connect the heart to the womb. This stage of the ritual is best carried out standing on the earth with your legs slightly apart, preferably wearing a skirt. In order to build the energy, we will first repeat the process that ensures a pure and steady connection between your womb and Mother Earth, from which you draw your feminine energy.

With your hands over the hara (fingertips together to create a downward-pointing triangle), imagine an umbilical cord that stretches between the root chakra deep within the earth and the sacral chakra. Beginning at the hara, inhale and then exhale slowly and deeply down along this umbilical cord and into the root chakra. Repeat the breath three times. At the end of the third exhalation, pause and experience a vast peace as you are washed in the waves of mystery, nothingness, and thousands of years of women's wisdom.

Now, inhale and draw the energy back up along the umbilical cord and back into your sacral chakra under your hands, repeating the process until your womb is full. Feel the strength and joy as the energy vitalizes and nurtures your energy field. Feel the inner power of knowing that you are eternally connected to the full creative force and wisdom of what it is to be a sacred woman.

Now place your right hand on the hara and your left on the heart chakra. See whether you can sense the rhythm or pulse of their energy fields, that of the hara often being slower and deeper. Imagine that you have a drinking straw that links these two chakras and signifies the masculine energy of the solar plexus.

Now imagine that you are located within the heart chakra, with one of the ends of the straw in your mouth. On inhalation, begin to draw the serpent energy, plus the gems of wisdom, up along the straw. On exhalation, allow it to fall back, but only by 30 percent. Repeat the process with deep inhalations and exhalations, until you feel the energy start to flow into your heart.

As it enters your heart you will sense a range of emotions including lightness, joy, laughter, and excitement. Using your imagination, see the energy in your heart chakra move between the breasts, mapping out a figure-eight design. In this way the Cow Mother churns the energy until essence becomes spirit. The process may even evoke memories of times when you have felt your heart opened spontaneously, the memories enhancing the experience until your heart is full with the expansive energy of joy, love, and a deep trust.

Finally, return your attention to the straw, which has become a divine passageway between the womb (your power) and the heart (joyful creativity and deep connection). To ensure this passageway stays open, with your hands still in place, inhale, moving your energetic awareness from the heart to the sacral chakra. Hold your breath for twenty seconds while you sense the power available to you to fulfill your dreams. Then exhale and follow the energy back into the heart. Repeat this five times. Then move the energy in the opposite direction. Start at the sacral chakra or womb and inhale into the heart, holding your breath for twenty seconds as you experience a lightness, enthusiasm, and joyfulness. Then exhale back to the womb and repeat five times.

Just as we need to maintain the connection between the root and sacral chakras, so we need to keep this passageway open, reminding us that the womb gives power to our words and the heart gives creative expression to our dreams.

PART FOUR

The Queen Bee

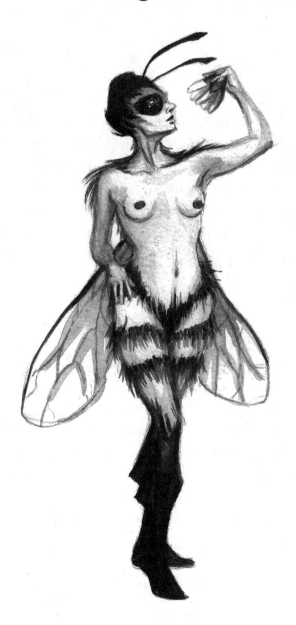

9

DEVELOPING WINGS TO FLY

It is now time to meet the Queen Bee, who rests on top of our crown chakra awaiting our arrival. Even though she is primarily linked to the activities of the tiny pineal gland, she appreciates that to gain perspective, we must first focus our attention on the whole brain. Unlike the fertility organs and the breasts, it is not initially obvious that there are any specific anatomical distinctions between the brains of men and women. It is true that a man's brain is 10 percent larger in volume, but research suggests this doesn't necessarily make him more intelligent; it is the extra neurons required to support the male's larger muscle mass that results in the brain's larger capacity.

Where differences between the brains of the sexes have been observed, with the help of modern imaging techniques, questions have been raised as to whether these differences should be attributed to genes, hormones, or the environment—the nature-versus-nurture debate. Since we now know that the brain's plasticity allows for new neuronal pathways to develop in response to the environment, even in adult life, it is no longer possible to say that a child's upbringing defines his or her subsequent brain activity. However, one study that looked at the influence of hormones in utero followed a group of girls who, because of an unusual disease found in their mothers, were bathed in high levels of testosterone while in the womb. These women were found to exhibit strong masculine tendencies.[1]

Many researchers still look at brain function through somewhat stereotypical perceptions. Men are seen as hunter-gatherers who require good navigational skills to hunt at distances many miles from their homes. They use intellectual, strategic skills to compete with other hunters and are happy to hunt alone, often in silence, to avoid scaring away their prey. Women are viewed as being more likely to stay around the home to nurture and ensure the survival of the family. They rely on strength in numbers and employ intuition and empathy to create community through constant communication. However, modern life is far less clear-cut; men increasingly stay at home with the family, and women take on the role of the hunter-gatherer. Although studies show that dissimilarities in brain activity do exist between the genders, it is clear that it is much more significant to look at whether the person expresses masculine or feminine tendencies rather than whether he or she is genetically male or female. Recently, it has been observed that fathers who spend more time with their children have significantly lower levels of testosterone than before they started a family, suggesting that men are biologically primed to be more caring and less aggressive when they are around the home.[2]

As we review the brain activity that is seen to be more prevalent in women, it is important to remember that the term *woman* here is equated with femininity.

THE INHERENT QUALITIES OF THE FEMALE BRAIN

Community

A woman's strength comes not from her muscle power, but from her ability to create community, which requires good communication skills and shared goals. To this end, women are known to have better social and verbal skills than men. This heightened desire to connect is reflected in the brain's structure: men have more neurons in their cerebral cortex, while women have more spaces between the neurons. These spaces are filled with dendrites and synapses that are essential for the exchange of information between the nerve cells—in other words, for shared communication.[3] This mirrors the tendency for women to gather and talk to one another when under stress rather than to activate the fight-or-flight response. UCLA psychologist Dr. Shelley Taylor calls this reaction "tend and befriend" and suggests that it arises as a result of increased levels of oxytocin released during stress. Oxytocin's effects are enhanced in the presence of estrogen, leading to a greater tendency for bonding, relaxation, and trust.[4] Testosterone, on the other hand, inhibits oxytocin, leading to the more classical response to stress: fight or flight. Notably, the sacral chakra, linked to estrogen release, is also associated with community, reciprocally rewarding relationships, and sharing. This suggests that women naturally gravitate to this center during times of stress. This reaction is often enhanced by sitting together in a group, often on the floor, which probably allows women to tap into the deeper wisdom of the Great Mother beneath their feet.

Communication

The two areas of the brain associated with language have been described as being larger in women than in men.[5] At the same time, women are more likely to communicate by telling stories and creating pictures to enhance their message rather than making direct statements.

Problem Solving

Whereas both genders can solve problems, men tend to achieve this by applying their analytical mind, whereas women access memories and past experience to reach a conclusion. A study found that when faced with a problem, women activate more of the white matter in their frontal lobes, while men rely on their gray matter from all over the brain.[6] Gray matter consists of nerve cells or neurons that initiate a thought or action, while white matter consists of myelinated axons, which run from the nerve cells and make connections all across the brain. The frontal lobes are associated with decision making and the ability to filter out what is important, allowing women to be excellent at multitasking when the process is not obscured by unnecessary details. Women are also able to extract themselves from the task and observe the bigger picture, while men tend to be totally focused on the one task and cannot possibly handle anything else!

There are also neural pathways that run from the frontal lobes to the limbic or emotional center, allowing a woman to decide which emotionally based memories are worth retaining, in accordance with social acceptability. This means that to solve a problem, a woman will access information far beyond the mere facts, providing her with the opportunity to make decisions that benefit the family and community as well as the individual.

Spatial Awareness

Although men are renowned for their ease at being able to turn images around in their minds and to read maps, women navigate themselves around the world using landmarks.[7] This emphasizes how natural it is for a woman to define herself in relationship to her surroundings, and it could explain why women are more likely to have a poorer sense of self than a man. Women also use other stimuli, such as shapes, smells, and sounds, to enhance their memory, tapping into the emotional memories of the limbic system.

Emotions and Empathy

Men and women are equally emotional, although women are more likely to *want* to show their emotions, especially through their facial expressions. It is noteworthy that increased levels of circulating prolactin in both men and women are thought to be the cause of the tears that well up in the presence of something beautiful.[8] Women are usually considered to be more empathic than men, readily able to pick up and act on subtle emotional clues, although this trait can also be seen in men whose feminine side is strong.

THE PINEAL GLAND

Esoterically, the various structures of the brain, including the cerebral cortex and the limbic system, are not regarded as the true origination point of our thoughts, actions, and emotions. They merely reveal a far deeper source of personal inspiration that is linked to our soul's purpose and is probably associated with a tiny pea-size structure called the pineal gland.

As we continue our journey into the mysteries of womanhood, we find ourselves looking at one of the biggest mysteries of the human body: the pineal gland, sometimes called the third eye. When I was a medical student, little was written about this tiny, pine-cone-shaped gland, apart from the fact that in many adults the gland is calcified.

For clarification, the pineal gland is about the size of your little finger's nail and is situated between the two hemispheres of the brain, toward the top of the head. It is not actually part of the brain; it sits outside the brain's natural defenses, also known as the blood-brain barrier. Several researchers, including Dr. Rick Strassman, clinical associate professor of psychiatry at the University of New Mexico

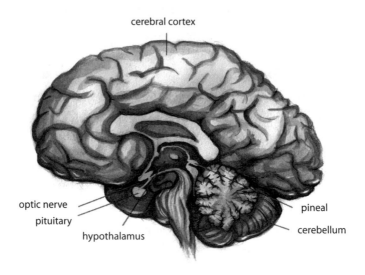

The pineal gland

School of Medicine and author of *DMT: The Spirit Molecule,* have remarked how interesting it is that the pineal is first seen in the fetus around the forty-nine-day mark, which is closely aligned to the time it is thought that the soul initially enters the physical body.[9] The gland is connected to the sympathetic and parasympathetic nervous systems and therefore is strongly influenced by the release of their neurotransmitters, including noradrenaline and adrenaline; it also has a profuse blood flow, second only to that of the kidneys. Its location, very close to the cerebrospinal fluid in the ventricles, allows its secretions easy access to all parts of the brain and nervous system. At the same time, because of its anatomical proximity, there is a strong connection between the pineal gland and the nerve impulses concerned with sound and light, as well as the emotions of the limbic system.

Calcification of the Pineal Gland

In 1985, scientists showed that adults with a calcified pineal gland were far more likely to have a defective sense of direction than those whose pineal gland was normal; similar results were also seen in homing pigeons.[10] This study clearly suggests that the pineal gland plays a major role in synthesizing information about our location within our environment; such input is gathered not only from our eyes and ears but also, it is believed, from the pineal gland's own sensitivity to electromagnetic wave patterns.

Another study carried out in 2008 showed that whereas calcification of the pineal gland is seen in 50 to 60 percent of Caucasians over the age of forty, it is extremely low in people of Africa, where the figures are between 2 and 5 percent.[11] When the pineal gland of black and white Americans was compared, the degree of calcification between the two groups was also found to be significant, with the gland of Caucasians showing far higher levels of calcification. There is clearly a cultural factor involved, requiring more detailed research.[12]

A 1997 study revealed that high levels of sodium fluoride from drinking water and toothpaste were found in the pineal gland, and the researchers hypothesized that this was a factor in pineal dysfunction and calcification.[13] Although calcium fluoride is naturally found in water, sodium fluoride is totally unnatural to the body and is in fact a by-product of the nuclear and pesticide industries. Despite the many attempts over the years to show it for what it is, medical and dental organizations insist that it is beneficial, which is certainly not the case for the pineal gland. While many European countries have banned its addition to water supplies, fluoride continues to be found in the water of 70 percent of the homes in the United States, in almost all of the drinking water in Australia, and in varying degrees in other countries. Adding sodium fluoride to the water in Africa is very unusual, on the other hand.

Apart from the damage fluoridation inflicts on the pineal gland, there are possibly other factors involved in the calcification process, although their involvement is less clear-cut. For a long time it was believed that aging had a part to play in the changes to the pineal gland, but in the aforementioned studies, where levels of calcification were seen to be low, they were low across all ages, decreasing the viability of this theory. In 1978, Mark Cohen, of the National Institute of Cancer, revealed that breast cancer is much more common in countries where calcification of the pineal gland is prevalent.[14] It is known that one of the pineal gland's hormones, melatonin, is particularly associated with the onset of menarche at puberty and probably influences a woman's menstrual cycle. Clearly, further research is required to clarify not only the link between calcification of the gland and breast cancer but also the link between calcification and the function of the pineal gland—in particular, its role in helping us access higher states of consciousness.

History and Esoteric Understanding of the Pineal Gland

The earliest records that speak of the pineal gland come from around the third century BCE. Its name comes from the Latin word *pineus,* meaning "pine." The French philosopher René Descartes was fascinated by the pineal gland, calling it the "seat of the soul" and the meeting place between the spiritual and the physical realms. Though his mystical beliefs in the gland were not questioned, many of his medical ideas were later disputed as knowledge of anatomy became more sophisticated.[15] Toward the end of the nineteenth century it was proposed that the pineal gland is a third eye, an idea that continues to flourish in many esoteric teachings. For this reason, the pineal gland is often linked to the third-eye chakra, while the pituitary gland is associated with the crown chakra. Nevertheless, I am in no doubt that the pineal gland belongs to the crown chakra, while the main role of the pituitary, or master gland, is to physically balance all the other glands in the body, which means it is related to the third-eye chakra.

This concept of the pineal being a third eye comes from the fact that in certain lizards and fish, a light-sensitive eye has been described. In *The Secret Doctrine* (1888), Madame Helena Blavatsky, the cofounder of the Theosophical movement, writes that in the early days, human beings had three actual eyes: two to look ahead and one to look behind. This suggests that the third eye was at the back of the head, which is in fact the position of the pineal gland. She goes on to say, "When men having fallen into matter, their spiritual vision became dim . . . the third eye commenced to lose its power."[16] According to Madame Blavatsky, as the third eye became buried beneath the hair and was petrified, inner vision had to be awakened by artificial stimuli (possibly mind-altering drugs), in processes known only to the sages Alice Bailey, the esoteric writer who followed Madame Blavatsky, writes in *Esoteric Healing* that "when the pineal gland returns to its full function, the divine purpose of humanity will work out."[17]

The Crown Chakra

This center preserves our link between the soul and its spiritual blueprint, also known as the higher self: the divine aspect of our being, which does not incarnate here on Earth. When we become dispirited, depressed, or exhausted, it is because, for some reason, the crown chakra has become closed and we are no longer able to receive inspiration and renewal for our soul. In my working experience, I commonly see this occur for those in the midst of grief. In the darkness of their despair, they find themselves questioning all their previously held beliefs about a God or the afterlife. I also intuitively perceive a cap or hands being placed over the crown, as if they are saying to their spiritual guides, "I'm not ready to receive any more insights or awareness; I just want to be left alone for a while." Such an instruction is well understood by those in the spirit world, who sometimes have to be reminded that we have to deal with emotions and the challenges of time in the physical world.

On other occasions I perceive the crown chakra is wide open, with energy flowing freely in both directions, and I see the person excited and fired up with new creative ideas. However, if there is no vessel suitable for the ideas, they will continue to just swarm around the head and never find a place to land. Since the feminine crown chakra is linked to the masculine base chakra, we need to be grounded in our body and fully committed to the venture to see our dreams become a reality.

The Endocrine Functions of the Pineal Gland
Melatonin

In 1958, the hormone melatonin was isolated from the pineal gland. It is derived from the alkaloid tryptamine and is metabolized from the neuropeptide serotonin, which is found in large quantities in the pineal gland. The secretion of melatonin is increased during darkness and decreased in the light, the highest levels being recorded between 2 and 3 a.m. In contrast, serotonin levels are higher during the day and lower at night. Melatonin is believed to regulate our circadian rhythms as well as our sleep patterns. Because of this, it is popularly used by those whose normal sleep patterns are disturbed by jet lag or who work the night shift, although it is not a panacea for all cases of insomnia and should be taken with care.

Melatonin inhibits the secretion of estrogen by the ovaries and hence ovulation. This is very important to all mammals, apart from humans, to ensure that vulnerable offspring are not born during the cold and dark winter months. Although it is commonly believed that the light, which affects our sleep patterns and circadian rhythms, reaches the pineal gland via the retina, some researchers believe that the pineal gland is itself light-sensitive, especially to the electromagnetic waves of celestial bodies such as the sun and moon.

DMT

For a long time, research on the pineal gland was totally focused on melatonin, with many believing that this hormone would provide confirmation of Descartes's hypothesis that the pineal gland is the seat of the soul. Yet despite its powerful connection to darkness and its natural contraceptive properties, melatonin didn't seem to have any deeper effects on the psyche.

Enter DMT, or N,N-dimethyltryptamine, a naturally occurring compound derived from tryptamine and its associated amino acid tryptophan. It is found in several plants as well as in the human body, especially in the brain, lungs, blood vessels, glands, and skin. DMT is a psychoactive or psychedelic drug, its main function being to alter perception and cognition. When we ingest it or it is released in the body, in particular from the pineal gland, we are transported from our three-dimensional world into a multidimensional universe, where our psyche becomes aware of a vast array of images and feelings held within the collective unconsciousness. Dr. Rick Strassman's research showed, when he gave intravenous DMT to volunteers, that it is not uncommon to meet sub-personalities, spirit guides, deceased loved ones, extraterrestrial beings, and even demons while under the influence of the drug. Despite DMT's ability to produce profound changes to our moods and perceptions, it is given an easy passage across the blood-brain barrier and into the brain, which can only be explained if it is understood to be nectar for the soul.

DMT is the primary psychoactive element in ayahuasca, a mainly South American spirit vine or plant medicine. In preparing the brew, the shaman will include parts of the plant that are known to inhibit the breakdown of DMT by enzymes in the stomach, allowing the drug to have its effects. In the same way, the pineal gland produces substances called beta-carbolines, which enhance the effects of DMT by preventing its breakdown by an enzyme known as monoamine oxidase.

According to Dr. Strassman, there are specific times in our lives when our body is flooded by DMT from the pineal gland. These include:

- When our spirit enters our physical body around the forty-ninth day after conception
- At the time of our birth
- During our moon time
- When giving birth
- In near-death experiences
- At the height of an orgasm
- During deep meditation

At other times, the levels are fairly stable. This is thought to be due to a protective mechanism that naturally isolates the pineal gland from daily fluctuating levels of the stress hormones adrenaline and noradrenaline. However, Dr. Strassman suggests that in patients with schizophrenia and other forms of delusional psychosis, these barriers are weakened, allowing higher than normal levels of DMT to be secreted, leading to many of the symptoms of psychosis.[18]

Occasionally, a sudden release of DMT from the pineal gland can occur during an uncontrolled spiritual awakening, when the energy of kundalini rises suddenly along the energy pathways and surges into the crown chakra. This may happen spontaneously, in association with shock, or when a person indulges in a spiritual practice for which he or she is ill prepared. The forces released often result in a "spiritual emergency," leading to both physical symptoms, such as involuntary jerking of the limbs and rushes of heat and insomnia, and mental changes. Along with visual and auditory sensations, some people experience fear, disorientation, and delusion, while others float in intense feelings of bliss and unconditional love.

Gateway to Higher Consciousness

I suspect it's easier for a woman to enter altered states of consciousness, without the need for mind-altering drugs, as her body is hormonally primed to shift its awareness, especially during her moon time, in childbirth, and after menopause. At such times, the secretion of DMT is potentially increased, although more studies are required to confirm this hypothesis. Meanwhile, research already suggests that when a woman is in labor, increased levels of DMT are released along with opiates, leading to the ecstatic feelings women so often report. During this time, the mother's body is naturally flooded with stress hormones such as adrenaline and noradrenaline, which breach the defenses of the pineal gland, leading to the release of high levels of DMT. The more the woman in labor is able to synchronize her breathing with the waves of contractions, the greater the blissful effect. As expected, these feelings are greatly reduced in the presence of an epidural or high doses of analgesia, as well as when the birth is via a C-section. Dr. Stanislav Grof, who carried out extensive research into the effects of psychedelic drugs on the psyche, commented that when a child is born by a C-section, it misses out on the ecstatic release that occurs during a vaginal delivery. He concluded that in his experience, such people have greater resistance to letting go of control and entering higher states of awareness, as they were not primed to DMT at the time of their birth.[19]

Dr. Grof, regarded as the father of holotrophic breath work, designed a specific technique to enhance self-development and wholeness. Through the use of this breathing technique, the person is encouraged to release her hold on everyday reality and allow her breath to carry her into altered states of awareness. On many occasions, music and visual imagery are added to bring the whole body, and especially the brain, into a state of higher resonance. At a certain point, the wave of resonance created by the cycling of the breath crests the defenses of the pineal gland, causing it to light up and start to produce increased levels of DMT. These same principles of using the breath, images, and sound, including chanting, to focus the mind and enter altered states of reality are seen in many forms of meditation. This is not a new practice but has been used for thousands of years by many cultures. Whether they used techniques like this in combination with mind-altering plant substances or not, ancient peoples knew that the portal to multidimensional worlds could be opened through activation of the pineal gland.

One story about the pineal gland that always fills me with a sense of truth comes from Jonathan Goldman, in his excellent book *Healing Sounds*. He shares a story about a visit to the underground tomb of Lord Pakal, in Palenque, Mexico. When all the lights were extinguished, he was guided to use his voice to tone, in ways in which he is truly gifted. Even though the room was completely dark, a diffuse light began to appear, which he suspects came from the pineal gland.[20] Physician Frank Barr concurs by showing that the pineal gland is rich in a substance known as neuromelanin, which has the ability to turn sound into light under certain circumstances.[21]

Whether through breath work, meditation, intuitive seeking, or the ingestion of psychedelic drugs, the key questions are the same: What is your highest intention? Why are you knocking on the door of your unconscious? Are you ready to see and take full responsibility for who you truly are? Most of the spiritual beings that were encountered during Dr. Strassman's studies were welcoming and kind, and they often appeared in the presence of bright lights and the sound of buzzing. This fanfare announces the arrival of the Queen Bee.

ENTER THE QUEEN BEE

I had never heard of the Queen Bee or even thought about bees until the early days of writing this book, when she came to call. As I was researching the various Venus figurines from 20,000 to 30,000 years ago, I happened to pick up an imitation statue of the Venus of Willendorf and held her in the cup of my hand. In many ways she is similar to all the other depictions of the fertility goddesses from those times, with large thighs, buttocks, and abdomen and voluminous breasts. She has no feet, and her thin arms are tucked into her sides. But what is most curious is that her head is wrapped in an intricate woven effect covering most of her face. It has been suggested by some researchers that the complete obliteration of her facial features is because as a fertility figure her face is less important. However, what is significant is that despite the rather crude features of the rest of her body, her head covering is well defined, suggestive of a cap or plaited hair.

When the head is examined in more detail we see the presence of seven circles, with two half circles at the neck and a rosette at the crown. The circles are transected by vertical grooves, causing some researchers to suggest that this is her hair, a symbol of great wisdom in many cultures. Yet despite this explanation, I was still not convinced, and so once again I looked down at the tiny figure for inspiration.

Almost instantly I recognized the image of a bee, and then a beehive, as I stared at the head covering. With my mind open, her appearance started to fall into place, the thin arms, the lack of feet, and the legs joined together all symbolizing the abdomen of a bee. According to Marija Gimbutas, there are many images of bees from the Sumerian, Minoan, and Egyptian cultures, and all show dancing figures with arms raised above their heads and what at first looks like a phallus between their legs, later to be recognized as the abdomen of the bee.[22]

Similarly, scholars had questioned why this figure was able to neither stand nor sit, suggesting that she was just meant to be held in the

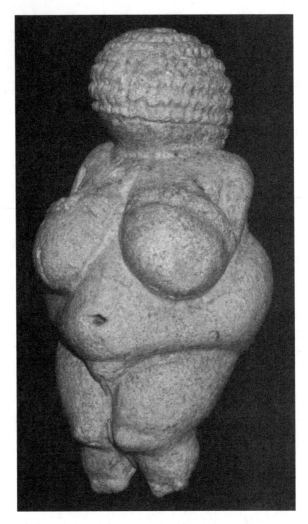

Venus of Willendorf, 22,000–24,000 BCE
(Natural History Museum, Vienna, Austria)

hand to bring comfort and sensuality. Yet her slightly curved form is far more suggestive of an insect, especially a bee.

Several other artists were able to capture the vibrancy of the bee, as seen in a honey-colored figurine of an Anatolian bee goddess found in Hacilar, Turkey, dated around 8000 BCE. As the honey appears to run off her body, she holds her breasts forward with her arms, while

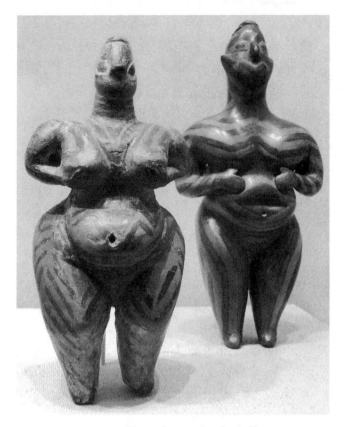

Bee goddess of Anatolia (at left)

her head is adorned with a beehive similar to that of the Venus of Willendorf.

Facts about Bees

Before delving further into the mythology of the bee, let's review a few facts about bees, in particular the honeybee (*Apis mellifera*), for honey has always been known as the nectar of the gods and goddesses. According to fossil records, the honeybee has been on this planet for at least thirty-five million years, and, like other bees, wasps, and ants, belongs to an order of insects known as Hymenoptera. This means that it is a bee that has two wings and a chewing mouthpiece, and it goes through a metamorphosis during its lifetime.

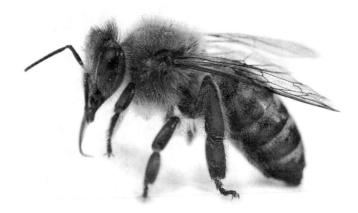

The honeybee

The honeybee is a social animal living in a colony or hive that holds between 50,000 and 60,000 individual insects; this includes one queen bee, approximately 50,000 sterile female worker bees, and approximately 500 to 1,000 male drones. Unlike the drones, the queen bee has a stinger, and unlike a worker bee, she is the only female that can mate.

There are three stages of honeybee development, known as the brood of the hive. These include:

The egg: This phase lasts until day three.

The larva: This stage lasts until around day nine. For the first three days a worker bee is fed with royal jelly, and then honey and pollen. On day nine, the wormlike larva creates a cocoon around itself, and the cell is capped by the female worker bees.

The pupa: During this phase, the larva undergoes an internal metamorphosis to acquire all the features of the adult bee. The process is completely internal, with the pupa inactive and well hidden within its cell. The timing of this phase varies depending on the type of bee; the queen emerges as an adult around day sixteen, a worker by day twenty-one, and a drone by day twenty-four.[23]

Honeybees show a natural form of epigenetics, where the environment influences the genes. Whereas the worker bee is fed royal jelly for only three days, a larva destined to be a queen is given it for six days. This triggers a cascade effect that acts on the DNA of the larva, which eventually results in a fully fertile queen bee.[24]

Wild bees build their hives inside anything that is dry, whether this is the hollow of a dead tree, a crevice in a rock formation, or the air space between the walls of a house. The shape we know as a beehive is a human construct, for as all apiarists know, the most practical shape for a hive is rectangular. Within the hive, each cell is hexagonal in design, the shape known to ensure strength and organization. Other than the Africanized honeybees, most species are not naturally aggressive unless the hive is invaded. Few animals would risk being stung by 50,000 bees in search of honey, except one, the bear, whose size and thick skin make his mission to taste this nectar of the gods so worthwhile!

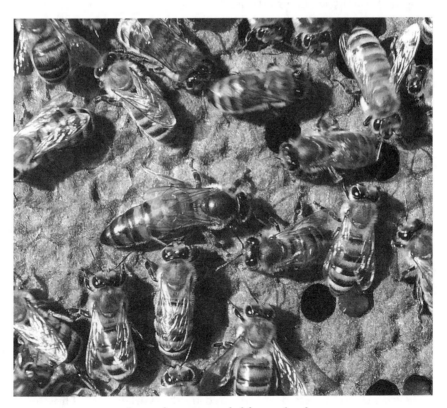

Queen bee surrounded by worker bees

Worker bees exemplify Chaucer's phrase "busy as a bee." They spend their whole life building, cleaning, cooling, and repairing the hive, as well as feeding the queen, drones, and larvae. They also collect pollen and nectar from flowers and make honey, beeswax, beebread, and royal jelly. Often traveling up to two miles a day in search of nectar, pollen, and water, they usually live about twenty days before dying of exhaustion. The nectar from plants is approximately 80 percent water and the rest is made up of complex sugars. Once the bee returns to the hive, the nectar is extracted from its "honey stomach." It is then mixed with enzymes to break down the sugars and spread throughout the honeycombs, where the excess water evaporates, aided by the beating of the bees' wings. Each worker bee has a barbed stinger, unlike the queen's stinger, which is curved and smooth. Once the stinger becomes lodged in its victim, it is often hard to remove, causing damage to the bee's own body and usually leading to its death.

Life for the drones, on the other hand, is fairly easy, as they are cared for entirely by the worker bees during their average seven-week life span. Their only purpose is to mate, and, if he is lucky, a drone's moment of glory will arrive when a new queen leaves the hive, releases her pheromones, and signals to the nearby drones that she is ready to mate. Mating occurs in flight, with drones seldom mating with a virgin queen from their own hive, thereby maintaining a healthy genetic diversity among honeybees. During mating, the abdomen of the drone becomes temporarily lodged in the queen, which leads to his sudden but happy death. Having mated with up to twenty drones, the new mother bee returns to the nest. As mating takes place generally in the warm weather, any excess drones still in the hive in the autumn are usually driven out of the nest to die so that there are fewer mouths to feed.

Mating is the only time the queen will sojourn into the outer world until she leaves for good. She retreats to the dark womb of the hive, carrying the sperm collected in a special pouch in her body. She starts to lay her eggs, up to 2,000 a day, in hexagonal beeswax-lined cells—the honeycomb—that have been prepared by the worker bees. Those eggs that are fertilized become worker bees and queens, while the unfertilized eggs become the male drones, the latter containing only a single expression of chromosomes, all from the queen. Therefore, as the only source of its genetic material comes from a queen, a bee colony is a true matrilineal society.

During her two- to four-year life span, a queen bee will lay 200,000 eggs, before she runs out of sperm and starts to lay unfertilized eggs, at which point the number of worker bees diminishes. This is a sign for the workers to start to feed the larvae of new queens with extra supplies of royal jelly, and for the old queen to prepare to leave the hive, taking with her about half of the worker bees. This process, known as swarming, makes space for a new queen to take over the hive. Since there can only be one queen, the virginal queen bees will attack and kill one another with their stingers until only one remains. A specific sound known as piping is emitted by each of the warring queens and is thought to be both a war cry and, based on the strength of her sound, a signal to the worker bees that she is a strong contender for their support.

Many scholars have looked at the intriguing question of how bees navigate and transmit information to one another. In 1973, Karl von Frisch won the Nobel Prize in Physiology or Medicine for his research in decoding the language of the bee. He described an intricate figure-eight dance, or waggle dance, which a bee performs at the entrance to the hive to let other bees know the location of the nectar. Through the position of the body of the messenger bee in relation to the sun, other bees are able to find the source of the nectar. In recent years, researchers have shown that the waggle dance is probably less important than originally thought, although it certainly shows a level of sophistication in terms of communication.

It is now believed that bees use a combination of skills to locate both the nectar and their hive. When a bee begins to forage, its path is irregular until it finds a suitable food source. Then it returns to the hive in a straight line, giving meaning to the phrase *to make a beeline.* Bees' navigation skills are still under investigation, although it is clear that they have the ability to discriminate colors and odors, to learn by association, to recognize the sun's position in the sky, and to detect the magnetic fields of Earth.

The honeybee has gained much more attention since 2007, when beekeepers observed a marked decline in bee populations because of a condition known as colony collapse disorder (CCD). Dependent as we are on flying insects such as bees to pollinate our fruit and other crops, this is a serious condition that could, in the long term, have devastating effects on our food supplies. CCD has mainly affected beehives in the United States and Europe, although there are signs of the disorder spreading across the world. Research shows that there are probably a number of factors involved, all of which weaken the bees' defenses, allowing viruses carried by mites and fungi to proliferate within the hive. Pesticides, genetically modified crops, and malnutrition have all been implicated, and all these factors arise from human activities. Particularly worrying is cell-phone radiation, which is known to disrupt the bees' navigation system, which relies on electromagnetic wave patterns. It has been shown that if you place a cordless phone system that uses microwaves near a hive, the bees from that hive will behave abnormally and are less likely to return to their hive.[25]

I suggest that this condition reflects a far greater problem: a reduction in the fertilization and expansion of human consciousness because of thousands of years of disconnection from our spiritual home and our multidimensional identity. I believe it is only through reverence and respect for the Great Mother, as Queen Bee, that we will start to repair the damage.

Bee Reverence

Throughout history and in cultures that have included the Maya, the Aboriginals of Australia, the Egyptians, the Sumerians, the Babylonians, the Cretans, and the ancient Greeks, gods and humans have paid reverence to the humble honeybee. Mythical stories stretching back over time speak of the strong links between this tiny insect and the mysteries of death and resurrection. Indeed, the mighty Greek god Zeus was said to have been fed honey as an infant because of its reputation as the nectar of the gods. Even in the past 2,000 years the bee has fascinated many famous families and individuals, including the French general Napoleon, the Merovingian dynasty, and Himmel, Hitler's deputy, reminding us of humankind's fascination with the acquisition of immortality. There are still many secret cults today that are linked to worship of the bee and its knowledge of life over death.

Honey

Humans have always prized the products of the hive, which include honey, beeswax, propolis, honeycomb, and royal jelly. Honey is particularly revered because of its natural antibiotic and preservative properties, which ensure it is always fresh and can be used as an antiseptic. In the past, it was used in many sacred rituals both as an offering to the gods and as the source of mead, a strong intoxicant and mind-altering substance. Indeed, the Egyptians, who were keen beekeepers, would use honey in the embalming process as well as leave pots of honey, honey cakes, and honeycomb as food for the souls of the dead.

Neith, the Egyptian Bee Goddess

Now that we have a better understanding of bees, let's return to the subject of the bee goddess. In Egypt, she was called Neith, although she has been known at other times and by other names.* The worship of Neith was prominent in the western Nile Delta during the First Dynasty (3050–2850 BCE), especially in the town of Sais, where the House of the Bee once stood. Some scholars believe the goddess Neith to be much older—indeed, pre-dynastic—emerging originally from the waters of the primordial mother, Nu, and in time giving birth to both Re (Ra), the sun god, and Sobek, the crocodile god of rebirth. Neith was worshipped as the goddess of war and hunting, similar to her

---

*To the Hebrews, she was Deborah; to the Greeks, Artemis; in the Minoan-Mycenaean cultures she was Potnia; and to the Phoenicians, she was Tanit.

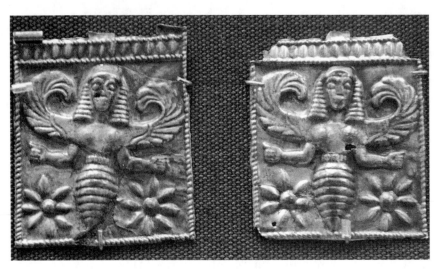

Bee goddess, perhaps associated with Artemis, seventh century BCE

Greek counterparts Athena and Artemis, with one of her symbols being a shield with crossed arrows positioned above her head.

It is important to distinguish between warfare and hunting when describing Neith's guardianship, for like Athena, who was unarmored before the arrival of the patriarchy, I sense the Egyptian goddess was masculinized to meet the needs of the day. The European honeybee is not naturally aggressive, using its sting only in defense of the hive. It does not attack other hives in an unprovoked manner, nor does it kill for pleasure, but only for survival of the colony, as seen in the expulsion of the drones before a hard winter.

Claas Jouco Bleeker, in his book *The Rainbow: A Collection of Studies in the Science of Religion,* comments that a similar shield hieroglyph, wherein the arrows are in front of the shield, suggests that Neith assisted in childbirth, thus mirroring one of the roles of her sister, the Greek goddess Artemis.[26] As any woman will confirm, childbirth is a time of death and rebirth, when a woman can find herself in the greatest pain and the greatest ecstasy simultaneously, as she undergoes a metamorphosis in order to accept this new being into her life. At the same time, the soul of the baby is making its final transition from the sacred waters of the womb before becoming fully incarnate—dying to one world before being born on Earth. This is a very vulnerable time for both mother and child and requires the assistance of midwives such as Artemis and Neith to hold open the interdimensional doorway to show the way.

Another image of Neith shows her holding the ankh, the key of eternal life, informing us that it is within her power to open the door so that we can experience the bliss of once again floating in the creative waters of the Great Mother. In her other hand, Neith holds a long stick with a hook on the end, which is known as a goad and is used to prod animals into action. The relevance of this symbol becomes clear in light of a story that tells of a lengthy debate between Horus and Set as to who should succeed Osiris as king of Egypt. With no decision made, the gods ask the goddess Neith, who is respected for her wisdom, to intercede in the matter. She sends back a reply that Horus must take up the position, and if he doesn't, "I shall become so furious that the sky will touch the ground." This suggests that Neith

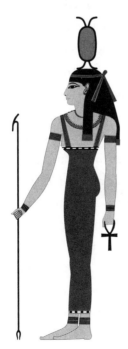

The bee goddess: Neith

is perfectly capable of sending a lightning strike to Earth using her goad if anyone dares stir her anger. Many of us can attest to her wrath when, having been stung by the barbed stinger of a bee, we experience waves of fiery pain pulsing through our body, with the release of the chemical histamine.

The goddess Neith is also commonly depicted wearing a weaver's shuttle on her head, synonymous with one of her epithets, Goddess of Weaving. She was believed to weave the wrappings and linens used in mummification, ensuring a safe passage for souls as they pass between the worlds. Doesn't this sound like the cocoon a larva must spin around itself before entering the pupa stage of its development? Clearly this is why the bee goddess was also given the title Guardian of Mortuaries: because of her understanding of the vulnerability a person faces as he or she transitions from one phase of consciousness to the next.

It is not surprising that several of the volunteers in the previously cited DMT study—like shamans and those who have near-death experiences— mention hearing humming and buzzing during their sojourns into other realms of reality; these are often accompanied by feelings of love and kindness, suggestive of the presence of the Queen Bee.[27]

Another epithet of Neith's is the Veiled Goddess, a title later ascribed to the goddess Isis. This comes from the fact that on the wall of Neith's home, known as the House of the Bee, there was said to be an inscription that read: "I am all that has been, that is, and that will be. No mortal has yet been able to lift the veil that covers me." Many different interpretations have been offered about the meaning of this inscription, although oftentimes without an accurate translation. According to Claas Jouco Bleeker, the word *veil* more accurately describes a weaving or web, which is appropriate since we know that Neith, the bee goddess, is associated with weaving. In ancient times, the web was the symbol of cosmic order and divine wisdom. This interpretation is much more in line with the inscription on the House of the Bee, which suggests that Neith applies her wisdom to spin order out of chaos. In this guise she is closely aligned with the Hopi Grandmother Spider and the Greek Ariadne, both of whom are seen as spinners of the universal fabric who act as intermediaries between the Creator and the people. Neith also mirrors Sophia's wisdom and insight, creating form or order from a place that is unbiased and kind. Based on Bleeker's translation, the final sentence would thus be interpreted as: "No mortal has ever disclosed or uncovered the mystery of my web."[28]

This web consists of many different frequencies of consciousness or light, each interconnected, from the tiniest grain of sand to the largest galaxy stretching out into the multidimensional universe. As mortals, it is impossible to see beyond our own small piece of the web; yet, as spiritual beings, we have wings by which we can fly beyond the reaches of our three-dimensional reality, and with the help of hormones such as DMT, which naturally comes from the pineal gland, we can travel the web, beyond the limitations of time and space.

The bee goddess is waiting for us to awaken to her presence and promises to aid us on our journey by:

- Handing over the key to eternal life
- Opening the doors and protecting us with her arrows as we pass between the worlds
- Goading us when we seem to falter or doubt ourselves
- Clothing us in soft garments of love at the most vulnerable times of our lives, when we are dying to the old ways and not yet fully reborn
- Humming softly to us, like a mother hums to her child
- Surrounding us in her web so that we will never feel lost, because wherever we are, she will be there
- Strengthening our core so that we can act like a lightning rod, bringing Heaven to Earth

Most importantly, she reminds us that she exists within each of us. We are each the spinner of our own reality; if we don't like the design or the fabric, it is within our power to change it, starting today.

The Greek Goddesses and the Melissae

Contemporaries of Neith are the Greek goddesses Artemis and Demeter, who were also revered as bee goddesses. As a triple goddess, each revealed three faces, appearing as:

- The intuitive Virgin, analogous to the bee that possesses the intuitive knowledge as to where to find the nectar by tapping into nature's signposts
- The Mother, who, as a bee, expresses herself through the fertility of the queen bee
- The Crone, who calls an end to one phase of life so that a new one can begin, much as the bee transforms through its different phases, from egg to adult

Often seen to accompany the goddesses, including the Anatolian earth goddess Cybele, were priestesses known as Melissae; they were perceived as nymphs, seen to be dancing around the queen with their hands held high. Such dancing certainly mirrors the constant activity of the worker bees around the queen, as they use their wings to cool and dry the hive. In Greek tradition, an unborn soul was known as a "bee-soul" or Melissa, reflecting a belief that souls emerge from the moon goddess Artemis, the goddess of rebirth, and travel to Earth as bees. A soul was said to be tempted by the sweetness of earthly delights, especially honey, which when eaten turns them into fully formed human beings. At the end of life, both the Greeks and Egyptians believed that it was through the transformation of the physical form back into a bee that the spirit was freed of all earthly restrictions.

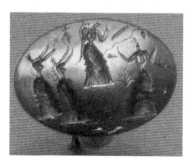

Gold ring from Isopata, showing the Melissae dancing around the Queen Bee (Archaeological Museum of Herakleion, Crete)

The Alchemy of the Bee

Throughout history, the bee has been associated with alchemical transformation, whereby a base substance, in this case the nectar of a plant, is transformed into the golden and immortal elixir known as honey. This process is, I believe, described in the following, written about 250 BCE: "In Egypt, if you bury an ox in certain places, so that only his horns project above the ground, and then saw them off, they say that bees fly out, for the ox putrefies and is resolved into a bee."[29] This piece of writing has intrigued historians for centuries, with various interpretations having been given, including one that implies that bees will gather around a rotting carcass. However, although wasps and flies enjoy the rotting meat of an ox, honeybees are vegetarian. Others have suggested that the ox represents the astrological sign of Taurus (April 21 to May 21), which in the Northern Hemisphere is certainly the month when bees become more active, as the aroma of various pollens fills the air.

However, I suggest that the inscription refers to a much more esoteric process: alchemy, especially as it relates to consciousness. The initial stages of this great work describe the successful transformation of a base idea into a manifested reality. However, it is the steps that follow that produce the rich rewards leading to self-realization, as any material success is transformed into fulfillment and the golden consciousness of enlightenment.

Just as exhalation always follows inhalation, at the height of any success we should always remember that the only reason for our experiences and the manifestation of our dreams is to extract the seeds of wisdom so they can eventually be offered to the Great Mother, allowing her consciousness to expand. At the same time, we metaphorically die to the old experience and, once again, like bees, fly to the Great Mother's source of no-thingness before being born with fresh inspiration.

The alchemical phase that begins the process to free our spirit is known as putrefaction and fermentation. During this stage, our story or experience—the ox—is broken down to release the pearls of wisdom. This phase often coincides with a dark night of the soul, when we undergo a metaphysical death as we release our hold on our outer identification and go within. This process is symbolized by the larva of the bee spinning a cocoon around itself, to become a pupa that will undergo a metamorphosis.

Like the pupa, as we pass through the darkness, we are lovingly wrapped in a cocoon woven by the Bee Goddess, who stands at the open door between the worlds. She gently goads us to disconnect from our old stories and prepare to fly free as the adult bee. I believe that the horns of the bull that are mentioned in the text from 250 BCE are referring to the uterus, the cauldron of death and the site of cleansing and purification in the transformational fire of the Dragon Queen. We are being reminded that the physical world is nothing other than a manifested dream, and therefore impermanent; success, victory, and accomplishment have no value in and of themselves. The true riches that arise from our manifestations come from the lessons learned and the expansion of self-awareness. Without allowing the uterus, the lower dantian, to break down our stories into those things that are of value and those things that need to be shed at the time of the dark moon, we will never know true spiritual fulfillment.

Many cultures honored this association between the ox and the bee, as depicted on ancient pottery, paintings, and carvings where bees are seen flying above images of the sacred cow. With the onset of patriarchal domination, we saw the role of the female cow being taken over by the male bull. The Greek bull god Dionysus was known as the "living spirit of wine" and as such could induce intoxication, ritual madness, and ecstasy—a classical description of the effects of DMT. Dionysus was also symbolized as a god of annual renewal and resurrection and was often depicted surrounded by a swarm of bees, believed to be souls released from the constraints of earthly life. Sacred rituals known as the Dionysian Mysteries used wine and honey-based mead, plus music and dance, to elevate participants to mystical states of consciousness.

This ritual mirrored the earlier Eleusinian Mysteries, which were created in honor of Demeter and her search for her daughter, Persephone, who was taken into the underworld. These sacred ceremonies, which began around 1500 BCE and continued until the fourth century CE, used music, mind-altering substances, and light to symbolically transport thousands of participants through their own dark night of the soul, until they reached enlightenment.

The next stage of the alchemical process is known as distillation or sublimation, where heat is applied to cause the essence, released from physical form, to rise up dissolved in water. In human terms, this means that once the meat of our stories has been broken down during putrefaction, i.e., inward reflection, the process of distillation allows our spirit to start to rise, carrying with it the pure wisdom of our experiences. During this time, we often find ourselves shedding tears, the water of which slowly washes away the details of the past, leaving a clean slate for future dreams to be created.

The vessel for the beginning of the distillation process is once again the uterus, with the hot breath of the Dragon Queen providing the heat.

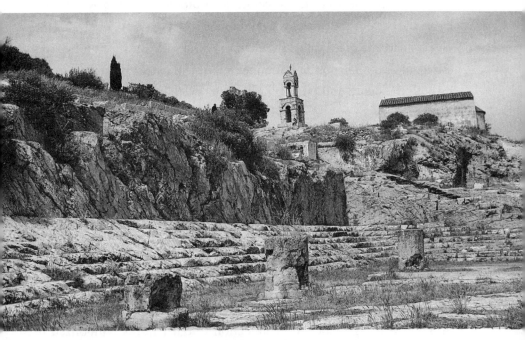

Eleusis, the site of mysteries for 1,800 years

As the vapors rise, carrying the spirit, they pass between the breasts and into the heart chakra, the middle dantian. Any persistent grief is reduced by the Mother Cow, who laces our tears with prolactin, enhancing our trust in the Great Mother and encouraging us to release our hold on the past, setting the volatile spirit free to rise up to the third eye. Here, like the pupa of the bee, our spirit is given wings to fly. This allows it to break free from the confines of its cell and soar out through the crown chakra, the upper dantian, as pure ethereal presence. This final stage of alchemy is known as coagulation, when the doorways open and we are propelled into the multidimensional universe of the Great Mother.

Many of us have had glimpses of such an existence through mind-altering activities like childbirth, sexual orgasm, meditation, ingestion of certain psychoactive drugs, or near-death experience. But as I will explain later, I believe that access to the multidimensional realms is limited due to conditions placed on our travel by the Queen Bee herself.

As the spirit is released, a sweet nectar is produced, amrita, which runs down the back of the throat. Likened to the secretions associated with the G-spot, and also often called the elixir of life, amrita consists, it is hypothesized, of a combination of hormones mixed with water, possibly secreted by both the pineal and pituitary glands. Its production has been the goal of deep meditation and sacred sexual practices for thousands of years, linked as it is with the blissful union with the divine Creator.

Reclaiming Our Sacred Name

In the Egyptian mystery schools, this entire alchemical process of transformation is known as the "raising of the djed" or the "raising of the dead"; it leads to the mastery of one's own energies, to the point where the person, in modern terms borrowed from the *Star Wars* universe, could be considered a Jedi knight. For women, the process is specifically about reclaiming our own sacred identity, which was taken from us 3,000 years ago. Such a reconnection to our truth is symbolized in the following story concerning the Egyptian goddess Isis and the patriarchal sun god Re (Ra):

Isis, wishing to regain the power of magic that was rightfully hers before the rise of Re, decides to trick Re into speaking his secret name, which holds the magic. She fashions a serpent out of Re's spittle and some clay and leaves it on the path that she knows the sun god takes each day. In time, Re is bitten by the snake, causing him to cry out in agony as the serpent's poison spreads throughout his body. In the midst of hot and cold sweats, he screams out in rage, causing the tears that flow from his eyes to turn into bees. There is only one person who can cure him, Isis, who does so after she has received Re's unspoken and secret name.

This story describes the symbols of distillation: the serpent represents the rising energy, the hot and cold sweats symbolize the heating and cooling process, and the tears that are transformed into bees represent the purified essence. And the sacred name? This is our own spiritual identity or essence that lives outside the confines of this temporal world. Are you ready, like Isis, to claim what is rightfully yours? Are you ready to grasp your own magical wand or lightning rod, which gives you magical powers over the cycles of birth and death? At this time, humanity and Earth herself need you to say yes, for we are created in the image of the Great Mother, and she cannot do this without us.

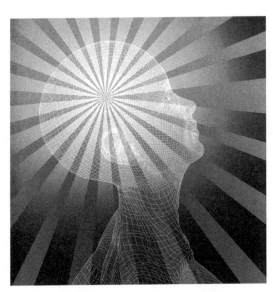

Our essence lives outside the confines of this temporal world.

The Atlantean Queen Bee

There is one last Queen Bee we need to meet to complete our journey. Last year, I was invited to lead a group to the beautiful Mediterranean island of Malta. Some believe its name came from the Greeks, who enjoyed the sweetness of the honey produced by its native variety of honeybees. Others say it comes from the Phoenician word for "shelter," or the Egyptian word *m'lita,* which means "the place with large stones." Another theory says it comes from the Sanskrit for "the place of magic."[30]

I knew little of the island except that it is said to be the location of some of the oldest megalithic sites in the world, a thousand years older than the Egyptian pyramids or Stonehenge. In addition, this tiny island of less than 122 square miles is believed to have originally housed over thirty-five temples, many of which are now hidden beneath the sea. Maltese historians are insistent that the first human settlers came to the islands from neighboring Sicily in 5200 BCE and immediately set about building the temples. Yet many contemporary historians, including Graham Hancock, question these dates, as there is no evidence of the construction of similar megalithic buildings on Sicily or in nearby Italy, where 7,000 years ago most of the inhabitants of those places were still simple farmers.[31]

There are also stories of strange-looking skulls and unusual teeth being found on the island, although the evidence of such artifacts has been either lost or discredited over time. A large number of skeletons from prehistoric animals have also been collected, suggesting that there was a land bridge between Malta and her sister islands and mainland Europe until around 13,500 years ago, when it disappeared under water, leaving the islands surrounded by the sea. If the animals used the land bridge, it is most probable that humans did too, making the megalithic sites much older than was previously thought.

Many of the surviving temples are specifically designed to align with the movements of celestial bodies, especially the sun and the moon, as is typical at other megalithic sites such as Stonehenge and Newgrange. However, with such a large number of temples involved, it

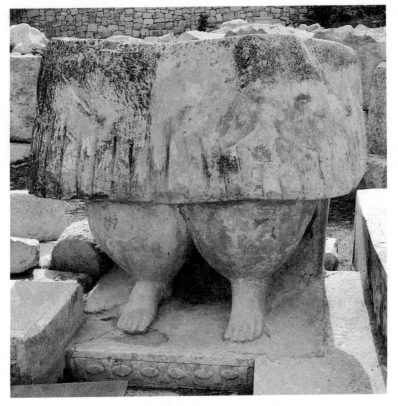

Fat lady of the Tarxien Temples

appears that Malta was once an important center, possibly going all the way back in time to the civilization of Atlantis, which, it is theorized, reached its peak around 20,000 BCE, before its power declined, until its final destruction in approximately 9600 BCE. According to Maltese visionary artist and writer Francis Xavier Aloisio, author of *Islands of Dreams,* during the days of Atlantis, Malta, Gozo, and Comino were three mountains in what he calls the Medi-terranean, or "middle of the land." These mountains were considered places where the confluence of telluric or dragon energy was extremely high. Hence they were chosen as sites for the downloading of cosmic energy onto Mother Earth via a pillar of spiraling energy—essentially a natural lightning rod. The various temples were designed to capture, store, or send this energy.[32] Indeed, in some of the temples, images of "fat ladies" have been found, each with only a hole where her head should be. It is believed that crystal rods were placed in these holes, which were then used to focus celestial light that came through slits in the temple walls, imprinting the archetypal consciousness of Heaven onto Earth.

According to Aloisio, one beautiful collection of temples on the island of Gozo was used primarily for the renewal and restoration of the soul. Designed in the shape of a woman, these temples are said to have been built by giants, and hence their name, Ggantija. It is easy to see how you would pass through the vulvar-shaped doorway, leaving behind the burdens and worries of the outer world. Passing along the narrow vaginal passageway, you would eventually reach each of three chambers. In the third and final chamber, in front of the holy of holies, your psyche would be opened through the use of the breath, sound, and images, so that your soul would be renewed and you would be bathed in the pure nectar of blissful love.

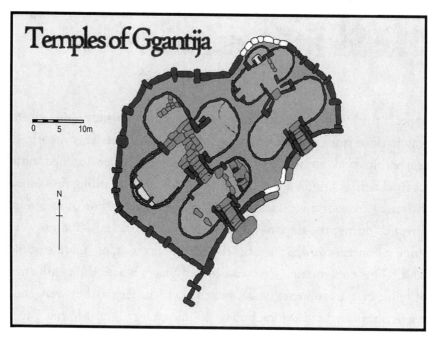

Ggantija temples on Gozo

What struck me as significant when I first visited these sacred sites was the extraordinary number of temples that revealed rows of small holes that had been carved into the walls, described by tourist books as evidence of wear and tear from rain. I instinctively knew we were in the presence of the Queen Bee, these dimples representing the cells of her hive. These temples were built not only for renewal, I suggest, but to receive the "eggs" of the Queen Bee, that is, the light of consciousness and inspiration. Nearly all the temples on the islands of Malta and Gozo are round and consist of the three curvilinear chambers. This convinced me that they were designed in the image of woman as she is and always has been—the source of fertilization on this planet. I suspect that as in the Minoan culture, certain women of these ancient islands were chosen to perform sacred rituals, acting as intermediaries between the Queen Bee and Mother Earth.

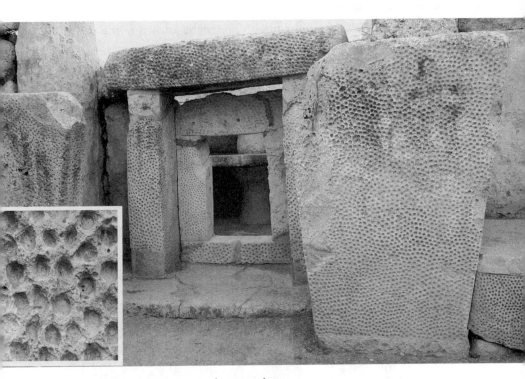

Beehive markings

One other site on Malta that deserves mention is the underground temple known as the Hypogeum. This honeycomb labyrinth of caves and passages extends far beyond the limits allowed to the average tourist. On its walls are faint red or black images, some of which we met in Crete, which depict an axe, a bull, and spirals interwoven with honeycombs. The central chamber has several small, rounded cubicles carved into its walls, similar to the cells in a beehive. Could it be that participants entered these cells to experience altered states of reality and connect with the multidimensional realms? It is clear that within these caves there would have been little or no outside sensory stimulation, allowing the awareness to be focused on the breath, similar to the shamans in the prehistoric caves. Notably, traces of the hallucinogenic substance ergot have been found in the chamber; similar to DMT, this plant substance would have opened the psyche to the supernatural world.

But the chamber was not entirely quiet, for in one of the walls a little way from the central chamber was a niche known as the oracle hole. It is known that when someone with a deep voice tones into the hole, the whole space resonates, especially if that person hum's like a bee. It has been suggested that the participants lying in their little cells would have heard a sound very similar to the heartbeat heard by a baby as it lies in the womb of its mother.

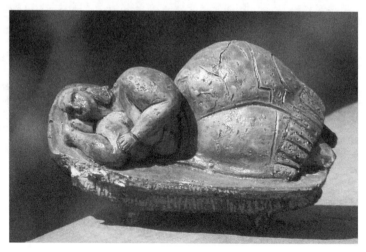

Sleeping lady found in the Hal Saflieni Hypogeum

To deepen the mystery, found in a pit of one of the chambers many years ago was a beautiful and delicate portrayal of a sleeping woman. Many believe that she symbolizes the meaning of the Hypogeum: a place to dream. She reminds us that we need to return to the womb to give birth to new consciousness. As we do so, we release our hold on external stimuli and cocoon ourselves, like the larva of the bee, in the trust, openness, and love of the Great Mother's heart. Only then are we ready to open ourselves to our own imagination and dreams.

Other researchers have suggested that the sleeping lady holds a far more important message for humanity. It is said that many thousands of years ago, the queen of Atlantis, a Queen Bee known as Astarte, made her home on the mountains of Malta. She acted as an intermediary between the worlds, giving birth to order out of chaos while holding open the door to humanity so it could ascend to explore the multidimensional universe. However, it soon became clear that humanity was not willing to be a mere spiritual traveler but wanted to possess the universal power for its own benefit, while also being unwilling to be responsible for its creations. To prevent further abuse of her gifts, the Queen Bee metaphorically fell asleep, thereby closing the door to the flow of new inspirations reaching Earth as well as preventing humanity from interfering with the natural order of the universe until we reach a level of conscious maturity. It is believed that her withdrawal from the world eventually led to the downfall of Atlantis, around 9600 BCE.

Bee-coming All That We Are

Whichever mythology we choose to follow, there is no doubt that along with our modern disconnection from the creative energy of the Dragon Queen and the love of the Mother Cow, we are also disengaged from the source of creation and inspiration accessed through the Queen Bee. As a result, the energy flow between the crown chakra and the star-child chakra is extremely limited. It is true that through meditation and visual imagery, often mediated by mind-altering hormones and drugs, we are able to travel into interdimensional realms. But the awareness that we can thus achieve often reaches only as far as our astral and mental bodies, wherein we encounter both the benevolent and malevolent forces of our imagination.

During the days of Atlantis, the Queen Bee's knowledge and wisdom taught humanity how to wield the magical wand or lightning rod to both manifest and dematerialize reality through creative intelligence. However, humanity did not appreciate that this could only occur in accordance with the Universal Laws, one of which basically states that for every action there is a reaction for which we need to take responsibility—the law of karma. Our unwillingness to be responsible for our creations was seen as unacceptable by all the other life-forms that share this multidimensional space. Therefore, the energy of our wand—dragon energy, or kundalini—was essentially neutralized, able to become active again only in the hands of those who are believed to be mature enough to handle the power of the wand. So far, few have achieved that right.

Since those days, we have continued to use part of our electromagnetic energy to create our reality, especially through the desire and will centers, which are the solar plexus and throat chakras, respectively. But outside serious behavioral infringements, we are rarely held accountable for our creations, and instead we expect sympathy for being the victim of our own circumstances rather than the creator. However pleasant it may be to have others reinforce our powerlessness, it does nothing to strengthen the power of our wand. Only when we own our creations will we have the power to make choices that will change our future.

If we also fail to understand that everything we perceive in the world is a manifested reflection of our own imagination, when we do enter altered states of awareness, the beings we meet will often appear alien to us, especially if they seem to be malevolent. We then seek to obliterate them or even forgive them in an attempt to extricate them from our awareness. Yet such actions could be seen as similar to cutting off an essential part of your body because you don't like the look of it.

In truth, such a journey into other realms of consciousness allows us to connect to all the possibilities of creation that exist within our small area of the collective unconsciousness, the imagination. Without taking ownership of what we manifest, the whole experience is merely phenomena-based, similar to watching a movie or playing a video game: when it finishes we simply switch it off and never wonder at its relevance to our life. Let me be clear: *If you have an emotional reaction to someone or some situation, you are being shown a part of your own creation that is awaiting integration.* If we are upset by poverty, where are we poor? If we fight against abuse, where are we abused? If we are trying to save the planet, what part of us needs saving?

The archetypal Queen will not awaken fully until we are willing to be accountable for our thoughts, words, and actions. In these present times of transformation, the Maya predict that in the new world to come, we will be increasingly sensitive to the effect of our actions on others and will feel these actions first within our own body. Perhaps that sensitivity will bring home to us the reality that a single thought can indeed affect the universal balance of consciousness.

Another extraordinary development presently enveloping Earth is that the veils between the dimensions of reality are falling away. This means that everything that was once hidden will now be revealed— the true meaning of the word *apocalypse*. This is the ultimate test for every member of humanity, for we will no longer be able to hide behind ignorance, subterfuge, or clever words, as everybody will see the source of our words and actions. There will be riots as governments, religious orders, and corporate institutions fall, their secrets spilling out for all to see. But remember, we are at the end of the Piscean Age, which means we no longer need leaders, gurus, and masters to follow; it is time for every single person, whatever his or her status, to become his or her own leader and master. Each of us must tap into our own wisdom and power, with respect and honor for all other life-forms that share our existence.

Every woman passes through the same stages as the tiny bee that moves from egg to adult:

- From infanthood to puberty, we are in the egg phase.
- From puberty to motherhood, we occupy the larva stage.
- During the reproductive years of motherhood, we experience the pupa stage as we cocoon ourselves inside the cells of our daily lives and mature.
- After menopause, we break out of our cell and develop the wings to fly.

The question to ask oneself is this: Do I want to be the worker bee or the Queen Bee?

ᕙ

RITUAL NO. 4
Receiving Inspiration from the Queen Bee

We will now reconnect the energies of the heart and crown chakras to create a powerful vessel that is open to receiving inspiration from the Queen Bee. This is best carried out on the third day of the dark moon, either standing or sitting with your back supported. Your head should be bent slightly forward so that your crown chakra is pointed toward the sky.

Begin at the heart chakra, allowing your breath to move in and out of this center, anchoring your awareness in love for ten breaths. Then inhale and deeply exhale, sending everything that you no longer wish to hold on to— thoughts, fears, concerns, anger, and shame—down into the root chakra and into Mother Earth, asking her with gratitude to transform these energies. Repeat at least six times.

Bob on the ocean of the Dragon Queen, holding your breath on exhalation, for as long as it takes to feel calm. Then with your hands on your sacral chakra, with the fingers touching and pointing toward the ground, allow the serpentine energy to first climb your legs and then pass through the vulvar opening up along the vagina before settling in the uterus. Take time to fill the uterus until the area feels warm.

Then place your right hand on the sacral chakra and your left on the heart chakra. Draw the serpentine energy, plus the gems of wisdom from past experiences, up to the heart using a straw. Allow the energy to be churned by the Mother Cow as she moves it between the breasts in a figure-eight movement. Enjoy the joy that builds as she continues this process. Now you are ready for the final step.

Move your awareness into the crown chakra. Hum softly to yourself by closing your lips and sounding a *ng* at the back of the throat. Imagine a straw that passes from the crown to the heart chakra, and, as you hum, suck the serpentine energy up into the crown chakra. You will start to feel your crown chakra tingle as the dragon/serpent energy stimulates the pineal gland to produce DMT and your spirit is given the wings to fly. Even though you may feel that your awareness is leaving your body, try to keep contact with the earth, as this will promote both grounding and a continual flow of energy.

With humility and gratitude, call on the Queen Bee to open the door. Offer her as gifts the gems of wisdom that you have carefully carried from past experiences, which will enhance the consciousness of the Great Mother. Assuming she grants you access into the multidimensional realms, let go of all expectations and experience the pure bliss of coming home at last, to the eternal oneness where all is known and everything exists in the no-thingness.

Remain here until you are ready to leave, and then imagine your crown chakra as a vessel and allow it to be filled with inspiration until it is full. Pour the energy gently into the heart, promising yourself that you will nurture and love these precious dreams and seeds of inspiration. Finally, pour them into the most powerful creative vessel, the womb, and allow your dreams to take seed and flourish until one day you feel the urge to push them out into the world for all the world to see.

CONCLUSION

THE CALL OF THE GREAT MOTHER

Recently I met up with a friend I hadn't seen for twenty-five years. As I attempted to consolidate the events of all those years into twenty minutes, I found myself repeatedly commenting, "Even though I love making plans and can spend many happy hours mapping out the future, most of the major events in my life have occurred because I was in the right place at the right time, often taking me in a completely different direction than the one I had planned or ever imagined." This was certainly true in the writing of this book. Who would have thought when I started my research that I'd end up writing about my own journey as I heal from breast cancer. It is clear that I just have to do the work to show up at the door and then hand over control to my higher self—for only it can see what is beyond the door and when the door will open.

You could say, as you read my story, that perhaps I could have learned the lessons sooner and therefore not had the experience of cancer. That's certainly true, but only a jolt of such a magnitude would have stirred up such deep emotions, causing me to release my hold on entrenched beliefs and attend to my needs. At the same time, I have a strong feeling that the tumor has helped me to write the book, so I can reach out to many more women who are just like me. Even though this is my story, I hope it resonates with others, giving them the courage to reach out for what is essentially their right as much-loved and sacred women.

As the book unfolded, I was amazed how much we, as women, have become separated from our divine identity; then I discovered my own disconnection. However, this disassociation between humankind and its spiritual nature hasn't merely affected women; it affects all of humanity. It is perfectly clear that men are suffering, but for their healing to occur, we women must lead the way, for we are the transformational vessel for all healing, not only for men but for the planet. With this in mind, I would like to share some of the inspiration I received from the archteypal consciousness of the Great Mother expressed as the wisdom of the Dragon Queen, the Mother Cow, and the Queen Bee.

HEAR THE FIERY AND EARTHY WISDOM OF THE DRAGON QUEEN

Nothing will change until women first choose to occupy, nurture, and accept their bodies, whatever their size and shape. Remember your ancestors, who for tens of thousands of years were revered for their curves, fertility, and voluptuousness. I can't image what they would think of the images of the "ideal" women flaunted in the media today. Corporate media makes its money by persuading and shaming women into believing that who they are is not okay. It is time to show the world that the Great Mother reveals herself in many ways, and we must celebrate these different images, whatever a woman's age, culture, or size.

Your body is your friend. It loves you so much it will even die for you. When you feel pain or disharmony or feel unusually emotional, listen to your body's wisdom, for its message is coming directly from your soul. If you do become ill, take time to review your life, knowing this is a golden opportunity for change if you just follow the signposts. Your beliefs and perceptions are not set in stone, nor is your genetic expression. If you are not enjoying your life, it's a sure sign that something needs to shift. On some level, you already know how you wish to feel, and when you embody those positive feelings and act as if you are already there, your perception of yourself will also begin to change.

Now I need to address the menstrual cycle and your covenant with the Great Mother. Everything in nature, including the sun and moon, the plants and the animals, accepts the wisdom of moving through phases of life in order to grow and thrive. Women are the bearers of this message for humanity. Nevertheless, the patriarchal fear of death and chaos has attempted to subvert these features from the lives of men and women, with disastrous results. There can be no creativity and productivity without releasing the old and allowing it to die. It is fear and jealousy of a woman's ability to naturally sit in the lap of the Great Mother and be transported into the blissful state of universal love and understanding every month, as well as during childbirth and menopause, that caused patriarchal leaders to retaliate by burning "witches," i.e., sacred women, and decrying anything that espouses the mysteries of womanhood. Remember, it is a woman's ability to walk through the valley of death without anxiety and come through unscathed that scares the patriarchy, for fear of death is a strong card they play in their desire for control.

As women have raised their voices in protest over the past few decades, they have also become seduced by offers of "equality" that have come at a cost: Give up your femininity and we will make you one of the boys. Why be bothered by "the curse?" We will provide you with drugs that mean you will never have to be inconvenienced by "female problems." *Women now speak the same language as men:* I'm far too busy to change, and I have all these responsibilities. I'll think about it when I retire. *But there is one thing women can never disconnect from, and that is the love of their children and grandchildren and their yearning for a sense of community. This kind of communion is naturally inherent in the blood mysteries, for every woman in the world is primed to experience these cycles. If mothers want to create healthy futures for their children, they can do this only by celebrating, with their sisters, what it is to be a woman, beginning with their own lives. It is time* to remove menarche, menstruation, pregnancy, and menopause from the realms of medical pathology and return them to the sacred events in a woman's life that they are, revered through rites of passage and sacred ritual. In this way, women are assured a continuous connection to my, the Dragon Queen's, power and wisdom.

This brings us to the matter of sex. There are only two processes in this world: sex, which moves a person from self-identity to unification; and birth, which moves the energy in the opposite direction. With such TV shows as Sex and the City, it is easy to imagine that every woman masturbates, has orgasms, loves the way her body looks, and has a drawer full of sexy underwear. But this isn't always the case. Sex is a normal and natural process, resulting in a blissful and healing union. Yet all too often it is portrayed as an act that follows dinner on a first date or something secretive and shameful that shouldn't be discussed in public. Sexuality and sensuality are also vulnerable to abuse, which is defined as any event that fails to honor and respect the sacredness of a woman's body. When a woman is sexually or emotionally abused, this affects the consciousness of every woman on the planet.

One of the ways to begin the healing is for women to start to speak more openly about their bodies and sensuality, as well as their sexual likes and dislikes, without feeling ashamed that they may be different from their sisters. On so many occasions it has been the cattiness of other women that has caused the girl-inside-the-woman to shut down, as she is called names by the very people she looks to for support. Today, the claws are not far beneath the surface of any interaction between women, even though our natural energy is not to be competitive. This feature emerged thousands of years ago as women started to lose their power and status within society, and it became necessary to compete with their sisters in order to survive the patriarchal paradigm. Remember, in reality, a field of cows needs only one bull to fertilize them; the bull is the lucky one, the one to be chosen. In ancient times, if a woman wanted to sleep with another woman's husband, she would first ask her "sister," who was often only too grateful for the rest! Perhaps this idea could be reinstated to help begin *to heal the wounds of betrayal that so many women still carry from their relationship with other women.*

Finally, I want to speak of reconnecting one's kundalini to my energy deep within the earth. This shouldn't be a laborious process, but rather something that emerges from pure joy.

Perhaps begin by enjoying the body through movement, song, and dance, allowing the hips to sway, thereby awakening the sacral and base chakras. The wearing of a skirt often facilitates the process, as it makes it easier for my dragon energy to pass through the vulvar doorway. Walk, stand, or lie on Mother Earth as often as you can, releasing all your sadness and grief when life has become heavy. Then fill your uterus or womb with my power and wisdom and speak from this place with confidence and love.

Now I will end and allow my other sisters to communicate.

HEAR WHAT THE MOTHER COW HAS TO SAY

I speak of love, the immortal nectar that transports every woman from a mundane place to one of ecstasy. Without love there is no connection, for love is the glue in every relationship. The greatest yearning in the world today is for love, with many women believing they are unloved or unlovable, despite all the love they give to others. But let me remind you, it is because of my love that you exist. I am not the same as a vengeful god who chooses who will receive his praise. I love all my children equally, and such love is represented by the softness and comfort of a woman's breasts—your breasts. These mountains that the ancient people knew flowed with the milk of immortality should be displayed with pride and respect, for nobody can reach enlightenment or become fulfilled except by surrendering their ego and their will at the altar of the breasts. Some have tried, but they have become driven by lust and madness as a consequence.

A woman's breasts, surrounding the heart chakra, are the intermediary between the spiritual realm of the Queen Bee and the earthly world of the Dragon Queen. Without the breasts and the power of love, the serpent-dragon and the owl-bee remain separate, and a woman will never be able to fully harness her sexual, creative power and spiritual inspiration. It's time for Lilith and other great goddesses such as Hera, Artemis, Isis, and Asherah to be reconnected to their full power so they can, once again, influence the natural rhythms of this Earth through every single woman who lives today. Healing must be brought to bear on the wounds of these divine beings, especially Hera, whose love of respectful and equal relationships is badly needed on this planet at this time.

But for a woman to master these powerful energies, she must first learn to love herself, incorporating the messages of the breasts: nurturing, trust, comfort, bonding, compassion, acceptance, and self-confidence. She cannot receive enough love from others if she first doesn't open her heart to be loved. Nor can she remain independent and oblivious to love, for such a sense of disconnection will eventually cause great inner sadness, for it was never meant to be that way. The first step is to let love in through spending time in nature, nurturing the body, and doing things you enjoy, before doing things you need to do. Surrounding yourself with bosom friends and family whose energy is soft and forgiving breaks down much of the conditioning that women have placed upon themselves. Remember, you are my beautiful, unique, and much-loved child, who doesn't have to do anything but be herself in order to be loved. When you love yourself, you can allow others to walk their unique path, joyful that there are times when you will meet, but not dependent on them for your existence.

NOW THE QUEEN BEE SPEAKS

My message is of pure essence and inspiration. I hold the door open to the Great Mother's void or primordial waters of no-thingness. When a woman enters this place, she experiences bliss almost beyond description. Yet today, few actually take time to revel in this ecstasy, and many never even make the journey, as their orgasms affect mainly the nervous system and not the consciousness. Women, in fact, have multiple opportunities to pass through the doorway between death and birth and to connect to universal oneness within the multidimensional realms. There is menses or moon time, childbirth, and postmenopause time. So few women, however, understand the importance of these sacred events for their health, for the health of their families, and for the health of the planet. Many see these events, especially the emotional and intuitive sensitivity that is heightened at these times as inconvenient; they prefer to take pills to dull their senses. Nevertheless, a woman's body has not forgotten how to move energy from the root chakra to the star child, and by following her breath, a woman can easily enter these altered states without the need for mind-altering drugs.

I, the Queen Bee, am holding the door open for you now. I don't want to use my goad if I can help it, but we have reached a moment of tremendous importance for humanity and for your soul's evolution. However, you will not be able to pass through the door unless you first surrender all thoughts of separation and enter the cocoon, much as the larva is sealed into its cell before becoming a pupa. It requires time and space away from the outer world. The cocoon was naturally woven into a woman's monthly cycle by the Great Mother, who expected that a woman would remove herself from family life during her moon time. Now, with most women ignoring the monthly call and with many women choosing to be sedated or drugged during childbirth, these precious moments to connect with the inspiration of the Great Mother are dwindling. As for postmenopausal women, few have been taught to set aside time each month to connect with the Mother's wisdom so that they can become the leaders and inspirational teachers they are meant to be and truly bear the title Grandmother.

But the great shift is under way, and it is time to birth a new world. To do this, women must once again be ready to open themselves to receive and give birth to waves upon waves of inspirational consciousness. Even though I, the Queen Bee, fell asleep thousands of years ago, I will awaken if enough women call to me, with their minds, hearts, and wombs ready to receive my messages. Together we can weave a new future, where responsibility, accountability, and, most of all, celebration of the Great Mother's gifts, without possessiveness, are experienced around the world. Remember that some of the easiest and most enjoyable ways to access the inspirational realms of the Great Mother are through song, dance, poetry, storytelling, and laughter.

This is our time. We are not alone. We are many: sisters, mothers, daughters, aunts, nieces, and grandmothers, plus the entire ancestral lineage of women. There are also many strong and loving men who are eager to support us as we step into our power. Linking together through our hearts, wombs, and minds, we are saying: *It is time for all women to be seen, loved, and healed, for this is the decree of the Great Mother.*

FULFILLING OUR DESTINY AS SACRED WOMEN

This final meditation links all the previous rituals together and is best carried out just before the new moon is seen in the sky.

᧐

RITUAL NO. 5
Giving Birth to New Waves of Consciousness

Find somewhere to stand, preferably barefoot, on the earth. Use your breath to calm your mind, gradually spending more time on the exhalation as you transfer any lingering thoughts into the ground.

Place your hands over your heart and inhale and exhale in and out of your heart. Imagine as you do that you are leaning your back against the bosom of the Great Mother, and, with each breath, your body is being filled with her love. Now, having previously spent some time separating the gems of wisdom from the past month's experiences from those things destined for the compost, leave the gems in the heart and move your awareness down to the sacral chakra.

Place your hands over your hara with your fingertips together and pointing downward. Imagine that your womb is a bottle or flask, with its neck directed toward the earth, and pour into the Mother all the emotions and beliefs you no longer wish to carry as well as everything you know is complete, both successes and unfulfilled dreams.

When this process is finished, focus your attention on the root chakra under your feet. Upon exhalation, hold your breath out for at least thirty seconds so you can bob on the ocean of the Dragon Queen. Feel the steady movement of the waves, which are filled with wisdom, love, and strength. Inhale and repeat the process until you feel calm.

When you are ready, begin to allow the Dragon Queen's energy to rise up along your legs, drawing it into the womb with the aid of the vaginal muscles. Feel the pulse of the dragon under your hands until the sacral chakra is warm and revitalized. You may include the tone of the sacral chakra—*oooo*—to enhance the experience as the womb fills.

It is now time to renew the connection between the womb and the heart. Place one hand on the heart chakra and the other on the sacral chakra, and suck the energy up from the womb to the heart until the heart is full. Now the Mother Cow takes over, gently churning the energy as it moves between the breasts until it is transformed into pure spiritual energy. Feel the waves of joy, excitement, and compassion increase as this process takes place, enhancing the experience, if you choose, with the soft tones of the heart—*ah-h-h*.

As we move to the next step, imagine your crown chakra as a third cup or container, and let the spiritual energy of the heart, plus the gems of wisdom, be drawn up into the downward-facing cup, using your breath to guide it. You will reach a moment when the cup overflows, and this will trigger the pineal gland to release DMT. With almost silent humming (creating a *ng* sound from the back of the throat with your lips closed), call in the Queen Bee, who opens the door, allowing your essence access to the multidimensional awareness of the Great Mother. Offer to the Great Mother, with love and gratitude, the gems of wisdom you extracted from your stories and experiences in the sacral chakra. As they are absorbed into the collective consciousness, remain in this blissful state for as long as you choose, without thought or desire.

When you are ready, turn the crown chakra's cup upward and collect the nectar of inspiration. Slowly pour this pure essence into the spiritual cup in your heart, where it is held between the breasts, as precious as a newborn child, receiving it with the gentle sound of *ah-h-h,* as you would welcome a loved one. Finally, imagine the womb as an upturned vessel and pour the spiritual seeds into its nurturing and succulent soil, toning *oooo* to embed the seeds. If you are able, sit on the earth and feel your womb and that of Mother Earth merge.

The next stage, pregnancy, may take a day, week, or months. As soon as you can, write in a journal or share any insights you may have received from the Queen Bee—although you may not be entirely clear on the details at this point. Water and feed the seeds regularly by nurturing yourself and making time to develop and give birth to any new ideas, especially around the full moon. As the moon starts to wane, be aware that the birth may now have to wait until the next moon cycle. As the dark moon approaches, take time to consider whether there are things in your life that may need to be released to make way for new life. Ask yourself, What am I holding on to that is complete? Repeat the whole process of cleansing and purification, renewal, surrender, inspiration, and nurturing at each dark moon. Be patient; you may need to repeat the process for several cycles before fully giving birth to your dreams, gaining strength and inspiration on each occasion.

Through this ritual your life will become richer, more fulfilling, and easier. But most importantly you will start to experience a sense of community unlike anything you have felt before as you connect not only to your spiritual ancestors and to the three faces of the Great Mother but also to millions of women across the globe who know that the time to embody the healing power of sacred woman has arrived.

HEALING THROUGH THE CHAKRAS

Here are some suggestions for bringing balance and health back into the chakras. The colors can be applied physically in the form of scarves or towels or can be brought into the energetic body through visual imagery, allowing intuition to choose the particular shade. The sounds or tones have been used since ancient times to reharmonize the energy body. I suggest toning each sound, starting at the base chakra, three times a day, being carefully to keep the *ay* and *ee* sounds soft and subtle. It is important that toning takes place in a sacred setting and not while driving or in some other mundane setting, as the whole experience, when done properly, will lead to a state of peace and bliss that can continue for about twenty minutes after the toning stops.

BASE CHAKRA

Color: All shades of red, from pale pink to deep blood red
Sound: *UH* (created by dropping the lower jaw and allowing a deep sound to vibrate the base chakra)

Complementary Healing Methods Include:

- Letting go of the need to be in control, perfect, and, in particular, "tight-arsed," by taking risks, being playful, and seeking spontaneity
- Dancing, especially when it is rhythmic and sensual and involves gyrations of the hips
- Drumming, especially in the company of others

SACRAL CHAKRA

Color: All shades of orange, from pale peach to the deep orange of the sun

Sound: *OO* (similar to cooing to an infant)

Complementary Healing Methods Include:

- Regular nurturing of self, including good food, massage, walks in nature, listening to music, and taking time to relax
- Learning to say yes when help is offered rather than the instinctual refrain "Oh no, I'm fine"
- Relaxing against something strong that offers support, such as the trunk of a tree, the warmth of a bath, a supportive, comforting pillow, or the arms of a loved one
- Allowing dreams to become reality by planting and nurturing your unique seeds of creativity

SOLAR PLEXUS

Color: All shades of yellow, from pale lemon to deep gold

Sound: *OH*

Complementary Healing Methods Include:

- Writing a list of past achievements, especially those that were personally challenging, and celebrating each one by awarding yourself a mini prize, e.g., flowers, chocolate, etc.
- Allowing time each day to talk about something that enhanced

your confidence without allowing anybody to interrupt you or burst your bubble

- Creating healthy boundaries, thereby recognizing which energy/ emotions belong to you and which belong to another person
- Imagining a mirror in front of you with the reflective surface pointing toward the person whose emotions sap your energy, allowing their energy to return to them

HEART CHAKRA

Color: All shades of green, from pale green through vibrant emerald to deep forest green
Sound: *AH*
Complementary Healing Methods Include:

- Asking your heart, What is the most loving thing I can do in this moment?
- Imagining sitting in a large, comfortable chair that is soft and supportive, where you can completely let go and trust
- Remembering everybody who loves you—past and present—and allowing that love to fill your heart
- Affirming to yourself daily: I am loved, I am lovable, and I am loving

THROAT CHAKRA

Color: All shades of blue, from pale sky blue to deep royal blue
Sound: *I* (as in *eye*)
Complementary Healing Methods Include:

- Singing or toning that releases any tension in the throat
- Quieting the chatter from the mind that usually exits in this chakra
- Speaking the truth of your feelings without swallowing what needs to be said
- Imagining standing on the top of a mountain and speaking with freedom to the wind

THIRD EYE

Color: Indigo; deep blue-purple as seen in deep water or a night sky
Sound: *AY* (rhymes with *say*, produced by almost closing the mouth so the sound comes from the back of the throat)
Complementary Healing Methods Include:

- Looking out into a clear night sky, allowing the muscles of the eyes to relax so they can take in the larger picture
- Breathing out, counting to ten, and settling the mind before reacting
- Learning to gather all the information before making a decision
- Asking your inner self, What is the wisest thing I can do in this moment?

CROWN CHAKRA

Color: All shades of violet, from soft lilac through lavender to deep purple
Sound: *EE* (produced by stretching the lips back and sounding from the back of the throat)
Complementary Healing Methods Include:

- Meditating in stillness while imagining the crown chakra receiving and sending light from the top of the head
- Writing down intuitive insights, then following through on the guidance received
- Asking for help from the spirit world, keeping the request simple
- Allowing the light that enters the top of the head to spread down through the whole body on the inhalation, and then letting it flow up and out on the exhalation
- Mindfully meditating, with your focus on feeling the ground under your feet when walking

NOTES

CHAPTER 1. WOMAN, KNOW THYSELF

1. Gimbutas, *The Goddesses and Gods of Old Europe*, 9.
2. Abma et al., "Teenagers in the United States," 14.
3. Mosher et al., "Sexual Behavior and Selected Health Measures," 21–22.
4. Watts and Zimmerman, "Violence against Women," 1232–37.
5. Unicef, *The State of the World's Children 2007*, 7.
6. Tjaden and Thoennes, "Full Report on the Prevalence, Incidence, and Consequences of Violence against Women," 3.
7. Ibid., 60.
8. Fisher, "Measuring Rape against Women."
9. Watts and Zimmerman, "Violence against Women," 1233.
10. United Nations Department of Public Information, "Women and Violence."
11. Ibid.
12. United Nations Global Initiative to Fight Human Trafficking, "Human Trafficking."
13. Watts and Zimmerman, "Violence against Women."

CHAPTER 2. MEETING OUR ANCESTRAL GRANDMOTHERS

1. Gimbutas, *The Goddesses and Gods of Old Europe*, 9.
2. Bednarik, "The Earliest Evidence of Palaeoart," 89–135.
3. Eisler, *The Chalice and the Blade*, 2.
4. Hancock, *Supernatural*, 7.
5. Taylor, "Uncovering the Prehistory of Sex."
6. Gardner, *Genesis of the Grail Kings*, 7–8.

7. Mellaart, *Catal Huyuk,* 181.

8. Stone, *When God Was a Woman,* 11.

9. Ibid., 31–35.

10. "Iroquois Women."

11. Sykes, *The Seven Daughters of Eve,* 54.

12. Lesnefsky et al., "Mitochondrial Dysfunction in Cardiac Disease," 1065–89.

13. Teitelbaum et al., "The Use of D-Ribose in Chronic Fatigue Syndrome and Fibromyalgia," 857–62.

14. Sykes, *The Seven Daughters of Eve,* 275.

15. Page, *2012 and the Galactic Center,* 8.

16. Gimbutas, *The Language of the Goddess,* 121.

17. Hodder, "New Finds and New Interpretations at Çatalhöyük," 6.

18. Eisler, *The Chalice and the Blade,* 29–41.

19. Gimbutas, *The Goddesses and Gods of Old Europe,* 186–87.

20. Eisler, *The Chalice and the Blade,* 29–41.

21. Gardner, *Genesis of the Grail Kings,* 51.

22. Ibid., 329–30.

23. Ibid., 59.

24. Stone, *When God Was a Woman,* 62–68.

25. Ibid., 191.

26. Bird, *Israelite Religion and the Faith of Israel's Daughters,* 107–8.

27. Stone, *When God Was a Woman,* 175.

28. Ibid., 214.

CHAPTER 3. LISTENING TO THE WISDOM OF THE BODY

1. Moynihan and Cassels, *Selling Sickness,* xi.

2. Prout and Fish, "Participation of Women in Clinical Trials of Drug Therapies."

3. U.S. Food and Drug Administration, "Women's Participation in Clinical Trials."

4. King and Brucker, *Pharmacology for Women's Health,* 60.

5. Arntz et al., *What the Bleep Do We Know!?*

6. Pert, *Molecules of Emotion.*

7. Lipton, *The Biology of Belief,* 15.

8. Talbot, *The Holographic Universe,* 98.

9. Lu, *A Woman's Guide to Healing from Breast Cancer,* 10.

10. Ibid., 3.

CHAPTER 4. VULVA, THE EXOTIC LILY

1. Ensler, *The Vagina Monologues*, 45.

2. Pereda et al., "The Prevalence of Child Sexual Abuse in Community and Student Samples."

3. International Center for Assault Prevention, "Statistics."

4. Birch, *Pathways to Pleasure*.

5. Reese et al., "Findings from the National Survey of Sexual Health and Behavior."

6. Camphausen, *The Yoni*, 21.

7. Ibid., 41.

8. Hodder, "New Finds and New Interpretations at Çatalhöyük," 6.

9. Ensler, *The Vagina Monologues*, 9–11.

10. O'Connell et al., "Anatomy of the Clitoris," 1189–95.

11. Chalker, *The Clitoral Truth*, 16.

12. Ibid., 36.

13. Darling et al., "Female Ejaculation," 29–47.

14. Camphausen, *The Yoni*, 72.

15. Gardner, *Realm of the Ring Lords*, 123.

16. Currie-McGhee, *Tattoos and Body Piercing*, 11.

17. Momoth, *Female Genital Mutilation*, 5.

18. World Health Organization, "Female Genital Mutilation."

19. Ibid.

20. Lightfoot-Klein, "The Sexual Experience and Marital Adjustment of Genitally Circumcised and Infibulated Females in the Sudan," 375–92.

21. Reese et al., "Findings from the National Survey of Sexual Health and Behavior."

22. Gerressu et al., "Prevalence of Masturbation and Associated Factors in a British National Probability Study," 266–78.

23. Winkel, "Male Circumcision in the USA."

24. Ibid.

25. O'Hara and O'Hara, "The Effect of Male Circumcision on the Sexual Enjoyment of the Female Partner," 79–84.

26. Maines, *The Technology of Orgasm*.

27. Treptow, "U.K. Government Encourages Teen Masturbation?"

28. Hutchins, *5 Minutes to Orgasm*.

29. Whalen and Roth, "A Cognitive Approach," 335–62.

30. Komisaruk and Whipple, "Elevation of Pain Threshold by Vaginal Stimulation in Women," 357–67.

31. Portner, "The Orgasmic Mind."
32. Ibid.
33. Akshoomoff and Courchesne, "A New Role for the Cerebellum in Cognitive Operations," 731–38.
34. Bartels and Zeki, "The Neural Correlates of Romantic and Maternal Love," 1155–66.
35. Marazziti et al., "A Relationship between Oxytocin and Anxiety of Romantic Attachment."
36. Anderberg and Uvnäs-Moberg, "Plasma Oxytocin Levels in Female Fibromyalgia Syndrome Patients," 373–79.
37. Turner et al., "Preliminary Research on Plasma Oxytocin in Normal Cycling Women," 97–113.
38. Brody and Kruger, "The Post-Orgasmic Prolactin Increase Following Intercourse Is Greater than Following Masturbation and Suggests Greater Satiety," 312.
39. Northrup, *Women's Bodies, Women's Wisdom*, 407

CHAPTER 5. SACRED SEXUALITY

1. Kenyon and Sion, *The Magdalen Manuscript*, 23.
2. Da Silva, "What Is Intercourse?"
3. Gimbutas, *The Language of the Goddess*, 105–6.
4. Stone, *When God Was a Woman*, 154–62.
5. George, *Mysteries of the Dark Moon*, 175–77.
6. Gardner, *Genesis of the Grail Kings*, 163.
7. Gardner, *Bloodline of the Holy Grail*, 310.
8. George, *Mysteries of the Dark Moon*, 177.
9. Silva, *Common Wealth*, 21–22.
10. Von Daniken, *Odyssey of the Gods*, 80.

CHAPTER 6. ENTERING THE CAVE
OF TRANSFORMATION

1. Prakasha and Prakasha, *Womb Wisdom*, 149.
2. Pregadio, *Awakening to Reality*, 8.
3. Van Lysebeth, *Tantra*, 330–40.
4. Northrup, *Women's Bodies, Women's Wisdom*, 293.
5. Aguilar and Mitchell, "Physiological Pathways and Molecular Mechanisms Regulating Uterine Contractility," 725–44.

6. Cutler, "Oophorectomy at Hysterectomy after Age 40?"

7. Smith and Judd, "Menopause and Post-menopause," 1030–50.

8. Fox, "Puberty Too Soon."

9. Crockett, *Healing Our Hormones, Healing Our Lives*, 57.

10. Ibid., 135.

11. Zhang et al., "Contemporary Cesarean Delivery Practice in the United States," 1–10.

12. Ray and Mandell, *Birth and Relationships*, 83.

13. Crockett, *Healing Our Hormones, Healing Our Lives*, 178.

14. Lu, *A Woman's Guide to Healing from Breast Cancer*, 137.

15. World Health Organization, "Cancer of the Cervix."

16. Northrup, *Women's Bodies, Women's Wisdom*, 273.

17. Antoni and Goodkin, "Host Moderator Variables in the Promotion of Cervical Neoplasia," 67–76.

18. Crockett, *Healing Our Hormones, Healing Our Lives*, 149.

CHAPTER 7. BREASTS, BEAUTIFUL BREASTS

1. Yalom, *A History of the Breast*, 3.

2. Russell, "Human Olfactory Communication," 520–22.

3. Rodgers, *Sex*, 102.

4. Storey et al., "Hormonal Correlates of Paternal Responsiveness in New and Expectant Fathers," 79–95.

5. McDowell, "Breastfeeding in the United States," 4.

6. Goodman, "Low Oxytocin Linked to Postpartum Depression."

7. Oddy et al., "Breastfeeding Duration and Academic Achievement at 10 Years," 3489.

8. Ford and Beach, *Patterns of Sexual Behavior*, 88.

9. Mead, *Male and Female*, 205.

10. Cole et al., *Breasts*, 158.

11. Walker, *The Woman's Dictionary of Symbols and Sacred Objects*, 303.

12. Yalom, *A History of the Breast*, 17–23.

13. Ibid., 93.

14. Foss and Southwell, "Infant Feeding and the Media."

15. Centers for Disease Control and Prevention, "Breastfeeding among U.S. Children Born 2000–2008."

16. Walker, *The Woman's Dictionary of Symbols and Sacred Objects*, 346.

CHAPTER 8. THE DISTRESSED BREAST

1. Chilnick, *Heart Disease,* 160.

2. Cancer Research UK, "Breast Cancer."

3. World Cancer Research Fund, "World Cancer Statistics: Breast Cancer."

4. American Institute for Cancer Research, "Stark Differences in Global Breast Cancer Rates Underscore Role of U.S. Lifestyle in Risk."

5. "US Breast Cancer Statistics."

6. Chlebowski et al., "Breast Cancer after Use of Estrogen Plus Progestin in Postmenopausal Women," 573–87.

7. MacRae, "Landmark British Study that Could Revolutionise Breast Cancer Treatment."

8. Susan G. Komen for the Cure, "Facts for Life."

9. Collaborative Group on Hormonal Factors in Breast Cancer, "Breast Cancer and Breastfeeding," 187–95.

10. American Cancer Society, "What Are the Risk Factors for Cancer?"

11. "Alcohol: A Woman's Health Issue."

12. Ness et al., "Infertility, Fertility Drugs, and Ovarian Cancer," 217–24.

13. Kerenyi et al., "Oncostatic Effects of the Pineal Gland," 313–19.

14. Ashizawa et al., "Breast Form Changes Resulting from a Certain Brassiere," 53–62.

15. "The British Study on Bra Wearing and Breast Pain."

16. Singer and Grismaijer, *Dressed to Kill.*

17. Eden et al., "Innersource Freedom Tips."

18. Michael et al., "Health Behaviors, Social Networks, and Healthy Aging," 711–22.

CHAPTER 9. DEVELOPING WINGS TO FLY

1. Collaer and Hines, "Human Behavioral Sex Differences," 55–77.

2. Gettler et al., "Longitudinal Evidence that Fatherhood Decreases Testosterone in Human Males," 16194–99.

3. Rabinowicz et al., "Gender Differences in the Human Cerebral Cortex," 98–107.

4. Wisniewski, "Forget Fight or Flight."

5. Harasty et al., "Language-Associated Cortical Regions Are Proportionally Larger in the Female Brain," 171–76.

6. University of California, "Intelligence in Men and Women Is a Gray and White Matter."

7. Kimura, "Sex Differences in the Brain."

8. Langseth and Frey, *Crying,* 135–39.

9. Strassman, *DMT,* 61.

10. Bayliss et al., "Pineal Gland Calcification and Defective Sense of Direction," 1758.

11. King, *Melanin,* 58–59; Murphy, "Carotid Cerebral Angiography in Uganda," 47–60.

12. Adeloye and Felson, "Incidence of Normal Pineal Gland Calcification in Skull Roentgenograms of Black and White Americans."

13. Luke, "The Effect of Fluoride on the Physiology of the Pineal Gland," 177.

14. Cohen et al., "Role of the Pineal Gland in Aetiology and Treatment of Breast Cancer," 814–16.

15. Lokhorst, "Descartes and the Pineal Gland."

16. Blavatsky, *The Secret Doctrine*, 289–306.

17. Bailey, *Esoteric Healing,* 160.

18. Strassman, *DMT,* 61.

19. English, *Different Doorway.*

20. Goldman, *Healing Sounds,* 106.

21. Barr, *What Is Melanin?*

22. Gimbutas, *The Goddesses and Gods of Old Europe,* 184.

23. Stone, "Overview of Bee Biology."

24. Maleszka, "Epigenetic Integration of Environmental and Genomic Signals in Honeybees," 188–92.

25. Kimmel et al., "Electromagnetic Radiation."

26. Bleeker, *The Rainbow,* 138.

27. Hancock, *Supernatural,* 382.

28. Bleeker, *The Rainbow,* 129.

29. Gimbutas, *The Goddesses and Gods of Old Europe,* 181.

30. Aloisio, *Islands of Dream,* 42.

31. Hancock, *Underworld,* 376.

32. Aloisio, *Islands of Dream,* 135.

BIBLIOGRAPHY

Abma, Joyce C., Gladys M. Martinez, and Casey E. Copen. "Teenagers in the United States: Sexual Activity, Contraceptive Use, and Childbearing, National Survey of Family Growth 2006–2008." Centers for Disease Control, *Vital and Health Statistics,* series 23, no. 30 (2010), www.cdc.gov/nchs/data/series/sr_23/sr23_030.pdf.

Adeloye, Adelola, and Benjamin Felson. "Incidence of Normal Pineal Gland Calcification in Skull Roentgenograms of Black and White Americans." *American Journal of Roentgenology* 122, no. 3 (1974).

Aguilar, Hector N., and B. F. Mitchell. "Physiological Pathways and Molecular Mechanisms Regulating Uterine Contractility." *Human Reproduction Update* 16, no. 6 (2010).

Akshoomoff, Natacha A., and Eric Courchesne. "A New Role for the Cerebellum in Cognitive Operations." *Behavioral Neuroscience* 106, no. 5 (Oct. 1992).

"Alcohol: A Woman's Health Issue." www.athealth.com/Consumer/disorders/womenalcohol.html.

Aloisio, Francis Xavier. *Islands of Dream.* San Gwann: BDL Malta, 2009.

American Cancer Society. "What Are the Risk Factors for Cancer?" www.cancer.org/Cancer/BreastCancer/DetailedGuide/breast-cancer-risk-factors.

American Institute for Cancer Research. "Stark Differences in Global Breast Cancer Rates Underscore Role of U.S. Lifestyle in Risk, Say Experts: Breast Cancer Rate in North America Twice That of South America." http://preventcancer.aicr.org/site/News2?abbr=pr_&page=NewsArticle&id=19381&news_iv_ctrl=1102.

Anderberg, U. M., and K. Uvnäs-Moberg. "Plasma Oxytocin Levels in Female Fibromyalgia Syndrome Patients." *Zeitschrift für Rheumatologie,* 59, no. 6 (2000).

Antoni, Michael H., and Karl Goodkin. "Host Moderator Variables in the Promotion of Cervical Neoplasia: Personality Facets." *Journal of Psychosomatic Research* 32, no. 3 (1988).

Arntz, William, Betsy Chasse, and Mark Vicente. *What the Bleep Do We Know!?* Deerfield Beach, Fla.: Health Communications, Inc., 2005.

Ashizawa, K., A. Sugane, and T. Gunji. "Breast Form Changes Resulting from a Certain Brassiere." *Journal of Human Ergology* 19, no. 1 (1990).

Bailey, Alice. *Esoteric Healing.* New York: Lucis Publishing Company, 1953.

Barr, Frank. *What Is Melanin?* Berkeley, Calif.: Institute for the Study of Consciousness, 1983.

Bartels, Andreas, and Semir Zeki. "The Neural Correlates of Romantic and Maternal Love." *Neuroimage* 21 (2004).

Bayliss, C. R., N. L. Bishop, and R. Fowler. "Pineal Gland Calcification and Defective Sense of Direction." *British Medical Journal* (Clinical Research Edition) 291, no. 6511 (1985).

Bednarik, Robert G. "The Earliest Evidence of Palaeoart." *Rock Art Research* 20, no. 2 (2003).

Birch, Robert. *Pathways to Pleasure: A Woman's Guide to Orgasm.* Stone Mountain, Ga.: PEC Publishing, 2000.

Bird, Phyllis. *Israelite Religion and the Faith of Israel's Daughters: Reflection on Gender and Religious Definition.* Cleveland: Pilgrim Press, 1991.

Blavatsky, Helena. *The Secret Doctrine,* vol. 2 (1888), www.theosociety.org/pasadena/sd/sd2-1-17.htm.

Bleeker, Claas Jouco. *The Rainbow: A Collection of Studies in the Science of Religion.* Leiden, Netherlands: Brill Archive, 1975.

"The British Study on Bra Wearing and Breast Pain." www.007b.com/bras_bare_facts.php.

Brody, Stuart, and Tillmann H. Kruger. "The Post-Orgasmic Prolactin Increase Following Intercourse Is Greater than Following Masturbation and Suggests Greater Satiety." *Biology Psychology* 71, no. 3 (March 2006).

Camphausen, Rufus. *The Yoni: Sacred Symbol of Female Creative Power.* Rochester, Vt.: Inner Traditions, 1996.

Cancer Research UK. "Breast Cancer." http://info.cancerresearchuk.org/cancerstats/world/breast-cancer-world/breast-cancer-world.

Centers for Disease Control and Prevention. "Breastfeeding among U.S. Children Born 2000–2008." www.cdc.gov/breastfeeding/data/NIS_data/index.htm.

Chalker, Rebecca. *The Clitoral Truth*. New York: Seven Stories Press, 2000.

Chilnick, Lawrence. *Heart Disease: An Essential Guide for the Newly Diagnosed*. Philadelphia: Perseus Books Group, 2008.

Chlebowski, R. T., L. H. Kuller, R. L. Prentice, et al. "Breast Cancer after Use of Estrogen Plus Progestin in Postmenopausal Women." *New England Journal of Medicine* 360 no. 6, 2009.

Chopra, Deepak. *Perfect Health*. New York: Harmony, 2001.

Church, Dawson. *The Genie in Your Genes: Epigenetic Medicine and the New Biology of Intention*. Fulton, Calif.: Elite Books, 2007.

Cohen, Michael, Marc Lippman, and Bruce Chabner. "Role of the Pineal Gland in Aetiology and Treatment of Breast Cancer." *Lancet* 2, no. 8094 (Oct. 1978): 814–16.

Cole, Ellen, Esther D. Rothblum, and Carolyn Latteier. *Breasts: The Women's Perspective on an American Obsession*. New York: Routledge, 1998.

Collaborative Group on Hormonal Factors in Breast Cancer. "Breast Cancer and Breastfeeding: Collaborative Reanalysis of Individual Data from 47 Epidemiological Studies in 30 Countries, Including 50302 Women with Breast Cancer and 96973 Women without the Disease." *Lancet* 360, no. 9328 (July 2002): 187–95.

Collaer, M. L., and M. Hines. "Human Behavioral Sex Differences: A Role for Gonadal Hormones during Early Development?" *Psychological Bulletin* 118, no. 1 (1995).

Crockett, Linda. *Healing Our Hormones, Healing Our Lives*. Winchester, England: O Books, 2009.

Currie-McGhee, Leanne K. *Tattoos and Body Piercing*. San Diego, Calif.: Lucent, 2006.

Cutler, Winnifred B. "Oophorectomy at Hysterectomy after Age 40? A Practice that Does Not Withstand Scrutiny." *Menopause Management: The Journal of the North American Menopause Society, for Health Care Professionals* 5, no. 5 (1996).

Darling, C. A, J. K. Davidson, and C. Conway-Welch. "Female Ejaculation: Perceived Origins, the Grafenberg Spot/Area, and Sexual Responsiveness." *Archives of Sexual Behavior* 19, no. 1 (1990).

Da Silva, Manuel Luciano. "What Is Intercourse?" www.dightonrock.com/what_intercourse.htm.

Demetra, George. *Mysteries of the Dark Moon*. San Francisco, Calif.: HarperCollins, 1992.

Dever, William. *Did God Have a Wife? Archaeology and Folk History in Ancient Israel.* Grand Rapids, Mich.: Wm. B. Eerdmans Publishing, 2005.

Diamant, Anita. *The Red Tent.* New York: Picador, 1998.

Eden, Donna. *Energy Medicine.* New York: Penguin, 1998.

Eden, Donna, Vicki Matthews, and Titanya Dahlin. "Innersource Freedom Tips." The Energy Medicine Handout Bank, www.energymed.org/hbank/handouts/is_freedom_tips.htm.

Eisler, Riane. *The Chalice and the Blade.* New York: HarperCollins, 1988.

Ellis, Lee. *Sex Differences: Summarizing More Than a Century of Scientific Research.* New York: Psychology Press, 2008.

English, Jane Butterfield. *Different Doorway: Adventures of a Caesarean Born.* Mt. Shasta, Calif.: Earth Heart, 1985.

Ensler, Eve. *The Vagina Monologues.* New York: Random House, 1998.

Feuer, G. M., and N. A. Kerenyi. "Role of the Pineal Gland in the Development of Malignant Melanoma." *Neurochemistry International* 14, no. 3 (1989).

Fisher, Bonnie S. "Measuring Rape against Women: The Significance of Survey Questions." www.ncjrs.gov/pdffiles1/nij/199705.pdf.

Ford, Clellan S., and Frank A. Beach. *Patterns of Sexual Behavior.* New York: Harper & Row, 1951.

Foss, Katherine, and Brian Southwell. "Infant Feeding and the Media: The Relationship between Parents' Magazine Content and Breastfeeding 1972–2000." *International Breastfeeding Journal* 1, no. 10 (2006).

Fox, Robin. "Puberty Too Soon." *Psychology Today* (April 2011).

Gardner, Laurence. *Bloodline of the Holy Grail.* Gloucester, Mass.: Fair Winds Press, 2002.

———. *Genesis of the Grail Kings.* Gloucester, Mass.: Fair Winds Press, 2002.

———. *Realm of the Ring Lords.* Gloucester, Mass.: Fair Winds Press, 2003.

George, Demetra. *Mysteries of the Dark Moon.* San Francisco, Calif.: HarperCollins, 1992.

Gerressu, M., C. H. Mercer, C. A. Graham, K. Wellings, and A. M. Johnson. "Prevalence of Masturbation and Associated Factors in a British National Probability Study." *Archives of Sexual Behavior* 37, no. 2 (Apr. 2008): 266–78.

Gettler, Lee T., Thomas W. McDade, Alan B. Feranil, and Christopher W. Kuzawa. "Longitudinal Evidence that Fatherhood Decreases Testosterone in Human Males." *Proceedings of the National Academy of Science* 108, no. 39 (2011): 16194–99.

Gimbutas, Marija. *The Goddesses and Gods of Old Europe*. Berkeley, Calif.: University of California Press, 1982.

———. *The Language of the Goddess*. New York: Thames and Hudson, 2006.

Goldman, Jonathan. *Healing Sounds*. Rochester, Vt.: Healing Arts Press, 1992.

Goodman, Brenda. "Low Oxytocin Linked to Postpartum Depression." www
.medicinenet.com/script/main/art.asp?articlekey=144314.

Gough, Andrew. *The Bee*. www.andrewgough.co.uk/bee1_1.html.

Hammer, Leon. *Dragon Rises, Red Bird Flies*. Wellingborough, U.K.: Aquarian Press, 1990.

Hancock, Graham. *Supernatural*. New York: The Disinformation Company, 2007.

———. *Underworld*. New York: Three Rivers Press, 2002.

Harasty, Jenny, Kay L. Double, Glenda M. Halliday, Jillian J. Kril, and Deborah A. McRitchie. "Language-Associated Cortical Regions Are Proportionally Larger in the Female Brain." *Archives of Neurology* 54, no. 2 (February 1997).

Hay, Louise. *You Can Heal Your Life*. Carlsbad, Calif.: Hay House Publishing, 2008.

Hodder, Ian. "New Finds and New Interpretations at Çatalhöyük." Çatalhöyük Archive Report, Catalhoyuk Research Project, Institute of Archaeology, 2005.

Hutchins, Claire. *5 Minutes to Orgasm: Everytime You Make Love*. Midlothian, Tex.: JPS, 2000.

Icke, David. *Human Race Get Off Your Knees: The Lion Sleeps No More*. Isle of Wight, U.K.: David Icke Books, 2010.

International Center for Assault Prevention. "Statistics." www.internationalcap.
org/abuse_statistics.html.

"Iroquois Women." In "Iroquois Confederacy and the U.S. Constitution." Portland State University, October 1, 2001, www.iroquoisdemocracy.pdx.edu/
html/iroquoiswoman.htm.

Janus, S., and C. Janus. *The Janus Report on Sexual Behavior*. New York: John Wiley & Sons, 1993.

Kaptchuk, Ted. *Chinese Medicine: The Web that Has No Weaver*. London: Rider, 1983.

Kenyon, Tom, and Judi Sion. *The Magdalen Manuscript*. Orcas, Wash.: ORB Communications, 2002.

Kerenyi, N. A., E. Pandula, and G. M. Feuer. "Oncostatic Effects of the Pineal Gland." *Drug Metabolism and Drug Interactions* 8, nos. 3–4 (1990).

Kimmel, Stefan, Jochen Kuhn, Wolfgang Harst, and Hermann Stever. "Electromagnetic Radiation: Influences on Honeybees (*Apis mellifera*)." www.hese-project.org/hese-uk/en/papers/kimmel_iaas_2007.pdf.

Kimura, Doreen. "Sex Differences in the Brain." *Scientific American* (May 13, 2002), www2.nau.edu/~bio372-c/class/behavior/sexdif1.htm.

King, Francis. *Tantra: The Way of Action*. Rochester, Vt.: Destiny Books, 1990.

King, Richard. *Melanin: A Key to Freedom*. Chicago, Ill.: Lushena Books, 2001.

King, Tekoa, and Mary Brucker. *Pharmacology for Women's Health*. Sudbury, Mass.: Jones and Bartlett Publishers, 2011.

Komisaruk, B. R., and B. Whipple. "Elevation of Pain Threshold by Vaginal Stimulation in Women." *Pain* 21, no. 4 (April 1985).

Krystal, Phyllis. *Cutting the Ties that Bind: Growing Up and Moving On*. York Beach, Maine: Red Wheel/Weiser Books, 1994.

Langseth, Muriel, and William H. Frey. *Crying: The Mystery of Tears*. Minneapolis, Minn.: Winston Press, 1985.

Latteier, Carolyn. *Breasts: The Women's Perspective on an American Obsession*. Binghamton, N.Y.: Harrington Park Press, 1998.

Lesnefsky, Edward J., S. Moghaddas, B. Tandler, J. Kerner, and C. L. Hoppel. "Mitochondrial Dysfunction in Cardiac Disease: Ischemia–Reperfusion, Aging, and Heart Failure." *Journal of Molecular and Cellular Cardiology* 3, no. 6 (June 2001).

Lightfoot-Klein, Hanny. "The Sexual Experience and Marital Adjustment of Genitally Circumcised and Infibulated Females in the Sudan." *Journal of Sex Research* 26, no. 3 (1989).

Lipton, Bruce. *The Biology of Belief*. Santa Rosa, Calif.: Mountain of Love, 2005.

Lokhorst, Gert-Jan. "Descartes and the Pineal Gland." In *The Stanford Encyclopedia of Philosophy*, summer 2011 ed., E.N. Zaita http://plato.stanford.edu/entries/pineal-gland/.

Lu, Master Nan. *A Woman's Guide to Healing from Breast Cancer*. New York: Avon Books, 1999.

Luke, Jennifer. "The Effect of Fluoride on the Physiology of the Pineal Gland." Ph.D. thesis, University of Surrey, Guildford, 1997.

MacRae, Fiona. "Landmark British Study that Could Revolutionise Breast Cancer Treatment: It Turns Out It's Actually TEN Different Diseases." *Mail Online*, April 18, 2012. www.dailymail.co.uk/health/article-2131616/Breast-cancer-treatment-British-study-classifies-disease-10-different-types.html.

Maines, Rachel. *The Technology of Orgasm: Hysteria, the Vibrator, and Women's Sexual Satisfaction.* Baltimore, Md.: The Johns Hopkins University Press, 1998.

Maleszka, R. "Epigenetic Integration of Environmental and Genomic Signals in Honeybees: The Critical Interplay of Nutritional, Brain and Reproductive Networks." *Epigenetics* 3, no. 4 (2008): 188–92.

Marazziti, D., B. Dell'Osso, S. Baroni, et al. "A Relationship between Oxytocin and Anxiety of Romantic Attachment." *Clinical Practice and Epidemiology in Mental Health* 2, no. 28 (2006).

Masters, William, Virginia Johnson, and Robert C. Kolodny. *Human Sexuality,* 5th ed. Boston: Allyn and Bacon, 1997.

McDowell, Margaret. "Breastfeeding in the United States: Findings from the National Health and Nutrition Examination Survey, 1999–2006." *National Center for Health Statistics,* no. 5 (April 2008).

Mead, Margaret. *Male and Female: A Study of the Sexes in a Changing World.* New York: Dell, 1971.

Mellaart, James. *Catal Huyuk: A Neolithic Town in Anatolia.* New York: McGraw-Hill, 1987.

Michael, Yvonne L., Graham A.Colditz, Eugenie Coakley, and Ichiro Kawachi. "Health Behaviors, Social Networks, and Healthy Aging: Cross-sectional Evidence from the Nurses' Health Study." *Quality of Life Research* 8, no. 8 (1999).

Momoth, Comfort. *Female Genital Mutilation.* Milton Keynes, U.K.: Radcliffe, 2005.

Mosher, W., A. Chandra, and J. Jones. "Sexual Behavior and Selected Health Measures: Men and Women 15–44 Years of Age, United States, 2002." *Advance Data from Vital Health and Statistics,* no. 362 (September 15, 2005).

Moynihan, Ray, and Alan Cassels. *Selling Sickness: How the World's Biggest Pharmaceutical Companies Are Turning Us All into Patients.* New York: Nation Books, 2005.

Murphy, N. B. "Carotid Cerebral Angiography in Uganda: A Review of 100 Consecutive Cases." *East African Medical Journal* 45, no. 2 (1968).

Myss, Caroline. *Anatomy of the Spirit: The Seven Stages of Power and Healing.* New York: Three Rivers Press, 1997.

Ness, Roberta, et al. "Infertility, Fertility Drugs, and Ovarian Cancer: A Pooled Analysis of Case-Control Studies." *American Journal of Epidemiology* 155, no. 3 (2002).

Northrup, Christiane. *Women's Bodies, Women's Wisdom: Creating Physical and Emotional Health and Healing*. New York: Random House, 2006.

O'Connell, Helen E., K. V. Sanjeevan, and J. M. Hutson. "Anatomy of the Clitoris." *Journal of Urology* 174, no. 4, part 1 (Oct. 2005).

Oddy, Wendy H., Jianghong Li, Andrew J. O. Whitehouse, Stephen R. Zubrick, and Eva Malacova. "Breastfeeding Duration and Academic Achievement at 10 Years." *Pediatrics: The Official Journal of the American Academy of Pediatrics* 127, no. 1 (Jan. 2011): e137–45.

O'Hara, K. O., and J. O'Hara. "The Effect of Male Circumcision on the Sexual Enjoyment of the Female Partner." *British Journal of Urology International* 83, suppl. 1 (January 1999).

Page, Christine. *2012 and the Galactic Center: The Return of the Great Mother*. Rochester, Vt.: Bear and Co., 2008.

———. *Frontiers of Health*. Saffron Walden, England: C. W. Daniel, 1992.

Pappolla, M. A., M. Sos, R. A. Omar, R. J. Bick, D. L. M. Hickson-Bick, R. J. Reiter, S. Efthimiopoulos, and N. K. Robakis. "Melatonin Prevents Death of Neuroblastoma Cells Exposed to the Alzheimer Amyloid Peptide." *Journal of Neuroscience* 17, no. 5 (1997).

Pereda, Noemi, G. Guilerab, and M. Fornsa, "The Prevalence of Child Sexual Abuse in Community and Student Samples: A Meta-analysis." *Clinical Psychology Review* 29, no. 4 (2009).

Pert, Candace. *Molecules of Emotion: The Science behind Mind-Body Medicine*. New York: Simon & Schuster, 1999.

Portner, Martin. "The Orgasmic Mind: The Neurological Roots of Sexual Pleasure." *Scientific American* (May 15, 2008), www.scientificamerican.com/article.cfm?id=the-orgasmic-mind.

Prakasha, Padma, and Anaiya Aon Prakasha. *Womb Wisdom: Awakening the Creative and Forgotten Powers of the Feminine*. Rochester, Vt.: Inner Traditions/Bear and Co., 2011.

Pregadio, Fabrizio. *Awakening to Reality: A Taoist Classic of Internal Alchemy*. Mountain View, Calif.: Golden Elixir Press, 2009.

Prout, Marianne N., and Susan S. Fish. "Participation of Women in Clinical Trials of Drug Therapies: A Context for the Controversies." *Medscape General Medicine* 3, no. 4 (Oct. 2001).

Rabinowicz, T., D. E. Dean, J. M. Petetot, and G. M. DeCourten-Myers. "Gender Differences in the Human Cerebral Cortex: More Neurons in Males, More Processes in Females." *Journal of Child Neurology* 14, no. 2 (February 1999).

Rako, Susan. *The Hormone of Desire: The Truth about Sexuality, Menopause, and Testosterone.* New York: Harmony Books, 1996.

Ray, Sondra, and B. Mandell. *Birth and Relationships: How Your Birth Affects Your Relationships.* Berkeley, Calif.: Celestial Arts, 1987.

Reese, Michael, D. Herbenick, and J. D. Fortenberry. "Findings from the National Survey of Sexual Health and Behavior." *Journal of Sexual Medicine* 7, suppl. 5 (Oct. 2010): 243–373.

Rodgers, Joann Ellison. *Sex: A Natural History.* New York: Macmillan, 2003.

Russell, Michael J. "Human Olfactory Communication." *Nature* 260 (April 8, 1976).

Silva, Freddy. *Common Wealth: Our Legacy of Sacred Sites and the Rebirth of Ancient Wisdom.* Portland, Maine: Invisible Temple, 2010.

Singer, Sydney, and Soma Grismaijer. *Dressed to Kill: The Link between Breast Cancer and Bra*s. Pahoa, Hawaii: ISCD Press, 1995.

Sitchin, Zecharia. *The Twelfth Planet: Book 1 of the Earth Chronicles.* New York: Avon Books, 1976.

Smith, K. E., and H. L. Judd. "Menopause and Post-menopause." In *Current Obstectric and Gynecologic Diagnosis and Treatment,* 8th ed., ed. A. H. DeCherney and M. L. Pernoll, Norwalk, Conn.: Appleton & Lange, 1994.

Stone, David M. "Overview of Bee Biology." www.uni.illinois.edu//~stone2/bee_overview.html.

Stone, Merlin. *When God Was a Woman.* Orlando, Fla.: Harcourt Brace, 1976.

Storey, A. E., C. J. Walsh, R. L. Quinto, and K. E. Wynne-Edwards. "Hormonal Correlates of Paternal Responsiveness in New and Expectant Fathers." *Evolution and Human Behavior* 21 (2000).

Strassman, Rick. *DMT: The Spirit Molecule.* Rochester, Vt.: Park Street Press, 2001.

Susan G. Komen for the Cure, "Facts for Life: Racial & Ethnic Differences." http://ww5.komen.org/uploadedFiles/Content_Binaries/806-373a.pdf.

Sykes, Bryan. *The Seven Daughters of Eve.* New York: W. W. Norton & Company, 2002.

Talbot, Michael. *The Holographic Universe.* New York: Harper Perennial, 2011.

Taylor, Shelley. *The Tending Instinct: Women, Men, and the Biology of Our Relationships.* New York: Henry Holt & Co., 2003.

Taylor, Timothy. "Uncovering the Prehistory of Sex." *British Archaeology,* no. 15 (June 2006).

Teitelbaum, Jacob, Clarence Johnson, and John St. Cyr. "The Use of D-Ribose in Chronic Fatigue Syndrome and Fibromyalgia: A Pilot Study." *Journal of Alternative and Complementary Medicine* 12, no. 9 (November 2006).

Tjaden, Patricia, and Nancy Thoennes. "Full Report on the Prevalence, Incidence, and Consequences of Violence against Women." U.S. Department of Justice (November 1998). https://www.ncjrs.gov/pdffiles/172837.pdf.

Treptow, Cornelia. "U.K. Government Encourages Teen Masturbation?" ABC News, July 14, 2009, http://abcnews.go.com/Health/MindMoodNews/story?id=8072314.

Turner, R. A., M. Altemus, T. Enos, B. Cooper, and T. McGuinness. "Preliminary Research on Plasma Oxytocin in Normal Cycling Women: Investigating Emotion and Interpersonal Distress." *Psychiatry* 62, no. 2 (1999).

UNICEF. *The State of the World's Children 2007.* New York: UNICEF, 2006. Available at www.unicef.org/sowc07/docs/sowc07.pdf.

United Nations. "Not a Minute More: Ending Violence against Woman." www.unifem.org/materials/item_detail.php?ProductID=7.

United Nations Department of Public Information. "Women and Violence." www.un.org/rights/dpi1772e.htm.

United Nations Entity for Gender Equality and the Empowerment of Women. "Violence against Women." www.unifem.org/gender_issues/violence_against_women.

United Nations Global Initiative to Fight Human Trafficking. "Human Trafficking: The Facts." www.unglobalcompact.org/docs/issues_doc/labour/Forced_labour/HUMAN_TRAFFICKING_-_THE_FACTS_-_final.pdf.

"United States Circumcision Incidence." www.cirp.org/library/statistics/USA.

University of California, "Intelligence in Men and Women Is a Gray and White Matter." UC Newsroom, January 20, 2005, www.universityofcalifornia.edu/news/article/6864.

"US Breast Cancer Statistics." www.breastcancer.org/symptoms/understand_bc/statistics.jsp.

U.S. Food and Drug Administration. "Women's Participation in Clinical Trials." www.fda.gov/ScienceResearch/SpecialTopics/WomensHealthResearch/ucm131731.htm.

Van Lysebeth, Andre. *Tantra: Cult of the Feminine.* York Beach, Maine: Samuel Weiser, 1995.

Von Daniken, Erich. *Odyssey of the Gods: The Alien History of Ancient Greece.* Boston: Element Books, 2000.

Walker, Barbara. *The Woman's Dictionary of Symbols and Sacred Objects*. San Francisco: Harper San Francisco, 1988.

Watts, Charlotte, and Cathy Zimmerman. "Violence against Women: Global Scope and Magnitude." *Lancet* 359, no. 9313 (April 2002).

Weil, Andrew. *Spontaneous Healing: How to Discover and Embrace Your Body's Natural Ability to Maintain and Heal Itself.* New York: Ballantine Books, 1996.

Whalen, S. R., and D. Roth. "A Cognitive Approach: Theories of Human Sexuality." In *Theories of Human Sexuality,* ed. J. H. Geer and W. T. O'Donahue, New York: Plenum, 1987.

Winkel, Rich. "Male Circumcision in the USA: A Human Rights Primer." www .drmomma.org/2010/02/male-circumcision-in-usa-human-rights.html.

Wisniewski, Linda C. "Forget Fight or Flight: It's All About Friendship." *Philly-Fit* (February–March 2005), www.lindawis.com/articles/01.php.

Witcombe, Christopher, L.C.E. "Art History Resources: Venus of Willendorf." http://witcombe.sbc.edu/willendorf.

Wolkstein, Diane, and Samuel Noah Kramer. *Inanna, Queen of Heaven and Earth: Her Stories and Hymns from Sumer.* New York: Harper & Row, 1983.

World Cancer Research Fund. "World Cancer Statistics: Breast Cancer." www .wcrf-uk.org/research/cancer_statistics/world_cancer_statistics_breast_cancer .php.

World Health Organization. "Cancer of the Cervix." www.who.int/ reproductivehealth/topics/cancers/en/.

———. "Female Genital Mutilation." www.who.int/mediacentre/factsheets/ fs241/en/index.html.

Yalom, Marilyn. *A History of the Breast.* New York: Alfred A. Knopf, 1997.

Zhang, Jun, James Troendle, Uma M. Reddy, et al. "Contemporary Cesarean Delivery Practice in the United States." *American Journal of Obstetrics and Gynecology* 203, no. 326.e (2010), www.advancedmfm.com/wp-content/ uploads/2010/05/ContemporaryCDGQ.pdf.

ILLUSTRATION CREDITS

Eran Cantrell: pages 1, 83, 95, 103, 108 (bottom), 113, 118, 125, 231, 233, 239, 240, 242, 245, 297, and 302

Christine Page: pages 30, 40, 41, 43, 44 (left), 45, 46, 48, 105, 106, 137, 145, 154, 159 (bottom), 160, 162, 163, 164, 165, 166, 167, 176, 188, 193, 203, 225, 251, 259, 264, 312, 327, 331, 333, and 334

Ramessos, courtesy of Wikimedia Commons: page 25

Jeff Dahl, courtesy of Wikimedia Commons: pages 44 (right) and 321

Rama, courtesy of Wikimedia Commons: page 250

Giovanni Dall'Orto, courtesy of Wikimedia Commons: page 253

Aeleftherios, courtesy of Wikimedia Commons: page 324

INDEX

225-26, 243, 294, 326–27, 338, 344

cancer of, 212

See also womb

Uxmal, 47–48

vagina, 22, 47, 84, 97, 99, 103. 108–15, 117–19, 121, 124, 126–27, 132, 134, 137, 170, 177, 179–87, 190, 203–6, 210, 227–28, 243, 309, 332, 338, 349

intercourse and, 102, 113

muscles of, 13, 127, 170, 182, 184–85, 227, 349

Venus, 20, 60, 65, 96, 258, 311

of Berekhat Ram, 20

of Hohle Fels, 24–25

of Laussel, 26–27

of Lespugue, 26

of Tan-Tan, 20

of Willendorf, 28, 311–13

vesica piscis, 103–4, 179

vulva, 22, 26, 84, 96–135, 146, 173, 179, 183–85, 227

shaped cowrie shells, 22, 106

See also yoni

womb, 17, 38, 42, 44, 46–47, 52, 65, 97, 107–8, 118, 136, 138, 141, 144, 148, 153, 162–64, 168–70, 172–73, 177, 179–80, 182, 184–89, 195, 201–2, 208–9, 211, 214–15, 217, 219–21, 223–28, 246, 272, 277, 295–96, 298, 316, 321, 334–35, 339, 344, 348–50. *See also* uterus

Yahweh, 37, 55, 57–58, 250

Yalom, Marilyn, 234

Yoni, 103

Yonimandala, 105

See also vulva

Zeus, 55, 61, 161, 163–64, 252–54, 256–57, 319

zygote, 141, 189, 201